Eating Disorders

THERAPY IN PRACTICE SERIES

Edited by Jo Campling

This series of books is aimed at 'therapists' concerned with rehabilitation in a very broad sense. The intended audience particularly includes occupational therapists, physiotherapists and speech therapists, but many titles will also be of interest to nurses, psychologists, medical staff, social workers, teachers or voluntary workers. Some volumes are interdisciplinary, others are aimed at one particular profession. All titles will be comprehensive but concise, and practical but with due reference to relevant theory and evidence. They are not research monographs but focus on professional practice, and will be of value to both students and qualified personnel.

Forthcoming titles

Eating Disorders

A guide for health professionals

Simon B.N. Thompson

Tatchbury Mount
Southampton, UK

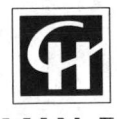

CHAPMAN & HALL

London · Glasgow · New York · Tokyo · Melbourne · Madras

Published by Chapman & Hall, 2–6 Boundary Row, London SE1 8HN

Chapman & Hall, 2–6 Boundary Row, London SE1 8HN, UK

Blackie Academic & Professional, Wester Cleddens Road, Bishopbriggs, Glasgow G64 2NZ, UK

Chapman & Hall Inc., 29 West 35th Street, New York NY10001, USA

Chapman & Hall Japan, Thomson Publishing Japan, Hirakawacho Nemoto Building, 6F, 1-7-11 Hirakawa-cho, Chiyoda-ku, Tokyo 102, Japan

Chapman & Hall Australia, Thomas Nelson Australia, 102 Dodds Street, South Melbourne, Victoria 3205, Australia

Chapman & Hall India, R. Seshadri, 32 Second Main Road, CIT East, Madras 600 035, India

Distributed in the USA and Canada by Singular Publishing Group Inc., 4284 41st Street, San Diego, California 92105

First edition 1993

© 1993 Simon B.N. Thompson

Typeset in 10/12 pt Palatino by Best-set Typesetter Ltd., Hong Kong
Printed in Great Britain at the University Press, Cambridge

ISBN 0 412 47420 4   1 56593 1823 (USA)

A catalogue record for this book is available from the British Library

Contents

Preface

Anorexia nervosa and **bulimia** are terms used to describe particular eating disorders. **Obesity** is a description of the Body Mass Index, a ratio involving body weight and height, and may be the result of an eating disorder. The purpose of this book is to guide the reader, whether a dietitian, speech therapist, clinical psychologist, psychiatrist, nurse (or nurse therapist), occupational therapist or other health professional, through the literature on eating disorders, beginning with the origins and epidemiology of anorexia nervosa.

The book may be read as a whole, providing a clear, comprehensive and practical guide to the disorders and their treatment, taking the reader in a step-by-step manner through causes, assessment, treatment and outcome, and finally to the research data. Alternatively, the book provides a detailed source of reference and is divided into four parts for this purpose: Chapters 1–3 are concerned with anorexia nervosa whilst Chapters 4–6 are concerned with bulimia and Chapters 7–9 concern obesity. Chapter 10 is a specialist chapter and examines the literature relating to eating and feeding disorders in people with learning disabilities. This layout allows the reader to refer to the sections relevant to his or her particular interests. A further reading section follows each chapter together with useful addresses, and a discussion, rather than a monograph of research, is presented as the last chapter of each section of the book. Finally, full references and a comprehensive index are included at the end of the book.

Chapter 1 begins with epidemiology of anorexia nervosa with a look at past and current theories including feminist views. Chapter 2 outlines the assessment procedures used, modern treatment approaches and outcome. Chapter 3 presents major topics of research in anorexia nervosa putting the reader in touch with up-to-date work in the area. The second part of the book presents the epidemiology of bulimia in Chapter 4; assessment, treatment and outcome in Chapter 5; and a selection of research topics in bulimia are presented and discussed in Chapter 6. The third part of the book presents the epidemiology of obesity in Chapter 7; assessment, treatment and outcome in Chapter 8; and research into obesity in Chapter 9. Finally, in the fourth part of the book, Chapter 10, the epidemiology, assessment, treatment and outcome of eating and feeding disorders in people with learning disabilities are presented and discussed. A selection of specialist research in this area is also presented and discussed at the end of this chapter.

Acknowledgements

The author would like to thank Dr Chris Freeman, Consultant Psychiatrist; Katherine Cheshire, Research Psychologist; staff and patients at the Cullen Centre, Royal Edinburgh Hospital, for their kind help during the research series. I am also grateful to my parents for their interest and support throughout; to G. Mitten, David J. Thompson (in exchange for the tiny bouncing crab-apples) and to Elisabeth, without whom life would be very dull. Finally, this book is for the many sufferers of chronic eating disorders who presented at our clinics; and in memory of a kind friend, Anne Christine Cornec, from Village-Morgat in Brittany, who tragically died as a result of anorexia nervosa.

Introduction

There has been much debate among researchers and health professionals concerning the differentiation of **anorexia nervosa** and **bulimia**. Indeed, the question constantly raised is whether or not bulimia is a subgroup of anorexia nervosa or the chronic form of anorexia nervosa on an acute to chronic continuum.

In order to explore these issues and others, it is important to begin by looking at the aetiology of anorexia nervosa. Several different standpoints have been presented in the past such as cultural, feminist, psychological and somatic. A vast body of literature has accumulated with competing theories not only concerning aetiology but also treatment approaches and, latterly, outcome studies. A few studies have examined eating and feeding disorders in people with learning disabilities. There are practical difficulties in conducting research into these areas especially when considering the nature of bulimia with the secrecy surrounding the bulimic's binge-eating episodes and the anorectic's constant combats with his or her inner conflicts. It is worth being cautious, therefore, when considering the results of such studies; it is often the differences between paradigmatic methodologies that have given rise to considerable academic debate.

On the other hand, it should not be overlooked that interest in the subject has grown with each decade with the establishment of anorexic aid groups and numerous articles appearing in both the academic and the popular press. Likewise, there are an ever-increasing number of 'weight-watching' groups concerned with avoiding or reducing obesity. It is beginning to look as if weight is also the fashionable obsession of the 21st century.

It is hoped that the considerable ground covered in past years will lead researchers and clinicians to focus universally on the efficacies of treatment approaches for the sufferers of these rather intractable 'diseases'.

1

Epidemiology of anorexia nervosa

DEFINITION OF ANOREXIA NERVOSA

Anorexia is a term used to describe the absence of appetite or desire (Sykes, 1977). The Greek prefix 'an' signifies being without, and the second part of the word, 'orexia', indicates desire for food. It can often accompany debilitating illnesses such as cancer, etc. (DeWys, 1977; Logue, 1906). Anorexia nervosa, on the other hand, is a syndrome characterized by the relentless pursuit of a thin body size (Bruch, 1973). Richard Morton (1689) has generally been credited with the publication of the first medical account of anorexia nervosa which he termed 'a nervous consumption', and there is abundant evidence that cases existed during the Middle Ages (Bliss and Hardin Branch, 1960).

Anorexia nervosa is associated with an exaggerated dread of weight gain and fat, often in spite of emaciation, and to the detriment of other physical and psychological aspects of the individual's life. The person with anorexia begins dieting in an attempt to lose weight. As Garfinkel and Garner (1982) suggest, over time, achievement of ever-decreasing weights becomes a sign of mastery, control and virtue. Anorexia nervosa is often considered to be a disorder in which the drive for a thinner shape is secondary to concerns about control and/or fears about consequences of achieving a mature shape. However, it has been shown that this hypothesis is not supported in every case. A large percentage of anorectics assume a sexuality before (45%) or during (37%) their illness (Buvat and Buvat-Herbaut, 1977). In the Buvat and Buvat-Herbaut (1977) study, it was suggested that specific problems related to sexuality did not have a causally important role in more than 22% of the anorectics. Considering these results with evidence from another study (Buvat-Herbaut *et al.*, 1983), it can be concluded that in the majority of cases, anorexia nervosa does not indicate an absolute rejection of the adult female body, although a fear or a refusal of sexuality can have a causal role in 20–40% of cases (Scott, 1988).

Not all patients with anorexia nervosa have exactly the same symptoms in the same degree or intensity. Not all cases present exactly the same symptoms as those elaborated in the American Psychiatric Association's (1987) *Diagnostic and Statistical Manual* (DSM-III-R). The DSM-III-R criteria are as follows:

1. refusal to maintain normal body weight;
2. loss of more than 25% of original body weight;
3. disturbance of body image;
4. intense fear of becoming fat;
5. no known medical illness leading to weight loss.

Some clinicians differentiate between primary and secondary anorexia (Rollins and Piazza, 1978; Brumberg, 1988), some favour a less stringent weight criterion, and some include hyperactivity (Kron *et al.*, 1978) and amenorrhoea – i.e. absence of menstruation (Halmi and Falk, 1983). There is also the matter of how anorexia nervosa is related to bulimia, the binge-eating syndrome.

According to Crisp (1977), anorexia can be divided into two phases, acute and chronic, and bulimia is the chronic or malignant phase of the illness. A similar opinion is held by Giuora (1967) who coined the term 'dysorexia' to represent the continuum with anorexia nervosa at one end and bulimia at the other end. Until 1980, when it was listed in DSM-III as a separate diagnostic entity, bulimia (from the Greek meaning 'ox hunger') was only a symptom, not an independent disease. But in 1985, in DSM-III-R, bulimia obtained independent disease status; according to the newest categorization, anorexia nervosa and bulimia are separate but related disorders. In the diagnosis of anorexia nervosa, there is increasing support for subtyping anorectic patients into those who restrict their dietary intake – 'restrictive anorectics' – and/or 'bulimarexics' (Harper, 1984). The bulimic anorectic is reported to be the most difficult to treat and the least likely to recover (Vigersky, 1977; Herzog and Copeland, 1985; Brumberg, 1988).

The sex ratio for sufferers of anorexia nervosa lies between 20:1 and 15:1 (Lambley, 1983; Lawrence, 1984; Welbourne and Purgold, 1984); clearly, females are predominantly at risk. The fact that 5–10% of all British anorexic sufferers are male (Welbourne and Purgold, 1984) also makes us doubt the idea that anorexia nervosa is solely a psychological and biological regression to avoid adult womanhood. Indeed, there is growing evidence to suggest that anorexia nervosa is not exclusive to females (Bloch, 1989; Merl, 1989; Slagerman and Yager, 1989; Hutson and Wald, 1990; Rosenvinge and Mouland, 1990). Furthermore, some adolescents who diet and control their weight successfully may become anorexic through an obsessional concern about food and weight control that has little to do with adolescence (Abraham and Llewellyn-Jones, 1984).

AETIOLOGY AND PREVALENCE

Since Lasègue's (1873) and Gull's (1874) descriptions, it has often been noted that anorexia nervosa is more common in females and usually develops during adolescence (Yates, 1970; Crisp *et al.*, 1974; Bemis, 1978; Bowden *et al.*, 1989; Cooper *et al.*, 1989; DiNicola *et al.*, 1989; Tolstoi, 1989; Yager *et al.*, 1989a,b). Theander (1970) described and followed 94 female patients in southern Sweden over a 30-year period; he calculated the overall incidence for women to be 0.24 per 100 000 population per year. But there was a sharp rise in incidence in the final decade of the study (1951–1960) to 0.45 per population. This was reflected in an increase from an average of 1.1 to 5.8 new cases per year in the area of Sweden that he studied. Kendell *et al.* (1973), using case registries from three areas (Camberwell, London; Monrose County, New York; north-east Scotland) found a comparable incidence from 0.37 in Monrose County to 1.6 per 100 000 in north-east Scotland. As with Theander, the study found a significant increase in the second half of the period under study (43 cases vs. 25 in the first half).

A ten-year computer search of medical and scientific journals shows that publications relating to anorexia nervosa increased from 59 per year in 1973 to 165 in 1982 (Butler, 1988). Clearly, interest in the subject has grown. Other studies have shown a steady increase in the number of cases of anorexia nervosa.

Another study used the psychiatric case register and hospital records from a major general hospital to estimate the incidence of anorexia nervosa in Monrose County between 1960–1969 and 1970–1976. They found that the number of diagnosed cases almost doubled (from 0.35 to 0.64 per 100 000) in the second time period of 1970–1976. Moreover, the increase occurred among females but not males and it was most prominent in the 15–24 year old group (Butler, 1988).

Anorexia nervosa rarely develops after the age of 25 years (Bhanji and Mattingly, 1988). However, Ryle (1936) reported 13 women who became ill between the ages of 31 and 59 years. He regarded the precipitating factors as multiple and varied, but they commonly included an operation, illness or the menopause. The physical and psychological findings were similar to those seen in younger individuals. Since there are many other causes of anorexia and loss of weight in the middle-aged and elderly, the diagnosis of anorexia nervosa should be made with caution and only after a thorough investigation has excluded organic disease and psychotic illness. For example, Bernstein (1972) describes the case of a 94 year old woman which Bhanji and Mattingly (1988) felt was in fact a depressive illness which responded to electroconvulsive therapy rather than one of anorexia nervosa. This poses the question of a differential diagnosis which will be discussed later in this chapter.

Although the condition known as anorexia nervosa has been most exclusively described within the European, North American and Australasian literature, it has also been recorded in other parts of the world and in other cultures; for example, Crisp (1980a) reports severe forms of the condition in the Arab/Moslem world. Clearly, the condition has crossed cultures as well as countries.

Psychological theories

The earliest psychiatric approach to anorexia nervosa derived from psychoanalysis. As Bhanji and Mattingly (1988) have stated, Freud did not publish any case histories of anorexia nervosa but did suggest that a neurotic fear of sexual activity occurred in some girls around the time of puberty and expressed itself as a loss of appetite (Freud, 1918). Nemiah (1959) suggested there were two types of psychoanalytical theory regarding anorexia nervosa: one stressed unconscious overt beliefs that impregnation could occur through the mouth; the other emphasized an intense, and sometimes mutual, dependency of the child on the mother, which was associated with the perpetuation of infantile attitudes and behaviour. Later theories placed emphasis on the family as a whole and not just the patient.

Hilde Bruch (1962) described three fundamental aspects of anorexia nervosa. The first of these is an inability to appreciate the need to be adequately nourished. The second is a disturbance of body image perception, which causes the patient to distort her perception of body thinness. Finally, there is an intense feeling of ineffectiveness. This latter aspect is seen as central to the disorder and may stem from the way in which the parents have treated their daughter: in selecting her friends, choosing her school regardless of her abilities, and giving her the things that they regard as best for her. In return, they have expected unswerving gratitude, loyalty and affection which results in her losing her sense of being an individual and feeling rather a part of her parents' private property. In anorexia nervosa, this is taken to the extreme where the girl adopts an attitude of self-control in that she critically governs her dietary intake.

Other clinicians and researchers regard anorexia nervosa as a means of the patient avoiding independence and its consequences (Waller *et al.*, 1989). Selvini Palazzoli (1974) and Minuchin, Rosman and Baker (1978), for example, have described families from a family therapy standpoint in which there are many covert alliances within the family system. These alliances may involve 'control' through sexual abuse or allegiance between one parent and the daughter over decisions that affect the daughter, other family members or the family system as a whole. Sometimes, it is the family's intention to create a healthy sense of mutual security; more often only dependence develops. Faced with the biological signals of impending adulthood and emancipation, the anorectic girl attempts to eradicate them by drastically reducing her body weight.

Crisp (1983) describes an alternative family theory where the relationship between parents is unsatisfactory and unsatisfying, and a divorce or separation may happen once the children are grown up. (Yet, according to Erichsen (1987) there is a remarkably low divorce rate in these families: 12% as opposed to 30% national average in Great Britain.) The daughter, sensing that the family situation is changing and uncertain, tries to remain a dependent child and finds that one way of maintaining this dependence on her parents is through starvation and the development of a weight phobia.

Some researchers have suggested that current social attitudes may explain not only the apparent increase in anorexia nervosa, but also its predilection for the adolescent middle class female (Bhanji and Mattingly, 1988). Indeed, society plays a great part in exerting pressures on individuals in many areas of life (Thompson, 1982; 1983b,c; 1984b; Thompson *et al.*, 1989; Copley, 1991; Scott, 1991). In particular, thinness in women has become equated with personal and professional success (Garner *et al.*, 1980). Many young women now have the option of a career instead of marriage and childrearing. Hence, examinations have become more important to them (see Mills (1978) and Mattingly and Bhanji (1982) on the relationship between pre-examination study and the onset of anorexia nervosa). Attitudes towards sexual activity are more permissive and means of contraception are more readily available, thus posing a threat to the sexually insecure young girl. Orbach (1985) has argued that the attitude of male dominated society towards women is not dissimilar to that of parents to daughters. That is to say that the constraints put on the daughter by her family in terms of what she can or cannot do and with whom she is allowed to associate may be similar to those constraints of a society that disallows personal growth or presents obstacles for women rather than career opportunities.

Somatic theories

The relationship between physical illness in general and anorexia nervosa has also been explored. Patton, Wood and Johnson-Sabine (1986) investigated over 300 cases and found that, in comparison with their control patients, the anorectics had a higher incidence of remote and recent severe physical disorders. The authors were not convinced of a direct causal association, but suggested that physical illness might increase the risk by generating an atmosphere of morbid concern within the family.

Particular interest has been devoted to hypothalamic or

midbrain tumours and chromosome abnormalities. The first account of anorexia nervosa arising in Turner's syndrome was that provided by Pitts and Guze (1963). Although a number of other reports have since appeared, it remains debatable whether or not the concurrence of these conditions is greater or less than expected through chance (Garfinkel and Garner, 1982). Whatever the final view, the possibility that chromosome abnormalities may predispose those afflicted towards anorexia nervosa has been further raised by reports of this condition in Down's syndrome (Cottrell and Crisp, 1984) and in a patient with Klinefelter's syndrome (Hindler and Norris, 1986).

Feminist views on anorexia nervosa

Obesity and overeating are central issues in the lives of many women today. In the United States, 50% of women are estimated to be overweight. Most women's magazines have a diet column; diet doctors and clinics are on the increase (Halle, 1992) and the names of diet foods are now an established part of our general vocabulary. 'Weight Watchers' has enrolled 8 million American women and each week across the United States, 12 000 classes are held, spreading and reinforcing cultlike behaviour. Wolf (1990a) has monitored its spread worldwide, with 37 million members entering 24 international cells over the past 25 years. While this preoccupation with fat and food has become so common that we tend to take it for granted, being fat, feeling fat and the compulsion to overeat are, in fact, serious and painful experiences for the women involved (Orbach, 1978).

According to the American Anorexia and Bulimia Association (Wolf, 1990b), each year 150 000 American women die of anorexia. This means that there are 17 024 more deaths from anorexia in the United States every 12 months than the total number of deaths from AIDS tabulated by the World Health Organization in 177 countries and territories from the beginning of the epidemic until the end of 1988. One survey puts the number of anorectics at between 5% and 10% of all American girls and women; while on some college campuses, 20% of women students are anorexic. *Ms* magazine reports that at least 50% of women on American campuses suffer from bulimia or anorexia (Wolf, 1990c).

In the United Kingdom, there were 3.5 million anorectics or

bulimics reported in 1989 (Wolf, 1990b): of these, 95% were female. Two generations ago, the average model weighed 8% less than the average American woman, whereas today she weighs 23% less. But the victory of the hunger cult against women's fight for equality is best illustrated by a 1984 *Glamour* magazine survey which found that an overwhelming majority of those interviewed chose losing 10 lb to 15 lb above success in work or in love (Wolf, 1990b).

Cross-culturally, from birth, girls have 10% to 15% more fat than boys. At puberty, the male fat-to-muscle ratio increases. The increased fat ratio in adolescent girls is the medium for sexual maturation and fertility. The average healthy 20 year old female is made of 28.7% body fat (Wolf, 1990a). By middle age, women cross-culturally are 38% body fat. A moderately active woman's calorie needs, again in contradiction to a central tenet of the myth, are only 250 calories less than a moderately active man's (2250 to 2500) or 2 oz of cheese! Weight gain with age is also normal cross-culturally for both sexes. Wolf (1990c) suggests that the body is evidently programmed to weigh a certain amount, which it defends.

Fat is sexual in women; Victorians called it affectionately their 'silken layer' (Wolf, 1990a). Twenty percent of women who exercise to shape their bodies have menstrual irregularities and diminished fertility. Fat tissues store hormones, so low fat reserves are linked with weak oestrogens and low levels of all the other important sex hormones as well as with inactive ovaries. It now seems that infertility and hormone imbalance are common among women whose fat-to-lean ratio falls below 22% (Wolf, 1990c). For this and other reasons, cosmetic surgery is the fastest-growing 'medical' speciality. More than 2 million Americans, at least 87% of them female, had undergone cosmetic surgery by 1988, a figure which had tripled in two years (Wolf, 1990b).

However, 'plastic' surgery is not free from complications and one of the first procedures used to remove fatty tissues, liposuction, has produced both interest and alarm amongst researchers. In France this technique has led to the death of nine women (Wolf, 1990b); the procedure involves the use of powerful suction devices which remove globules of tissue together with nerve networks, dendrites and ganglia. It is extremely difficult to obtain accurate or objective information about cosmetic surgery as figures for mortality rates are not routinely kept by American cosmetic surgeons. The British Association of Aesthetic Plastic Surgeons has also said that statistics are not available (Wolf, 1990c); but one cosmetic surgery in America has admitted to one death in 30000, which must mean at least 67 American women dead up to 1990 (Wolf, 1990b).

Yet being fat isolates and invalidates a woman (Boskind-Lodahl, 1976). Almost inevitably, the explanations offered for fatness point a finger at the failure of women themselves to control their weight, control their appetites and control their impulses. Women suffering from the problem of compulsive eating endure a double anguish: feeling out of step with the rest of society, and believing that it is all their own fault. Self-starvation, resulting in anorexia nervosa, is often regarded as a reflection of a culture that praises thinness and fragility in women. Many women pinpoint the onset of their anorexia as an exaggerated response to dieting and teenage ideals of femininity. As Orbach (1978) says, compulsive eaters like anorectics sense something amiss at adolescence and seek the answer in their individual biology. Their bodies change, become curvy and fuller and take on the shape of a woman. They change in a way over which they have no control. They do not know at the time whether or not they will be small-breasted and large-hipped or whether their bodies will eventually end up as stereotyped teenagers.

These distresses render in young women feelings of confusion, fear and powerlessness. Their changing bodies are associated with a changing position in their worlds at home, at school and with their friends. A curvy body meant the adoption of a teenage girl's sexual identity. This is the time, as Orbach (1978) comments, for intense interest in appearance, the time when girls learn the tortuous lesson about not revealing their true selves to boys whether on the tennis court or in school, or in discussing affairs of the heart. These rules and regulations governing behaviour, and the explosive changes taking place, are quite out of tune with what has previously been learned and the feelings they generate are enormously complicated.

Several women have said, on looking back on their adolescence – a time when they were growing and yet effectively stopped eating – that they felt so out of phase with all that was going on that withdrawal from food was an immensely satisfying way to be in control of the situation (Orbach, 1984). In transcending hunger pangs they were winning in one area of the struggle with their apparently independently developing bodies. They were attempting to gain control over their shapes and their physical needs. They felt their power in their ability to ignore their hunger.

However, this power to overcome hunger results in a contradiction because in her very attempt to be strong, the anorectic becomes so weak that she becomes less independent, more dependent. She needs more care and concern from others because of her weakened physical state. This adaptation poses yet another dilemma. As Parker and Mauger (1976) write, 'For a great many women manipulation of their own bodies is too often their only means of gaining a sense of accomplishment. The link between social status and slimness is both real and imagined. It is real because fat people are discriminated against; it is imaginary because the thin, delicate ideal image of femininity only increases a person's sense of ineffectualness'. Furthermore, in the distortion of body size that follows the manipulation of hunger feelings, the anorectic and the compulsive eater powerfully indict sexist culture. The young woman takes herself out of the only available arena and worries that should she express her sexual feelings her whole world will crack (Orbach, 1978).

In the retreat from a sexual identity the anorectic young woman is pointing to the difficulties of the various aspects of womanhood (Friar Williams, 1977), and sexual identity is an aspect of gender identity so that in rejecting models of sexuality one is simultaneously rejecting models of femininity. This is the dilemma that faces many women and is expressed both through the symbolic meanings of being thin and food refusal for the anorectic.

CHARACTERISTICS OF THE FEMALE ANORECTIC

Both relative overweight and underweight are accompanied by an increased risk to health and to life. All the eating disorders are associated with increased illness because both anorectics and, to a lesser extent, bulimics are underweight. In addition to the complications associated with bulimia (which will be discussed in Chapter 4), the anorectic, because of extreme weight loss, suffers from cessation of menstruation (Stewart *et al.*, 1990), cold intolerance, dry skin often covered by fine body 'lanugo' hair – soft, downy hair on the nape of the neck and forearms – cold and blue extremities, peripheral oedema, bradycardia (slowing of the heart rate to less than 50 beats per minute) and hypotension (low blood pressure). Depression more extreme than that usually associated with bulimia often occurs (Agras, 1987); about half the fatalities due to anorexia nervosa are caused by suicide. Any intercurrent illness, such as pneumonia, also carries more risk than it does for the individual who is at normal weight.

Patterns of eating in established anorexia nervosa may take two broad forms. The more common pattern is usually known as **abstinent anorexia nervosa** (Palmer, 1982). Almost every anorectic begins with this pattern and most continue to behave in this way throughout their illness. Some, however, may develop other behaviour patterns as time passes such as purging themselves of food after a meal. The eating behaviour of the abstinent anorectic resembles ordinary slimming in the inappropriate context of an abnormally low body weight. The anorectic works hard at limiting her diet and weight even though she is already very thin. Typically she will avoid all foods which she considers to be fattening, particularly high carbohydrate foods. However, she may allow herself to eat substantial amounts of bulky low calorie foods such as celery, crispbread or cottage cheese. Sometimes her diet will come to be only very small in amount but also quite eccentric in its constituent foods (Kay and Shapira, 1972; Palmer, 1982). A few anorectics take on a yellow skin pigment through eating large numbers of carrots but little else. The whole gamut of slimming activity may be present although it often seems charged with a frantic force which is absent from such behaviour when slimming is an appropriate response to obesity. As Palmer (1982) suggests, what to the commonplace slimmer may be a struggle or a chore, to the anorectic may seem a source of morbid fascination.

In terms of the total calorific value of food eaten, an abstinent anorectic will characteristically exist on an average daily intake of under 1000 calories, compared with the norm of two or three times this amount. The anorectic is struggling to keep up her position of abstinence in the face of not only her sensations of hunger but also the demands of a truly undernourished body. Although her behaviour resembles normal slimming, the context is quite different. Most anorectics will initially deny that they are hungry. Some probably do truly lose their appetite, but will later admit that they were experiencing a strong desire to eat. Many sufferers become preoccupied with food. They are, for instance, eager to prepare other meals which they will not eat themselves. Likewise, most anorectics have some lapses of their control and eat more from time to time. When the strong self-control breaks, an eating binge may follow. At times, the amount of food eaten during one binge may be very large. It seems that for some individuals the struggle to control their weight by abstinence alone becomes too much and they find additional mechanisms. Palmer (1979) suggests these individuals are those in whom the hunger drive is greatest or the control of impulses is least developed. It is these individuals who go on to the second broad pattern of eating behaviour which is characterized by overeating, self-induced vomiting and often by the abuse of laxatives and other drugs.

The onset of self-induced vomiting is a considerable complication in primary anorexia nervosa. (Primary anorexia nervosa is generally considered to be a disease of young people; secondary anorexia, sometimes called 'anorexia tardive', occurs at any age after puberty.) The habit of vomiting will often start when an abstinent anorectic feels bloated and uncomfortable after she has for once 'let go' and eaten more than usual. She then vomits to relieve the discomfort and perhaps also the guilt which she feels about having indulged her appetite. Later, however, she may realize that vomiting is a kind of insurance policy against the effect of overeating because it interferes with the otherwise inevitable link between eating and weight. The fear of weight gain then no longer serves as a brake upon the impulse to eat and overeating may become both substantial and regular. The vomiting which started as a response to unwelcome inner feelings may become premeditated. Anorectics often develop a considerable facility for vomiting. An individual may come to be able to vomit at will without, for instance, the need to stick her fingers down her throat.

Sometimes vomiting may allow the person to return to a

more regular pattern of eating whilst avoiding weight gain. Thus some individuals may achieve a kind of stability combined with an apparently unremarkable diet. Two or three meals are eaten each day; but two or three meals are vomited up again in secret shortly after they are eaten. It is possible for this pattern to continue for months or even years and yet for the anorectic to successfully conceal her vomiting from those near to her. Certainly some women with 'mysterious' thinness and 'mysterious' amenorrhoea accompanied by an apparently good appetite and diet are chronic covert vomiters. However, the stability of this pattern is more apparent than real since the individual is now involved in a balancing act. On the one hand, she has her eating behaviour which may be linked to a routine of social expectations but is always more or less disrupted by impulses to overeat. On the other hand, she must vomit up sufficient of what she eats to keep her weight down but not so much as to render herself physically ill. Not surprisingly the seesaw usually begins to wobble and only in a few cases can a kind of fragile stability be maintained for long. Sometimes the balance swings in favour of weight gain and occasionally this gain may provide the individual with the opportunity for recovery. Unfortunately, it is more usual for the individual to panic as her weight increases and drastically cut back her food intake once more. Even chronic vomiters have their times when they return to a predominantly abstinent pattern. However, the temptation to eat and then vomit is seldom resisted for long.

THE MALE ANORECTIC

It would appear that a substantial proportion of general practitioners do not believe that anorexia nervosa occurs in males (Bhanji, 1979). In part this stems from insistence on amenorrhoea before the diagnosis can be made, and in part from a conviction that the underlying psychopathology is specific to the female. Palmer (1982) nevertheless states that in the definite case the individual's low weight, odd eating and his attitude to both will be enough to make a clinical diagnosis possible. Investigation can also reveal similar patterns of hormonal change to those which underlie the amenorrhoea in the female.

Beumont, Beardwood and Russell (1972) reviewed the literature and traced a total of 250 alleged male cases of anorexia nervosa. The authors were left with only 25 instances of probable anorexia nervosa, to which they added six of their own. In the same year, a further 13 cases were described by Crisp and Toms (1972). The majority view today is that this disorder does occur in adolescent males but is uncommon. The main clinical features are unexplained loss of weight and profound constipation.

Richard Morton's (1689) first reported anorectic was a male who had similar symptoms to an 18 year old female patient of Morton's who would be diagnosed as anorexic by today's DSM-III-R criteria. Mintz (1983) also provides descriptions and case histories of five anorectic males and Wilson, Hogan and Mintz (1983) cite several studies reporting male anorectics from 1689 to 1978. However, Bruch (1975) emphasizes the rareness of the condition in males and reported only ten male patients out of a series of 70 anorectics treated between 1942 and 1970. A number of authors have reported on the most outstanding features of this illness in males (Falstein, Feinstein and Judas, 1956; Crisp, 1967; Bruch, 1971; Taipale *et al.*, 1972; Deneux *et al.*, 1977; Hasan and Tibbetts, 1977; Screenivasan, 1978; Hay and Leonard, 1979; Ollendick, 1979; Fichter and Keeser, 1980). Premorbid features include childhood obesity, parental overprotection, excessive obedience and a family setting with considerable strife and instability. Usually the anorectic managed to maintain a precarious psychic equilibrium until the stresses of pre-adolescence and adolescence proper destabilized it. Mintz (1983) comments that obesity and excessive preoccupation with food in family members were not unusual.

Several reasons have been put forward for the low incidence of male anorexia nervosa. For instance, Dally, Gomez and Isaacs (1979) suggest that in Western society today slimness is pursued enthusiastically by young women. Male adolescents, on the other hand, do not generally have a strong desire to be slim. In fact, they like to be muscular and well built. Nylander's (1971) Scandinavian study showed that 50% of 18 year old girls considered themselves too fat, compared with 7% of 18 year old boys.

Other reasons include the fact that the female figure changes during puberty in such a way that a girl cannot help but be aware of it. Many girls with anorexia nervosa are upset, not so much by menarche as by their growing breasts and enlarging hips, and what these signify. Starving minimizes these changes or reverses them, and at the same time reduces libido. It is significant that the fear that female patients have of becoming fat so often centres around their hips and thighs. Male hips remain slim, and although chests may enlarge this is not because of fat and it is usually welcomed as a sign of masculinity. The fear of fatness expressed by male anorectics usually concerns their bodies as a whole; it is not focused on a particular body area.

Lastly, male anorexia nervosa may of course be more common than it appears. Female anorexia nervosa is widely recognized today. A relatively small loss of weight, cessation of menses for two or three months, and the girl is usually referred to her general practitioner. But a male can lose a considerable amount of weight and excite no comment; or, as Andersen and Mickalide (1983) suggest, they may be too embarrassed to report their symptoms to doctors. The incidence of male anorexia nervosa is therefore difficult to assess.

Certainly many researchers have reported that male anorectics present with similar symptoms to their female counterparts (Seaver and Binder, 1972; Tunbridge and Fraser, 1972; Dally, Gomez and Isaacs, 1979) with reasons for not eating ranging from being too fat to the belief that food was liable to cause tiredness and impair mental concentration. It would seem, though, that male anorectics exhibit slightly more obsessive–compulsive behaviour than female anorectics (Wiener, 1976; Dally, Gomez and Isacs, 1979) and may become very rigid in their daily routines.

DIFFERENTIAL DIAGNOSIS OF ANOREXIA NERVOSA

Organic disease must be considered and excluded in every patient with anorexia nervosa. In most cases, and certainly those with primary anorexia nervosa, this is not difficult. Nonetheless, mistakes are still made, particularly in secondary cases with atypical features, complicated by purging and vomiting or the abuse of drugs and laxatives. Anorexia and loss of weight are common symptoms during the course of many illnesses. Vitamin and iron deficiencies are virtually never seen in primary anorexia nervosa (Bruch, 1965; Crisp, 1977;

Dally, Gomez and Isaacs, 1979), although they can develop in secondary anorexia nervosa. Their presence should immediately raise doubts about diagnosis.

Infectious diseases such as tuberculosis (a common complication in the past) or brucellosis are still sometimes encountered today with anorexia nervosa. Tuberculosis, which used to account for many of the deaths reported in the past, is more likely to follow starvation than cause it (Thompson and Morgan, 1990). Mononucleosis (a condition in which the blood contains an abnormally high number of mononuclear leucocytes) sometimes occurs a few months before the onset of primary anorexia nervosa; glandular fever is not uncommon in adolescence and may sometimes be the trigger that fires off anorexia nervosa.

Gastrointestinal disorders may rarely be confused with anorexia nervosa and then only in the older atypical cases. Characteristically, patients with anorexia nervosa are constipated. Only those with secondary anorexia nervosa who abuse laxatives, or whose diet is largely composed of nuts, present with diarrhoea or steatorrhoea. A history of childhood coeliac disease (where the small intestine fails to digest and absorb food, a sensitivity to the protein gliadin contained in the gluten of wheat germ) is occasionally encountered, but often turns out to be dubious on close investigation. Dally, Gomez and Isaacs (1979) reported that of 400 patients seen over the past 20 years, none had coeliac disease or signs of malabsorption at the time of onset of weight loss.

Crohn's disease (in which segments of the alimentary tract become inflamed, thickened and ulcerated) and ulcerative colitis (a condition of unknown cause in which the rectum as well as a varying amount of colon become inflamed and ulcerated) have been reported to occur with anorexia nervosa; abdominal pain occurs in about 10% of patients and sometimes paralytic ileus and gastric dilation are possible complications, especially of bingeing after starvation.

The blood sugar levels in anorexia nervosa may be extremely low in severe starvation and it is not uncommon for emaciated patients to be admitted to hospital with a blood sugar of 1.4 mmol per litre (normal range is 3.5 to 5.5 mmol per litre). Hypercholesterolaemia is also a common finding, with levels as high as 13.25 mmol per litre (normal range is 3.7 to 6.9 mmol per litre), and sometimes hypercarotenaemia. However, it is now recognized that anorexia nervosa does not resemble Simmond's disease (characterized by loss of sexual function, loss of weight and other features of hypopituitarism); although there is certainly an endocrine disturbance in anorexia nervosa, as manifested by amenorrhoea, it is clear that the anterior pituitary itself is normal and that it is the hypothalamus, influencing the pituitary, which is disturbed (Dally, Gomez and Isaacs, 1979; Bhanji and Mattingly, 1988).

Apart from physical symptoms there are often psychiatric overlays with anorexia nervosa. Obsessional and phobic anxiety symptoms (Thompson, 1989) are occasionally so prominent that the features of anorexia nervosa are missed. Depression of mood, disturbance of sleep and other symptoms and signs which can accompany depression are by no means rare. Suicidal gestures are common among those who binge (Bruch, 1978); but suicide itself occurs in 2% of patients with long-standing anorexia nervosa (Dally, Gomez and Isaacs, 1979), from despair and eventual loss of hope of recovery. Carrier (1939) considered depression to underlie many of his cases of anorexia nervosa although, like Dally, Gomez and Isaacs (1979), he recommended that eating disorders associated with obvious depressive illness should not be termed anorexia nervosa.

Several writers, including Kraepelin (1920), have tried to equate anorexia nervosa with manic depressive illness. Decourt (1951) argued that some of his patients were depressed and described cyclothymic swings in one patient. Carrier (1939), too, quoted a case of a girl who had repeated episodes of anorexia nervosa between the ages of 18 and 32 years; from 28 years onwards she developed mania which alternated with depression. Manic depressive illness has been seen in association with anorexia nervosa-like behaviour (Dally, Gomez and Isaacs, 1979); but patients with such a combination should not be diagnosed as suffering from anorexia nervosa.

It has also been suggested in the past that schizophrenia can be related to anorexia nervosa (Dubois, 1913); Nicolle (1938) also supported this view. Using Bliss and Hardin Branch's (1960) very broad diagnostic criteria for anorexia nervosa, it can be seen that schizophrenia could be related; however, these views are very much in the minority amongst researchers and clinicians and it is generally accepted that anorexia nervosa may be distinguished as a disorder in its own right as defined by the DSM-III-R criteria.

FURTHER READING

General

Bhanji, S. and Mattingly, D. (1988) *Medical Aspects of Anorexia Nervosa*. Wright, London.

Hill, A.J., Oliver, S. and Rogers, P.J. (1992) Eating in the adult world. The rise of dieting in childhood adolescence. *British Journal of Clinical Psychology*, **31**, 95–105.

Mehrabian, A. (1987) *Eating Characteristics and Temperament: General Measures and Interrelationships*. Springer-Verlag, New York.

Nielsen, S. (1992) Seasonal variation in anorexia nervosa – some preliminary findings from a neglected area of research. *International Journal of Eating Disorders*, **11**(1), 25–36.

Palmer, R.L. (1982) *Anorexia Nervosa: A Guide to Sufferers and their Families*. Penguin Books, Harmondsworth.

Raich, R.M., Rosen, J.C., Deus, J., Perez, O., Requena, A. and Gross, J. (1992) Eating disorder symptoms among adolescents in the United States and Spain – a comparative study. *International Journal of Eating Disorders*, **11**(1), 63–72.

Feminist literature

Barrow McBride, A. (1978) *Living with Contradictions: A Married Feminist*. Hamlyn, London.

Orbach, S. (1984) *Fat is a Feminist Issue 2: How to Free Yourself from Feeling Obsessive about Food*. Hamlyn, London.

Parker, R. and Mauger, S. (1976) Self-starvation. *Spare Rib*, **28**, 7.

2

Assessment, treatment and outcome of anorexia nervosa

Assessment of anorexia nervosa differs from that of obesity and most cases of bulimia in that the prospective patient is often poorly motivated for treatment and is being brought for consultation by an alarmed family. The major diagnostic features of anorexia nervosa are: a weight less than 25% of actual or expected bodyweight, a very restricted eating pattern often accompanied by excessive exercise, a fear of gaining weight, and amenorrhoea (in women). Use of the questionnaire together with a clinical interview will usually quickly lead to the correct diagnosis, although it should be remembered that physical illness may mimic anorexia nervosa, and that a concurrent investigation by the medical team is essential for correct diagnosis.

Assessment usually consists of three phases:

1. Completion of a screening questionnaire that allows much of the basic information concerning the problem to be easily obtained in a systematic manner.
2. Interview to clarify the basic history of the problem and to make an accurate diagnosis of the main disorder and any associated psychological problems.
3. Self-monitoring of the problem behaviour for several days forms the last element in a detailed assessment so that therapeutic recommendations can be made followed by treatment.

Patient's name ....

Date ....

It would be helpful for us to know how you have been feeling about your appearance during the last *four weeks*. Please answer all of the following questions by carefully reading each of them and circling ONE number to the right of each question.

	NEVER	RARELY	SOMETIMES	OFTEN	VERY OFTEN	ALWAYS
1. Have you felt happiest about your shape when your stomach has been empty?	1	2	3	4	5	6
2. Have you pinched areas of your body to see how much fat there is?	1	2	3	4	5	6
3. Have you been afraid that you might become fat or fatter?	1	2	3	4	5	6
4. Have you worried about your thighs spreading out when sitting down?	1	2	3	4	5	6
5. Has thinking about your shape interfered with your ability to concentrate?	1	2	3	4	5	6
6. Have you imagined cutting off fleshy areas of your body?	1	2	3	4	5	6
7. When in company, have you worried about taking up too much room?	1	2	3	4	5	6
8. Has worry about your shape made you feel you ought to exercise?	1	2	3	4	5	6
9. Has feeling bored made you brood about your shape?	1	2	3	4	5	6
10. Have you avoided running because your flesh might wobble?	1	2	3	4	5	6

Figure 2.1 Eating behaviour questionnaire (adapted from a similar scale used at the Cullen Centre, Royal Edinburgh Hospital).

Screening questionnaires

Standard eating disorders questionnaires have included the Eating-Related Characteristics Questionnaire (ECQ) and the Supplementary Eating-Related Characteristics Questionnaire (SECQ) which has 142 items covering lack of appetite, secret bingeing, preoccupation with and fear of gaining weight, dieting, etc. (Mehrabian and Riccioni, 1986; Mehrabian, 1987).

	NEVER	RARELY	SOMETIMES	OFTEN	VERY OFTEN	ALWAYS
11. Have you felt so bad about your shape that you have cried?	1	2	3	4	5	6
12. Have you worried about other people seeing rolls of flesh around your waist or stomach?	1	2	3	4	5	6
13. Have you been so worried about your shape that you have been feeling that you ought to diet?	1	2	3	4	5	6
14. Have you felt that it is not fair that other women are thinner than you?	1	2	3	4	5	6
15. Has eating even a small amount of food made you feel fat?	1	2	3	4	5	6
16. Have you avoided wearing clothes which make you particularly aware of the shape of your body?	1	2	3	4	5	6
17. Has eating sweets, cakes or other high calorie food made you feel fat?	1	2	3	4	5	6
18. Have you thought that you are the shape you are because you lack self-control?	1	2	3	4	5	6
19. Have you not gone out to social occasions because you have felt bad about your shape?	1	2	3	4	5	6
20. Has seeing your reflection made you feel bad about your shape?	1	2	3	4	5	6
21. Has being naked, such as when taking a bath, made you feel fat?	1	2	3	4	5	6
22. Have you been particularly self-conscious about your shape when with others?	1	2	3	4	5	6
23. Has feeling full after a meal made you feel fat?	1	2	3	4	5	6
24. Have you compared yourself to other women and felt fat in comparison?	1	2	3	4	5	6
25. Have you felt ashamed of your body?	1	2	3	4	5	6

Figure 2.1 *Continued*

Other tools used by clinicians in the screening process include questionnaires such as the Eating Attitudes Scale (Garner and Garfinkel, 1979) and the Stanford Eating Disorders Questionnaire (Agras, 1987). This latter questionnaire is used routinely

Treating anorexia nervosa

Please place an 'X' under the column which applies best to each of the numbered statements. Most of the questions directly relate to food or eating although other types of questions have been included. Please answer each question carefully. Thank you.

	ALWAYS	VERY OFTEN	OFTEN	SOMETIMES	RARELY	NEVER
1. Like eating with other people.	…	…	…	…	…	…
2. Prepare foods for others but do not eat what I cook.	…	…	…	…	…	…
3. Become anxious prior to eating.	…	…	…	…	…	…
4. Am terrified about being overweight.	…	…	…	…	…	…
5. Avoid eating when I am hungry.	…	…	…	…	…	…
6. Find myself preoccupied with food.	…	…	…	…	…	…
7. Have gone on eating binges where I feel that I may not be able to stop.	…	…	…	…	…	…
8. Cut my food into small pieces.	…	…	…	…	…	…
9. Aware of the calorie content of foods that I eat.	…	…	…	…	…	…
10. Particularly avoid foods with a high carbohydrate content (e.g. bread, potatoes, rice, etc.).	…	…	…	…	…	…
11. Feel bloated after meals.	…	…	…	…	…	…
12. Feel that others would prefer if I ate more.	…	…	…	…	…	…
13. Vomit after I have eaten.	…	…	…	…	…	…
14. Feel extremely guilty after eating.	…	…	…	…	…	…
15. Am preoccupied with a desire to be thinner.	…	…	…	…	…	…
16. Exercise strenuously to burn off calories.	…	…	…	…	…	…
17. Weigh myself several times a day.	…	…	…	…	…	…
18. Like my clothes to fit tightly.	…	…	…	…	…	…
19. Enjoy eating meat.	…	…	…	…	…	…
20. Wake up early in the morning.	…	…	…	…	…	…
21. Eat the same foods day after day.	…	…	…	…	…	…

Figure 2.2 Eating Attitudes Test (EAT 40; Garner and Garfinkel, 1979).

	ALWAYS	VERY OFTEN	OFTEN	SOMETIMES	RARELY	NEVER
22. Think about burning up calories when I exercise.	...	...	...	...	...	...
23. Have regular menstrual periods.	...	...	...	...	...	...
24. Other people think that I am too thin.	...	...	...	...	...	...
25. Am preoccupied with the thought of having fat on my body.	...	...	...	...	...	...
26. Take longer than others to eat my meals.	...	...	...	...	...	...
27. Enjoy eating at restaurants.	...	...	...	...	...	...
28. Take laxatives.	...	...	...	...	...	...
29. Avoid foods with sugar in them.	...	...	...	...	...	...
30. Eat diet foods.	...	...	...	...	...	...
31. Feel that food controls my life.	...	...	...	...	...	...
32. Display self-control around food.	...	...	...	...	...	...
33. Feel that others pressure me to eat.	...	...	...	...	...	...
34. Give too much time and thought to food.	...	...	...	...	...	...
35. Suffer from constipation.	...	...	...	...	...	...
36. Feel uncomfortable about eating sweets.	...	...	...	...	...	...
37. Engage in dieting behaviour.	...	...	...	...	...	...
38. Like my stomach to be empty.	...	...	...	...	...	...
39. Enjoy trying new rich foods.	...	...	...	...	...	...
40. Have the impulse to vomit after meals.	...	...	...	...	...	...

Figure 2.2 *Continued*

for anorexic patients but is lengthy to administer, asking some 52 questions of the patient. It is a proven tool for use in research but alternatives may be sought in the first instance for clinical assessment (see Figures 2.1 and 2.2).

The first item of the Stanford Eating Disorders Questionnaire asks for identifying information from the patient and infor-

Name .... Age .... Date of birth ....

Address .... Telephone ....

.... Occupation ....

General practitioner ....

Address .... Telephone ....

....

Next of kin .... Religion ....

Address ....

.... Marital status ....

Telephone ....

Referred by .... Date first seen ....

Date referred ....

Referral diagnosis ....

Medication .... Laboratory results:

.... Bloods ....

.... Other (specify) ....

....

....

Detailed history

Psychological:

Social:

Physical:

Onset:

Development:

Precipitating factors:

Relieving factors:

Help given to date:

Reasons for seeking help now:

Availability of support:

Figure 2.3 Structured diagnostic interview.

Impact of problem on:

Job:

Leisure/hobbies:

Relationships:

Own views of:

Problems:

Expectations of treatment:

Comments on past treatment:

Family history: age, occupation, amount + quality of contact, health problems of family

Father:

Mother:

Brothers + sisters:

Husband/wife/partner:

Children:

Relevant others:

Current family circumstances:

Home atmosphere:

Personal history

Infancy + childhood:

General health + nervous traits:

Personality:

School (age started, standard reached, attitude to school + schoolmates):

Work (age started, number of jobs, reasons for change, satisfaction level, ambitions):

Social life/network:

Intake of alcohol .... tobacco .... drugs ....

street drugs .... caffeine (coffee, tea, coke) ....

Leisure/hobbies:

Sexual history (menstrual history, how information gained, early sexual experience, distressing sexual experience, other sexual experience):

Life events:

Relevant topics not covered:

Clinician .... Date ....

Figure 2.3 *Continued*

mation about the present occupation, schooling and living situation. The questionnaire then addresses weight, asking for present weight, ideal weight and satisfaction with body image, as well as the attitudes of family and friends towards the patient's weight. A chart is appended, allowing for a detailed lifetime history of weight changes, including the patient's assessment of how over- or underweight they were at various periods of their life, as well as the ways in which they attempted to alter their weight. This section is followed by detailed questions pertaining to binge-eating and purging, followed by an assessment of activity levels. Finally, a medical history and brief family history are requested.

The diagnostic interview

Both the patient and family members should be interviewed during the diagnostic process and it is usually best to see each individual separately first in order to gather as much independent information as possible. There is sometimes a considerable difference between information presented from family and patient, often exhibiting exaggeration of events due to a difference in interpretations (see Thompson and Gittins (1989a) for a discussion of parents' and staff's opinions). This is common in many psychiatric disorders. It is often useful to conduct a structured interview covering topics in a particular order (Figure 2.3).

When a diagnosis has been reached, feedback should be given to the patient and family together so that each person involved hears the same message and has an opportunity to discuss the issues raised by the diagnosis. Such feedback should include the diagnosis, prognosis and an outline of the treatment plan. For most cases of anorexia nervosa, inpatient treatment aimed at restoration of normal body weight will be needed. This recommendation will often raise protests from the patient, which is an area in which family support is very much of benefit. The aim of the clinician is to aid the family in confronting the prospective patient on the need for hospitalization, focusing upon the interpersonal processes involved. The clinician should not, however, become involved in persuading the patient to enter a hospital, because this will tend to enmesh the clinician in the family problem.

During the interview it is also important to assess the patient's mood because many patients with eating disorders have associated depression or dysphoria. This may be carried out by either administering a questionnaire, such as the Beck Depression Inventory (Beck *et al.*, 1961), or by structuring the interview by systematically questioning the patient using the questions in the inventory (Figure 2.4). This is best conducted by a clinical psychologist who is able to make recommendations for treatment based on interpretations made from the results of the inventory. An assertiveness inventory (Gambrill and Richey, 1975) is also sometimes a useful tool to use during the interview to assess the patient's personality traits.

Clinical experience strongly indicates that social factors are important in the development of eating disorders (Gordon, 1990), and these should be addressed in the diagnostic interview. However, it is difficult to demonstrate conclusively that such factors are critical and to discern which ones are most influential. The process of interviewing may take one or several sessions, depending upon the degree of resistance to treatment and the willingness of the family to confront the issues. A formal diagnosis can then be made using the criteria set out in the *Diagnostic and Statistical Manual of Mental Disorders* – DSM-III-R (as discussed in Chapter 1 under *Epidemiology*). This should not be confused with Feighner's criteria (Feighner *et al.*, 1972) which have commonly been used in the past for the purposes of research, though they have not been adopted for clinical use because of their broader categorization of the disorders.

It is often helpful to have the patient and family members visit the inpatient unit to demystify this aspect of treatment, although some would argue that such hospitals may give a frightening impression to the would-be inpatient, especially since a one-off visit cannot provide a representative impression. Once the patient has indicated a willingness to enter the hospital, an initial behavioural contract should be worked out, detailing the role and responsibilities of the patient and the consequences for gaining or losing weight. This contract should be negotiated with the patient, thus introducing this form of interchange. The different kinds of therapy – reinforcement of weight gain, group meetings, family therapy – should be carefully explained to the entire family and their expected role and participation in these activities made clear.

Patient's name .... Date ....

Clinician ....

Instructions: This is a questionnaire. On the questionnaire are groups of statements. Please read the entire group of statements in each category. Then pick out the one statement in that group which best describes the way you feel today, that is, *right now*! Circle the number beside the statement you have chosen. If several statements in the group seem to apply equally well, circle each one.

Be sure to read all the statements in each group before making your choice.

1. 0 I do not feel sad
   1 I feel sad
   2 I am sad all the time and I can't snap out of it
   3 I am so sad or unhappy that I can't stand it

2. 0 I am not particularly discouraged about the future
   1 I feel discouraged about the future
   2 I feel I have nothing to look forward to
   3 I feel that the future is hopeless and that things cannot improve

3. 0 I do not feel like a failure
   1 I feel I have failed more than the average person
   2 As I look back on my life, all I can see is a lot of failures
   3 I feel I am a complete failure as a person

4. 0 I get as much satisfaction out of things as I used to
   1 I don't enjoy things the way I used to
   2 I don't get real satisfaction out of anything any more
   3 I am dissatisfied or bored with everything

5. 0 I don't feel particularly guilty
   1 I feel guilty a good part of the time
   2 I feel quite guilty most of the time
   3 I feel guilty all of the time

6. 0 I don't feel I am being punished
   1 I feel I may be punished
   2 I expect to be punished
   3 I feel I am being punished

7. 0 I don't feel disappointed in myself
   1 I am disappointed in myself
   2 I am disgusted with myself
   3 I hate myself

8. 0 I don't feel I am any worse than anybody else
   1 I am critical of myself for my weakness or mistakes
   2 I blame myself all the time for my faults
   3 I blame myself for everything bad that happens

9. 0 I don't have any thoughts of killing myself
   1 I have thoughts of killing myself, but I would not carry them out
   2 I would like to kill myself
   3 I would kill myself if I had the chance

10. 0 I don't cry any more than usual
    1 I cry more than I used to
    2 I cry all the time now
    3 I used to be able to cry, but now I can't cry even though I want to

Figure 2.4 Beck Depression Inventory (BDI; Beck *et al.*, 1961).

11. 0 I am no more irritated now than I ever am
    1 I get annoyed or irritated more easily than I used to
    2 I feel irritated all the time now
    3 I don't get irritated at all by the things that used to irritate me

12. 0 I have not lost interest in other people
    1 I am less interested in other people than I used to be
    2 I have lost most of my interest in other people
    3 I have lost all of my interest in other people

13. 0 I make decisions about as well as I ever could
    1 I put off making decisions more than I used to
    2 I have greater difficulty in making decisions than I used to
    3 I can't make decisions at all any more

14. 0 I don't feel I look any worse than I used to
    1 I am worried that I am looking old or unattractive
    2 I feel that there are permanent changes in my appearance that make me look unattractive
    3 I believe that I look ugly

15. 0 I can work about as well as before
    1 It takes an extra effort to get started at doing something
    2 I have to push myself very hard to do anything
    3 I can't do any work at all

16. 0 I can sleep as well as usual
    1 I don't sleep as well as I used to
    2 I wake up 1–2 hours earlier than usual and find it hard to get back to sleep
    3 I wake up several hours earlier than I used to and cannot go back to sleep

17. 0 I don't get more tired than usual
    1 I get tired more easily than usual
    2 I get tired from doing almost anything
    3 I am too tired to do anything

18. 0 My appetite is no worse than usual
    1 My appetite is not as good as it used to be
    2 My appetite is much worse now
    3 I have no appetite at all any more

19. 0 I haven't lost much weight, if any, lately
    1 I have lost more than 5 pounds
    2 I have lost more than 10 pounds
    3 I have lost more than 15 pounds
    I am purposely trying to lose weight by eating less.
    Yes ...   No ...

20. 0 I am no more worried about my health than usual
    1 I am worried about physical problems such as aches and pains, or upset stomach, or constipation
    2 I am very worried about physical problems and it is hard to think of much else
    3 I am so worried about my physical problems that I cannot think about anything else

21. 0 I have not noticed any recent change in my interest in sex
    1 I am less interested in sex than I used to be
    2 I am much less interested in sex now
    3 I have lost interest in sex completely

Figure 2.4 *Continued*

When weight loss has not reached extreme proportions (less than 15% weight loss) outpatient treatment may be indicated. The same process of feedback should be used as with inpatient treatment and the potential necessity of hospitalization, if weight is not gained, should be explained to the patient and family; acceptance of this should be made an integral aspect of treatment. Many patients will try to gain weight to avoid hospitalization and the prior agreement for hospital care removes a potential problem from the clinician should the patient not gain weight. A treatment contract should be worked out and signed by the patient and clinician.

Self-monitoring

The methods by which therapeutic progress will be monitored also form an aspect of initial assessment because baseline measures should be obtained at this time in order to make comparisons with later measures. Particularly for anorexia nervosa, the determination of weight under standard conditions will form one of the main outcome measures. Such weights should be obtained using a balance scale resting upon a hard surface (as soft surfaces may lead to inaccurate weights) calibrated to zero. Both the therapist (clinical psychologist and/or dietitian and also possibly the nursing staff on the hospital ward) and the patient should maintain a simple weight chart. However, whilst very useful, self-monitoring is often difficult to maintain with anorectics because of their resistance to treatment, making essential information almost impossible to obtain during the assessment phase.

A typical self-monitoring form for use with anorectics (and also for bulimics) is shown in Figure 2.5. The rationale behind self-monitoring is that the patient becomes objectively aware of his or her patterns of eating through the process of routinely recording eating habits. Typically, each instance of food intake is recorded together with the time of day, type of food, quantity of food, type of preparation and length of each eating episode. In addition, speed of eating is estimated on a 1–7 scale from slow to fast; hunger is rated in a similar manner and moods and thoughts are also recorded. The rationale for the use of self-monitoring should be carefully explained to the patient, pointing out that accurate data concerning the problem needs

Food record to be completed daily						
Day, time	Place (e.g. home)	With whom	Extent of hunger before (0–10)	Is it a binge? (Y/N)	Type, quantity of food	Activity during eating

Extent of feeling full after eating (0–10)	Use of vomiting, laxatives? (Specify)	Feelings after vomiting, laxatives

Figure 2.5 A typical self-monitoring chart for outpatient anorectics and bulimics.

to be collected so that both patient and clinician can know which behaviours should be addressed. It should also be emphasized that patients who continue to monitor their behaviour tend to progress better than patients who do not do so (Agras, 1987). There is also a need to explain the method for collecting the data which can be summarized thus:

1. Complete the self-monitoring record immediately after the behaviour has been engaged rather than at the end of a day.
2. A detailed record is required. It is debatable whether or not the patient should be supplied with a completed record as an example. There is always the possibility of being influenced if an example is given whereas the nursing staff can check to see if the patient is recording items correctly or has not fully understood the record form.
3. The usefulness of the record to the patient should also be emphasized in terms of behavioural change and the planning of meals.

After discussing this procedure, therapy can then be undertaken. There are several alternative theories and procedures which will be discussed later in this chapter.

SOME ETHICAL CONSIDERATIONS

It is important to be cautious about identifying the source of problems as being within the patient when they might more appropriately be attributed to social situations or cultural factors (Strasser and Giles, 1988). Perhaps the most difficult ethical dilemma, often unavoidable in patients with anorexia nervosa, concerns the problem of free will versus determinism. An anorexic patient is usually brought to the general practitioner's surgery unwillingly by agonized parents who are alarmed by her physical condition. When faced with an emaciated anorectic showing signs of potentially fatal consequences of severe weight loss, the physician's first responsibility is to save the patient's life. But, as in the case of suicidal tendencies, intervention can become the subject of controversies revolving around such topics as the right of self-determinism, the sanctity of life and the responsibility to self and others. Difficult questions arise concerning the right to refuse treatment versus the enforcement of treatment on individuals who are considered dangerous to themselves. When an anorexic patient claims she has freely chosen to become thin, it is debatable whether or not she has the right to stay that way. Beumont, Burrows and Casper (1987) suggest that the patient in this condition no longer has that freedom when she loses control over her pursuit of thinness.

The psychological nature of the eating disorder – the paralysing sense of ineffectiveness (Bruch, 1973) – makes the situation still more complicated. At the centre of the therapeutic relationship lies the tension between protection and confrontation, medical paternalism and patient autonomy. In many cases, the clinician may feel forced to act on behalf of the patient while recognizing that one of the patient's basic problems is her lack of self-determinism. Imposed treatment is justifiable if it has the potential of giving the patient in the long term a greater psychological freedom than the one she is losing in the short term by being treated against her will.

However, imposed treatment should seldom mean compulsory detention. Treatment may also be imposed by the use of psychological forces from the patient's natural milieu. We can ask the parents or spouse to help persuade the patient to accept treatment if necessary, and thus make the family share responsibility in the decision-making process. Sometimes parental failure is the essential obstacle for treatment. If parents are unable or unwilling to ally themselves with treatment, the clinician's responsibility includes the obligation to act accordingly. Interventions may range from the educational (instruction and confrontation appealing to the parental responsibility) to the institution of legal procedures, e.g. transfer of custody; compulsory detention. Sometimes the clinician cannot avoid the dilemma of confronting the patient with a disturbed family system or protecting her against deleterious family influences (Harper, 1983).

Whatever the stage of illness the patient presents, the physician has to widen his or her medical diagnostic scope to a kind of psychosocial assessment on which further treatment planning must be based. Even when faced with medically acute situations, the clinician must pay attention to the psychological dimensions of his or her decisions and interventions. But it is equally important that non-medical therapists learn to recognize the somatic complications of starvation and collaborate with medical personnel in the treatment of eating disorders.

Treatment of anorexia nervosa is not a matter of correcting laboratory abnormalities and restoring emaciated bodies, nor is it just a question of getting access to the psychological world of the patient. We are in fact treating sensitive and fragile human beings where existence is both psychologically and physiologically distorted (Beumont, Burrows and Casper, 1987). Each decision for active intervention should be made by weighing the potential benefits of a treatment procedure against its possible risks, both from a psychological and a physiological point of view (Thompson, 1987e,f; Thompson and Coleman, 1988b; 1989). As Francis and Clarkin (1981) have suggested, 'Our first obligation is to follow the injunction *primum non nocere*; second is the identification of patients we neither help nor hurt; third, and sometimes most difficult, is to allow patients on their way to spontaneous improvement to recover without us'. The greater the rescue fantasies a clinician has, the greater the risks of ill-considered therapeutic activism. The problem is that we know little or nothing about the 'natural' course of anorexia nervosa or bulimia. Since primary prophylaxis of eating disorders is still a theoretical concept, we must confine ourselves to secondary prevention, i.e. tracing and treating patients as early as possible (Vandereycken and Meermann, 1984a).

Another difficult issue concerns the clinician's right to refuse treatment. After several unsuccessful treatment attempts and after having discussed the situation of therapeutic *impasse* with other colleagues in order to rule out unrecognized counter-aggressive reactions, the therapist may feel compelled to render an ultimatum about whether or not treatment can continue. Refusing treatment or referring the patient elsewhere may be justified because of the clinician's lack of experience. The central problem remains that of differentiating the treatable from the untreatable (Hall, 1982). Sometimes it is best to consider whether or not the patient is better off without an eating disorder in the long term and whether or not the patient has the necessary resources, both internal and external, to cope with the process of recovery. The balance of advantages and disadvantages of the disorder and its eventual treatment may only be accessible during or after some therapeutic trial. In other words, it is important to offer the patient a chance to change.

DECIDING WHEN TO HOSPITALIZE

Once the diagnosis has been made, with the exception of medical emergency indications, the decision to hospitalize a person with anorexia nervosa is usually based on a combination of criteria (Hodas, Liebman and Collins, 1982; Pierloot, Vandereycken and Verhaest, 1982). These include: medical criteria (which concern, in particular, a serious and potentially life-threatening deterioration of the patient's health); psychosocial criteria (referring to a seriously disturbed life situation that may not be cause and consequence of the eating disorder); psychotherapeutic criteria (especially in patients with a poorer prognosis – longer duration, late onset, occurrence of bulimia, vomiting or purging, etc.) (Figure 2.6).

In many referrals for hospitalization, the clinician is often expected to play the authority figure. This position can be much more comfortable when realizing that the patient and his

Medical criteria
- Dangerous alterations in vital signs, such as bradycardia, postural hypotension, hypothermia and electrolyte balance (hypokalaemia).
- Suicidal tendencies or attempts, psychotic reactions.
- Severe acute or unremitting extreme weight loss (more than 25% below normal weight – some researchers use stricter criteria, e.g. 30% below normal weight: Beumont, Burrows and Casper, 1987).
- Intercurrent infection in a cachectic patient (i.e. patient with abnormally low weight, weakness and general bodily decline).

Psychosocial criteria
- Abnormal social isolation with avoidance of interpersonal contacts or inability to engage in study or work.
- Marked family disturbance inaccessible to treatment.

Psychotherapeutic criteria
- Need for an intensive psychotherapeutic milieu which can induce a change process that otherwise would take a longer time to obtain.
- Previous treatment failures, such as refusal to engage in outpatient therapy, lack of motivation, etc.

Figure 2.6 Criteria for hospitalization for a patient with anorexia nervosa.

or her family should not abdicate their responsibilities; that an alternative to hospitalization is referral to an outpatient facility (although usually less successful in terms of therapeutic success – Beumont, Burrows and Casper, 1987); and that a good compromise between hospitalization and outpatient treatment is a day treatment programme with or without partial hospitalization. In the end, it is generally considered that the best guarantees of success in therapy are a constructive patient/family–clinician relationship and an explicit but consistent treatment plan. But the degree of success also depends very much on the style of the therapeutic approach and on the clinician personally.

HOW TO TREAT

Over the years there have been numerous types of treatments for anorectics. However, only three of these have gained sufficient research evidence for their use clinically. These are behavioural, cognitive (and often cognitive–behavioural) and pharmacological. As Agras and Kraemer (1983) have pointed out, the relative rarity of anorexia nervosa has retarded the development of a scientifically based approach to treatment because between-group outcome studies with sufficient statistical power are extraordinarily difficult to carry out. Thus, although there have been studies of the treatment of anorexia nervosa, all have been short-term and directed towards the restoration of normal weight. Longer term treatment is based entirely upon clinical experience. Few well-documented treatment approaches to this phase of therapy exist. Nonetheless, using analogous approaches to the treatment of bulimia, a cognitive–behavioural approach to the treatment of anorexia nervosa has been described in some detail (Garner and Bemis, 1982).

Behaviour therapy

The behaviour therapy approach dismisses unconscious conflict as the cause of mental illness and requires that symptoms are treated in their own right and not as the superficial manifestations of something else. The existence of an unconscious region of the mind is not disputed, but rather its significance. The behaviourist believes that people are as they are because they have learned to be that way.

This learning process takes two forms, the first being by classical, or Pavlovian, conditioning. Thus, if meals happen to coincide with an unpleasant event, such as a family argument, an aversion to food may develop and persist long after the coincident event has ceased to occur. The other form of learning depends on operant conditioning. Here the important factor is not the concurrence of stimuli, but the effect of a particular response. If the response results in pleasurable events it is more likely to be repeated than if something unpleasant happens. An adolescent girl may one day be off her food; her mother reacts with solicitous attention and so refusing food comes to have its rewards. If drastic dieting ensues and the concern aroused serves to re-unite a previously divided family, there is further inducement to continue. The disappearance of an unpleasant consequence is just as potent a reinforcer as the arrival of a pleasing one. The girl who is no longer teased because she is overweight may be sorely tempted to continue to diet even though her weight is now normal.

The major behavioural approach to the treatment of anorexia

nervosa uses reinforcement theory in an inpatient setting to motivate patients to gain weight. This method was first described in 1965 (Bachrach, Erwin and Mohr, 1965). These workers treated a severely emaciated 37 year old woman who weighed 21.4 kg on admission to hospital, a drop of some 32.2 kg from her normal adult weight. Social reinforcement that included attention, conversation and praise was made contingent upon eating. To enhance the effects of reinforcement, the patient was placed in a hospital room devoid of amenities such as television, books or frequent visits from the nursing and medical staff and visitors. Reinforcer deprivation of this sort has been shown to enhance the effects of contingent reinforcement on performance.

The first procedure used consisted of the clinician sitting with the patient at every meal and conversing with her only when she ate. Conversation and praise were used to shape an approximately normal eating rate. Other reinforcers, such as going for walks or visits from relatives, were also made contingent upon satisfactory eating behaviour. The patient gained some 7 kg with this regimen and then her weight levelled off. At this point, the clinicians suspected that she was vomiting her food after eating. Reinforcement then was made contingent upon weight gain, rather than upon eating behaviour. This is evidently a superior contingency because it insures both a reasonable caloric intake and the reduction of self-induced vomiting. Unfortunately, the effect of this change in contingencies was not clear because the patient was discharged too soon after it was introduced to evaluate its effectiveness (Agras, 1987).

Subsequent case reports appeared to confirm the finding that reinforcement contingencies applied to weight gain were successful in helping anorectics to gain weight. For the most part, privileges of various kinds have been made contingent upon small increments of weight gain over the previous highest weight. Some interesting variations have, however, been reported. In one study, the well-known reinforcing properties of physical exercise for the anorexic patient were used to advantage (Agras and Kraemer, 1983). These investigators made access to physical activity contingent upon weight gain, reporting marked success in three patients. In yet another variation on this theme, the activity of another anorexic patient was restricted by using chlorpromazine in sedative doses. Increments of drug dose were removed, dependent upon weight gain, thus allowing increases in activity levels contingent upon weight increase.

Despite these initial successes in uncontrolled case studies, the first experimental analysis of the use of positive reinforcement in anorexia nervosa revealed some rather puzzling results (Agras *et al.*, 1974). In this experiment, an anorexic patient was served 6000 calories per day, divided into three meals and an evening snack. Meals lasted for 30 minutes and were eaten alone, being served and removed without comment regarding the amount eaten by the nursing staff. Three experimental phases were held: a baseline condition, a reinforcement phase and a return to baseline. During the baseline condition, in order to have the patient attend to the process of recovery and to feel motivated, she was asked to record the number of mouthfuls of food that she ate at each meal and to plot these data on a graph kept on the wall of her room.

Reinforcement consisted of praise and social attention for eating more (for details of this type of procedure, see Thompson and Gittins, 1989a,b), as measured by mouthfuls and by caloric intake. In addition, pleasurable activities such as time outside her room and walks with a nurse were made contingent upon small increments of weight gain. The introduction of reinforcement led to rapid increases in caloric intake and a corresponding increase in weight. Reinforcement was then removed in a return to baseline conditions. Remarkably, caloric intake remained stable and weight gain continued despite the absence of reinforcement. Two replications of this experiment with different patients revealed similar results. These findings suggested that although contingent reinforcement was responsible for the beginning weight gain, another variable was responsible for continued weight gains.

On inquiry, each of these patients claimed that once they realized that they could gain weight, they continued to eat in order to be able to leave hospital, an environment that they had come to dislike because of the various restrictions on their behaviour. This, of course, is an example of negative reinforcement, in which an individual behaves in a particular way in order to remove an aversive event or situation from their personal environment. To nullify the effect of negative reinforcement in subsequent experiments and to examine the effect of positive reinforcement uncomplicated by negative reinforcement, a contract was negotiated with the participant and her parents, such that the participant would remain in hospital for 12 weeks for the purposes of research, whether or not she gained weight during that time. In this way, the effect of negative reinforcement was removed, because it was not possible for the patient to leave hospital by gaining weight.

The effects of this new contingency were quite clear. In contrast with the previous experiments, when positive reinforcement for weight gain was removed the patient's caloric intake and weight dropped. By removing the obscuring effect of negative reinforcement, the effect of removing positive reinforcement was clarified. It is therefore possible to conclude that both positive and negative reinforcement lead to weight gain in the anorexic patient.

Another observation during these experiments led to the delineation of two further therapeutic factors. During the baseline condition of the previous experiments, patients tended to increase their caloric intake and weight, yet positive reinforcement had not yet begun. During this phase the patient was served large meals in order to be able to measure caloric intake accurately and was given feedback about her weight each day, the number of mouthfuls that she ate at each meal and her daily caloric intake. Either of these two factors, the large meals or feedback, or both, might have had therapeutic effects.

To investigate the effect of informational feedback, a potentially powerful procedure in behavioural change (Thompson, 1984a; 1985; 1986), a new baseline condition devoid of both feedback and reinforcement was instituted. Caloric intake under this condition seemed to be stable. When positive reinforcement was begun in the next phase, without the addition of feedback, no effect was observed on caloric intake or weight. When feedback was added in the next phase, the patient began to eat more and to gain weight. Removal of feedback led to weight loss. Thus, neither feedback (as shown in the baseline phases of previous experiments) nor reinforcement by themselves lead to major weight gain. It is the combination of reinforcement and feedback that has the best therapeutic effects. (The reader is directed to the following papers detailing the effects of informational feedback, in a variety of therapeutic settings, including the use of computer graphics to effect behavioural change in patients: Hards, Thompson and Bate, 1986; Thompson, Coleman and Yates, 1986; Thompson, Hards and Bate, 1986; Thompson, 1987a,b,c,d; Thompson and Coleman, 1987a,b,c; 1988a; Morgan and Thompson, 1989; Thompson, 1990a.)

Finally, the effect of serving large meals was also investigated. It was found that the intake of anorexic patients was always lowered by some 500 calories per day when smaller meals were served, even though the anorexic never ate all the food served to her at any one meal (Agras *et al.*, 1974; Elkin *et al.*, 1973). These four procedures, positive and negative reinforcement, informational feedback and the serving of large meals, form the basis of a therapeutic approach to the inpatient treatment of anorexia nervosa. Later in this chapter, inpatient and outpatient treatment of anorexia nervosa will be discussed.

In 1979, Eckert *et al.* described a large-scale clinical trial of the effects of behaviour therapy as compared to milieu therapy. This study involved 81 anorexic women who participated in the experiment for 35 days. Only the initial effects of the different treatments were investigated in this study: 40 patients were allocated at random to behaviour therapy and 41 to milieu therapy. The weight gains at 35 days were not significantly different between these two groups. It did appear, however, that patients who had received no previous outpatient therapy responded better to behaviour therapy than those who had been previously treated. This finding suggests that behaviour therapy might be particularly applicable to the less complicated case of anorexia nervosa.

Systematic desensitization

Systematic desensitization involves treating anorexia nervosa as a phobia of eating and utilizes techniques used to allay other irrational fears. The anorectic is gradually exposed to the aversive stimulus, being helped to feel relaxed and calm at each stage. Eventually a state of panic is replaced by one of equanimity – exposure to the stimulus may be in the real situation (*in vivo*) or one that resembles it (*in vitro*) or may take place in the patient's imagination by the clinician 'planting' suggestions (imaginary). The clinician may rely on talking the patient into being relaxed or on a short-acting tranquillizer.

Systematic desensitization is most effective when the phobia is for a specific object or situation. Because of this its effectiveness in anorexia nervosa has been limited and most clinicians who favour behaviour therapy use operant conditioning as this is more appropriate to the alteration of complex behaviour patterns (Bhanji and Mattingly, 1988).

Operant conditioning

It is important that operant conditioning is carried out with the full consent of the patient and her family. It is also important to remember that rewarding appropriate behaviour is more effective than punishing undesirable acts (Bhanji and Mattingly, 1988), which are best ignored. The ultimate target (signalling the completion of treatment) and all rewards should be agreed in advance. Once a goal has been achieved the reward should follow as soon as possible. Targets are usually drawn up by those carrying out the treatment; rewards are chosen by the patient and are then administered in inverse order of preference as successive targets are reached. A stipulated rate of weight gain is the commonest target, but in some programmes it is the amount of food consumed. The successful application of operant conditioning calls for constant vigilance, as patients are adept at surreptitiously disposing of food or may enhance their weight by drinking copious amounts of water or concealing weights in their clothes. Some will also obtain rewards independently; a fairly easy matter in the case of cigarettes.

Excessive exercising, commonly found in anorexia nervosa, has received virtually no attention in the behavioural literature. Mavissakalian (1982) has described the use of an operant conditioning programme in which reinforcement was contingent both on eating a meal within 30 minutes of presentation and on a one hour rest period following a meal. In addition, there was reinforcement for weight gain. Two patients with anorexia nervosa were treated in this way and both became overweight following discharge. No data were reported on the patient's level of exercising following treatment.

In spite of its disadvantages, operant conditioning can result in rates of weight gain better than those obtained by psychotherapy alone and comparable to those achieved by medical means. Unfortunately, long-term benefits are as disappointing as with any other treatment. An early review of operant conditioning in anorexia nervosa was provided by Bhanji (1979) and a later discussion presented by Garfinkel and Garner (1982). However, one of the main criticisms of behaviour therapy, particularly operant conditioning, is that it ignores the personal factors which led to the anorexia nervosa. Furthermore, by taking control over the patient the clinician runs the risk of perpetuating the loss of individuality and sense of ineffectiveness which is so often a feature of this disorder.

Behaviour therapy produces rapid weight gain but ignores the wider issues. Psychodynamic therapy on the other hand is directed at what many psychiatrists regard as the cause, but takes much longer to carry out. Often the two approaches are combined and psychotherapy substituted for behaviour therapy once the patient has regained weight; it has often been said that psychotherapy may be the final incentive in a behavioural programme.

Cognitive therapy

Cognitive therapy used for the treatment of anorexia nervosa is based on the work of Beck and colleagues (1979) in the treatment of depression. Cognitive therapy has been used extensively and described since by a number of authors (Garner and Bemis, 1982; Garfinkel, 1985; Mizes and Klesger, 1989; Blackburn and Davidson, 1990). Four stages may be distinguished in cognitive therapy in which an attempt is made to modify dysfunctional thoughts:

1. Identification of dysfunctional thoughts;
2. Examination of these thoughts;
3. Identification of underlying dysfunctional beliefs and values;
4. Examination of these beliefs and values.

Dysfunctional thoughts are identified by self-monitoring, particularly at key times, for example when patients are reluctant to adhere to agreed behavioural instructions. In addition, the clinician may elicit thoughts by asking patients to imagine what would pass through their mind if, for example, they were asked to weigh themselves or if someone commented on their appearance. Having identified dysfunctional thoughts, patients are taught to question their validity. Particular emphasis is placed on getting patients to specify exactly what they think and on **operationalizing** ill-defined notions. For example, some patients think 'I'm getting fat' if they start to gain any weight whatsoever. In this circumstance the notion 'getting fat' is examined and operationalized. Patients are asked to consider such questions as 'At what stage does a person become fat?', 'Can "fatness" be reduced to a specific weight or shape?', e.g. clothes size, and 'Am I actually approaching this clothes size?'. Arguments and evidence to support or refute the thought are then marshalled.

Generation of counter-arguments is an important process and patients are asked in this stage to consider what others would think given the particular situation; whether they are applying one set of standards to themselves whilst applying another less rigorous set to others; and whether their style of reasoning may be dysfunctional. In addition, behavioural experiments are sometimes used to obtain further information relevant to the thought under scrutiny. The aim is to help patients reach a carefully reasoned conclusion which should then be used to govern their behaviour. For example, if a patient concludes that, although gaining weight made her think 'I am getting fat', the balance of evidence failed to support this view, it would not be appropriate for her either to chastise herself or to go on a diet.

The next stage is to address the dysfunctional beliefs and values. These cannot be identified using the technique for eliciting dysfunctional thoughts. This is because these beliefs and values are so much part of these patients' conceptual scheme that they are unable to stand back and analyse them. Instead, they have to be inferred from the patients' behaviour (e.g. from their avoidance of so-called fattening foods) and from the nature of their dysfunctional thoughts (e.g. 'I feel fat'). The technique for questioning these beliefs and values is similar to that used when examining patients' thoughts except that more of the work has to be done in treatment sessions (Beumont, Burrows and Casper, 1987). The clinician tries to help the patient examine the significance and validity of their underlying attitudes (Garner and Bemis, 1982). It involves not only the questioning of these attitudes, but also an examination of their development and maintenance.

Other clinicians working with anorectics have chosen to

classify dysfunctional schemas (i.e. thoughts and beliefs) in a different way (e.g. Palmer, 1982):

1. Specific ideas: 'If I eat 1 kg of food, I will gain 1 kg in weight' (i.e. ideas related to weight or to eating).
2. Non-specific ideas: 'Nobody likes a person who loses their temper all the time' (i.e. ideas that a non-anorectic could hold as well as an anorectic).
3. Linking ideas: 'If I gain lots of weight, everyone will think I'm ugly' (i.e. ideas which have references to both weight and/or other issues).

However, whichever classification is chosen, the methods remain similar in getting the patient to expose their thoughts and beliefs and to search for evidence to support or refute them.

Cognitive–behavioural therapy

Garner and Bemis (1982) proposed a cognitive–behavioural approach to the treatment of anorectics after confirming the significance of distorted thinking patterns in the maintenance of the anorexic syndrome. While some still conceptualize anorexia nervosa as having a unitary cause, there is still a growing recognition that the disorder is multidetermined in the sense that it may develop from the complex interaction of different predisposing factors within different individuals (Lucas, Duncan and Piens, 1976; Strober, 1980; 1983; Casper, 1982; Hollin and Lewis, 1988). It has been argued that a particular advantage of a cognitive–behavioural understanding of anorexia nervosa is that it is not necessarily incompatible with other models that view the origin of the disorder as related to early developmental defects (Garner and Bemis, 1982). Regardless of the theoretical orientation, most researchers would accept that at some point, causal factors converge at the patient's belief that 'It is essential that I be thin'. Thus, much of the apparently bizarre and irrational behaviour observed in anorexia nervosa is the direct result of a set of beliefs, attitudes and assumptions about the meaning of body weight.

Much of the speculation regarding the pathogenesis of anorexia nervosa conforms to an avoidance paradigm, which assumes that the probability of a behaviour increases following negative reinforcement, i.e. the removal or offset of an aversive stimulus (Garner and Bemis, 1982). This model accounts for much of the anorectic's stereotypical behaviour such as dieting, exercise, vomiting and the use of purgatives to avoid the feared stimulus, i.e. fatness. It is also compatible with the conceptualization of anorexia nervosa as an adaptive disorder where the 'weight phobia' represents a threat from feared circumstances associated with psychosexual maturity (Crisp, 1980b; Lacey, 1983).

It is well recognized that avoidance behaviour is resistant to extinction because it insulates the individual from recognizing when aversive contingencies are no longer in operation. Cognitive variables may contribute to this process. Beck (1967; 1976) has observed that avoidance behaviour may be perpetuated by hyperactive cognitive sets, which may eventually operate in an autonomous fashion. A belief system develops to which incoming information is shaped to fit; data that are inconsistent with the system are either disregarded or distorted in the interest of the predominant belief. However, anorexia nervosa may be distinguished from a simple phobic disorder since symptoms are maintained by positive as well as negative reinforcement. Weight loss provides not only a solution for avoiding the feared situation of 'fatness', but also a sense of gratification in its own right. Social reinforcement, though, does not adequately account for the development of anorexia nervosa, since the emaciated state achieved by most is well beyond the societal standards for shape. Rather, the relentless dieting is maintained by potent cognitive self-reinforcement from the sense of mastery, self-control and competence derived from successful dieting. For the anorectic, hunger is no longer simply an aversive stimulus. It acquires a new meaning because it is associated with a higher accomplishment. As Garner and Bemis (1982) have aptly suggested, the anorectic's extraordinary attempts to control her appetite provide a long-coveted sense of mastery within the context of lifelong feelings of incompetence.

Assessment of cognition, affect and behaviour is largely dependent upon self-report data, and therefore the accuracy of the information derived will be predicated upon the establishment of a trusting, cooperative relationship between patient and clinician. In its absence, the patient is understandably reluctant to reveal vital aspects of thinking and may consciously falsify her experience. If cognitive therapy is the treatment of choice, then this aspect of the assessment phase is particularly important. The cognitive–behavioural approach to anorexia nervosa may be distinguished by its explicit concern with beliefs, values and assumptions as well as the patient's behaviour. The key issues which it should address may be summarized under the following 11 points:

1. **Articulation of patient's beliefs**. Many anorexic patients exhibit obsessional behaviour in performing daily routines in a sometimes particularly superstitious manner. Obsessive–compulsive disorder may be manifested in the anorectic and needs to be addressed during the treatment phase. Exposure to situations in which the patient feels compelled to perform in an obsessional manner and then preventing their response from happening (**response prevention**) is a way in which the disorder is treated. However, the reader is referred to documentation elsewhere concerning the complex issues surrounding the disorder and its treatment (Rachman, Hodgson and Marzillier, 1970; Roper, Rachman and Hodgson, 1973; Stern, Lipsedge and Marks, 1973; Marks, Hodgson and Rachman, 1975; Rabavilas, Boulougouris and Stefanis, 1976; Beech and Vaughan, 1978; Foa, 1979; Rachman *et al.*, 1979; Cobb, 1983; Salkovskis and Warwick, 1985).

2. **Reattribution techniques**. The reattribution technique has been applied to several areas of bodily experience that provide feedback inconsistent with recovery. Garner and Bemis (1982) explain that rather than directly modifying the body image misrepresentation frequently observed in anorexia nervosa (Slade and Russell, 1973; Dally and Gomez, 1980; Whitehouse, Freeman and Annandale, 1988; Warah, 1989), clinicians may assist patients in altering their interpretations of their self-perceptions (see also, Garner and Garfinkel, 1981; Garner and Bemis, 1982). Since the anorectic's refractory perception of herself as too fat is instrumental in maintaining dieting efforts, she must begin to question the validity of her subjective experience of her body. This may be accomplished by interrupting or overriding self-perceptions of fatness with counter-arguments

such as 'I know that people with this disorder cannot trust their own size perception' (Garner and Bemis, 1982).

3. **Hypothesis testing**. Garner and Bemis (1982) have described this application in detail. Specific testable hypotheses may be generated such as:
   (a) Do others really believe that thinner people are more desirable?
   (b) Is this relationship linear, i.e. the thinner you are, the more desirable and more competent you are?
   (c) Are there really just a few people who accept this current trend in fashion uncritically?
   (d) Do most people actually think of 'thinness' when they think of the words 'desirable' or 'competent'?

4. **Challenging the patient's beliefs through behavioural exercises**. Personal experiments may provide valuable corrective experiences that promote belief change. These may be targeted at idiosyncratic eating patterns or at the beliefs underlying social avoidance or excessive dependence on parents (Garner and Bemis, 1982). By practising self-initiated behaviour, patients can generally provide evidence to contradict their conviction that they are incompetent.

5. **Decentring**. This is a strategy for viewing a particular belief from a different perspective in order to evaluate its validity more objectively. It is particularly useful in combating patients' egocentric conviction that either they or their behaviour are central to other people's attention (e.g. 'I am worried that other people will notice that I have gained 2 kg'. The clinician can reply to this comment: 'Do you really notice when other people gain or lose small amounts of weight?'). Through the technique of decentring, the clinician may be encouraged to develop for the patient a more realistic idea of the impact that most behaviour has on others.

6. **Decatastrophizing**. This technique was originally proposed by Albert Ellis (1962) for combating anxiety resulting from magnification of the negative consequences of a particular event. It involves translating vague and implicit predictions of calamity into more realistic expectations. Such questions asked by the clinician may be: 'If the feared situation did occur, would it be as devastating as you imagine?'. As Ellis (1962) suggests, the **catastrophizing** in which patients

engage often inadvertently results in the very condition that is most feared. The anorectic who demands thinness of herself in order to be happy is in fact anxious when she considers herself as being fat. This anxiety remains, even at a low weight, since she is constantly aware of the risk of regaining weight.

7. **Challenging the patient's 'should' statements**. Horney (1950) declared that the 'tyranny of the shoulds' is the cornerstone of neurotic disturbance. This is the extreme thinking reflected in catastrophizing and dichotomous (black–white) reasoning and has been indicated in the anorectic's excessive reliance on the words 'should', 'must', 'ought' in directing her actions. This tendency has also been observed in many psychological disorders (Ellis, 1962; Beck, 1976). Vertes (1971) has suggested that the legitimate uses of such words may be easily distinguished from the inappropriate applications; Beck *et al.* (1979) has suggested that response prevention may be used to provide empirical evidence that 'shoulds' can be ignored without dire consequences. Indeed, a variation of response preventions may be effective in modifying the anorectic's attendant cognitions as well as her compulsive behaviour; the rigid rules of the following may be revised slowly as she is exposed to contradictory evidence, e.g. 'I must perform my exercise routine and eat the same safe food every day or I will gain weight uncontrollably'. Since successful response prevention may elicit intense anxiety, it is important for the clinician to be both aware and sensitive to the conflict imposed by resisting the 'shoulds'.

8. **Palliative techniques**. As Garner and Bemis (1982) have suggested, patients are often unable to employ more sophisticated cognitive techniques to challenge maladaptive thoughts for a variety of reasons; 'parroting' or 'distraction' (Thompson, 1983a; Thompson and Morgan, 1990) may avert destructive behaviours that could sabotage weeks of therapeutic progress. If overwhelming anxiety related to food or shape interferes with reasoning, the anorectic may be taught to parrot coping phrases to help her through the experience, such as 'I will finish each bite of my meal; I will not get fat'. Essentially these techniques involve forcefully 'changing the cognitive channel' (Garner and Bemis, 1982)

rather than attempting to modify beliefs through challenging, disputing or examining evidence in a systematic way. Indeed, parroting adaptive beliefs may be useful for patients who become ensnared in protracted debate and indecision about whether or not they are 'fat' or whether they adhere to their plan for gaining weight.

9. **Challenging cultural values regarding shape.** One of the major obstacles in encouraging the anorectic to relax her intense striving for thinness is that this therapeutic objective is in opposition to prevailing standards for physical attractiveness of women within Western society (Garner *et al.*, 1980). The anorectic's vulnerability to external influence increases the impact of these social pressures. It has even been argued that anorexia nervosa has acquired a not altogether unfavourable social connotation which may interfere with motivation towards recovery (e.g. Branch and Eurman, 1980; Garner and Bemis, 1982; Garner, Garfinkel and Olmsted, 1983).

10. **Patient's self-esteem.** As most researchers and clinicians would agree, the typical anorectic is highly self-critical and experiences herself as inadequate in most areas of personal or social functioning. A number of studies have provided evidence of this extreme form of self-disparagement (Casper, Offer and Ostrov, 1981; Garner and Garfinkel, 1981); the anorectic's negative self-evaluation appears to precede weight loss and is not ameliorated by simple renourishment. It would seem that the poor self-esteem occurs despite excellent objective performance and apparently normal or even ideal childhood (Garner and Bemis, 1982). Early research on persuasibility found that subjects with low self-esteem were more responsive to influence from the media and individual social interactions. These subjects also perceived themselves to be more vulnerable to the exercise of power over them in various situations (Cohen, 1959).

Guidano and Liotti (1983) have argued that the most striking quality of the sense of ineffectiveness is that 'it is usually expressed as a general expectation of failure' which is not necessarily attributed to personal responsibility or precise external events. This may contrast with the state of the depressed patient, who is predisposed to assume an 'emptiness in personal identity', as if there is nothing inside to which success or failure could be attributed. There is remarkable similarity between Bruch's (1977; 1979; 1980) descriptions of the ineffectiveness dimension and Lefcourt's (1966) definition of the locus of control (internal–external) construct. Lefcourt defines external locus of control as 'the perception of positive and/or negative events as being unrelated to one's own behaviours in certain situations and therefore beyond personal control' (p207).

Continual assessment and re-assessment are required to determine possible functions served by the patient's weight-related self-evaluation, i.e. the meanings attached to pursuing thinness and avoiding fatness. Patients must gradually understand that their belief system makes their disorder functional; yet at the same time it is dysfunctional in the broader sense in that it confines the patient to a restricted and obsessional lifestyle.

11. **Patient's self-awareness, body sensations and perceptions**. For many years, researchers have described deficits in self-awareness in anorexia nervosa (Wall, 1959; Jessner and Abse, 1960; Frazier, 1965; Bruch, 1978; Selvini Palazzoli, 1974). These deficiencies may, in part, be mediated by self-esteem; however, they may develop from and be maintained by distorted beliefs or assumptions about stimuli arising in the body. Distorted beliefs related to physiological states pose unique problems for which specific treatment strategies are indicated. Cognitive distortions may be identified that are specifically related to aspects of internal experience, such as the identification and responsiveness to beliefs; identification and expression of affect; identification and responsiveness to bodily sensations and perceptions.

Confusion and mistrust related to bodily sensations in particular have been clinically observed in anorexia nervosa (Whitehouse, Freeman and Annandale, 1988; Bowden *et al.*, 1989; Warah, 1989). Patients very often report doubts or distorted beliefs about internal states and display little confidence in the reliability or validity of bodily sensations. It may be that these cognitions are secondary to fundamental interoceptive disturbances, or that the anorectic's poor overall self-concept results in her questioning the reliability of all aspects of her experience. The confusion in the area of bodily functioning may be responsible for the anorectic's compensatory overcontrol of natural biological processes, as well as her reliance upon 'rules' and intellectual strategies to determine what is happening inside her body. These issues will be discussed in the next section.

BODY IMAGE AND ITS DISTURBANCE IN THE ANORECTIC

The perception of body shape is affected by cultural and social factors (Leon, 1982) and there have been many reports relating an alleged increase in the prevalence of anorexia nervosa to societal pressures of a similar kind (Boskind-Lodahl, 1976; Bruch, 1978; Garner *et al.*, 1980; Garfinkel and Garner, 1982). However, why certain individuals within a culture develop anorexia nervosa while others do not has yet to be determined.

The original and primary source of information on body image was derived from the neurology literature and the first documented account of body image disturbance was reported by Ambroise Pare, a seventeenth century surgeon. He described how patients who had a limb amputated would often report an illusory feeling of continued presence of the missing member or 'phantom limb' (McCrea, Summerfield and Rosen, 1982), hence, **phantom limb phenomenon**. References to the body image concept are frequently reported in the literature. Contexts include neurological disease (Kolb, 1975), psychiatric disorders (Schilder, 1935), hypnotic phenomena (Klemperer, 1954), drug effects (Savage, 1955), fatigue, stress and just before falling asleep (Federni, 1926), sensory deprivation (Azima, Lemieux and Azima, 1962) and psychotherapy (Fisher and Cleveland, 1958). Traub and Orbach (1964) commented that experiences of body perception have been observed in diagnostic classification of patients including those under the effects of hallucinogenic drugs. This breadth of coverage has subsequently resulted in vague, equivocal definitions; for example, in psychiatric terms, the concept of body image has included surface attitudes, emotions and personality reactions of individuals towards their bodies. Because of the lack of any precise operational definition, it has been variously referred to as body schemata, postural model, perceived body ego and body boundaries percept (Gellert, Girgus and Cohen, 1971). Bennett (1960) provided an operational definition of body image, describing it as a set of phenomena named by individuals when asked to describe their own bodies, respond to a questionnaire about their bodies or draw a picture of them.

One of the most often quoted definitions of body image is '. . . the picture of our own body which we form in our mind, that is to say, the way in which the body appears to ourselves' (Schilder, 1935). Schilder recognized the important relationships among social, psychological and physiological factors in body image formation and claimed that body image has both a conscious and unconscious component.

Hilde Bruch (1962) described three key symptoms which she regarded as having causal significance in the development of anorexia nervosa:

1. A disturbance of delusional proportions in the body image and body concept.
2. A disturbance in the accuracy of perception or cognitive interpretation of stimuli arising in the body, with a failure to recognize signs of nutritional need (the most prominent deficiency of this type).
3. A paralysing sense of ineffectiveness.

Her clinical observations have stimulated considerable interest in investigating body image perception in patients with anorexia nervosa (McCrea, Summerfield and Rosen, 1982; Garfinkel and Garner, 1984).

Bruch was particularly impressed by the lack of concern shown by anorectics regarding their state of emaciation. She was intrigued by the finding that despite the denial of their cachectic physiques, they often acknowledged that their arms were too thin and would become acutely embarrassed when their arms were exposed in public. Bruch was of the firm conviction that unless patients with anorexia nervosa changed their attitudes concerning their body image, their immediate outcome would be unfavourable. The second characteristic which Bruch identified was a disturbance in the accuracy of perception (perceptual disturbance) and cognitive interpretation (conceptual disturbance) of stimuli arising within the body. She maintained that anorectics were unable to recognize sensations of hunger and patients would often deny or fail to recognize it, even in the presence of stomach contractions. Yet patients would complain of acute abdominal discomfort after consuming only a small quantity of food.

Assessing body image disturbance in anorectics

Investigation into the body image disturbance phenomenon can be conducted at the assessment phase. However, since it is also used as an assessment of therapeutic progress as well as in research, it will be discussed here in the context of treatment and treatment tools.

The search for an objective measurement of body image has continued since the 1900s with a variety of variables being investigated including body dissatisfaction and preferred body proportions (Jourard and Secord, 1955), body anxiety (Secord, 1953), concept of body size (Fisher, 1951), plasticity of body schema (Schneiderman, 1956) and position of body image in space (Witkin *et al.*, 1954). Essentially three different techniques have been used, namely projective techniques, self-report questionnaires and experimental techniques. The latter have included visual size estimation, image marking procedures, the distorting photograph technique and the distorting television image procedure.

Movable caliper technique

Slade and Russell (1973) first used this technique after modifying a visual size estimation method developed by Reitman and Cleveland (1964) to assess body image perception in schizophrenic patients. The technique allows body contours to be projected onto a screen and enables the estimated figure to be directly contrasted with the size of the actual figure. The apparatus consists of two movable lights mounted on a horizontal bar which was set at eye level. The lights can be adjusted to indicate perceived widths of specific body regions or parts. Subjects are usually seated in a dark room and asked to estimate the dimensions of body regions as well as the size of an inanimate object. The data obtained are compared with the actual dimensions recorded previously. Measures of body perception accuracy are then derived for each body region using the following formula:

Treating anorexia nervosa

$$\frac{\text{Perceived size}}{\text{Real size}} \times 100$$

Slade and Russell (1973) confirmed that anorectics over-estimated their body dimensions (face, chest, waist and hips) when compared to a normal control group who were remarkably accurate in establishing their body widths. However, the tendency of patients to overestimate their body widths did not extend to inanimate objects (e.g. blocks of wood). Patients became more accurate in their judgement as they regained weight. Also, those patients who continued to overestimate their body size at discharge were the most likely to relapse after hospital.

Image marking method

An unsophisticated, inexpensive and more basic approach for assessing body image perception was developed by Askevold (1975). The patient stood in front of a sheet of paper, which was attached to a convenient wall, and was asked to imagine that she was standing in front of a mirror and could see her reflection. She was requested to mark the points which corresponded to various body regions or parts. A further requirement was to mark the point which corresponded to the top of the head which gave an estimation of perceived height.

This procedure has been reported to differentiate anorectics from controls (Pierloot and Houben, 1978; Wingate and Christie, 1978; Bowden *et al.*, 1989). However, this finding was not confirmed by Strober (1980) who reported that both patients with anorexia nervosa and an age-matched psychiatric inpatient population overestimated body size during admission and six months after discharge. Slade (1985) has combined the data from published studies using this method and concluded that both anorectics and neurotic controls overestimate their body widths but that the anorectics do so to a greater extent. This finding was also supported by Touyz and Beumont (1985) and Whitehouse, Freeman and Annandale (1988). As the latter authors suggest, the finding of Freeman *et al.* (1985), of over-estimation of body size in anorexia nervosa and controls, is probably due to methodological differences.

Distorting photograph technique

Glucksman and Hirsch (1969) developed this technique to assess total body size perception in a small group of obese patients as well as in a control group. Images of the subjects were projected onto a screen using a slide projector and the subjects were able to distort the photograph along the horizontal axis. They were able to distort the image in either direction to make themselves up to 20% thinner or fatter than reality. The researchers also asked the subjects to accurately assess the dimensions of a symmetrical vase, as well as the weight of an anonymous male and female. The undistorted images were initially projected for ten seconds and were then distorted and the subjects were required to make the screen image correspond to the initial, undistorted one.

Garner *et al.* (1976) applied this technique to assess body size perception in patients with anorexia nervosa and obesity. They found that half of the anorectics showed a marked tendency towards overestimating their physiques and that this was positively related to measures of introversion and lack of self-control. Garner *et al.* (1976) also found that the tendency to overestimate physiques did not generalize to other people or objects. Bruch's (1962) earlier prediction was confirmed that those patients who overestimated their own physiques had a poor prognosis (Garfinkel, Moldofsky and Garner, 1977).

Distorting television image technique

Utilizing the advancements in technology, Allenbeck, Hallberg and Espmark (1976) developed a sophisticated technique which made use of a specially modified video monitor which enabled the individual to look thinner or fatter. Deviations from the actual body size of the individual were displayed using electrical instruments. This technique has been reported to have several advantages including the availability of the apparatus, instant feedback and a high quality image.

The procedure involves taking a photograph of the subjects using an instant Polaroid camera. While being photographed the subjects stand on a rotating platform, on which an outline of two feet placed 95 mm apart at the heels and pointing at an angle of 25° has been painted. They pose in a standardized position, feet on the imprints, arms by the side and slightly adducted and eyes fixed on a point one metre above the camera. The photographic print is scanned by a video camera, using a zoom lens. The signal from the video camera is fed into two monitors arranged in tandem. One is set up for viewing by the experimental subject; the other is attached to a camera and is used to take photographs of the images the subjects choose. An adjustable control alters the shape of the image being projected through the mechanism of the zoom lens. The images can be varied only in the horizontal plane so as to give an 'endomorphic', 'mesomorphic' or 'ectomorphic' figure without distorting height. The control knob is graduated on a linear scale, a setting of 100 indicating 100% accuracy in the judgement of body image and a setting of 50 an underestimation of body size by 50%.

Typically these tasks for each orientation are required of each subject: an estimate of her own physique (subjective image), a setting corresponding to the physique she considers ideal (ideal image) and a setting corresponding to the least favoured physique (least desired image). The subject is then shown an image in a random manner and is asked to adjust the image to correspond to the impression they have of what an average, normal weight individual would look like. They are then confronted directly with the 'model' and asked to match the image on the screen with the contours of her body.

Using this method, Whitehouse, Freeman and Annandale (1988) found a positive correlation with the Drive for Thinness subscale of the Eating Disorders Inventory (Garner, Olmsted and Polivy, 1983) among normal controls but not among anorectics. Bowden *et al.* (1989) found all their subjects demonstrated consistently less distortion on the video technique than on either the image marking or a visual size estimation technique. Several authors have concluded that although anorectics tend on average to overestimate their body size more than controls, the tendency is not unique to anorexia nervosa and therefore has no specific diagnostic relevance. It would also seem that this particular method has produced inconsistent evidence for the size overestimation effect in anorectics.

MEDICAL MANAGEMENT OF ANOREXIA NERVOSA

During the 1900s numerous somatic remedies have been advocated at various times for the medical treatment of anorexia nervosa (Bemis, 1978). These have included implanted calves' pituitary, testosterone, L-dopa, thyroid extract, vitamins, antipsychotic (neuroleptic) drugs, corticosteroids, ACTH (adrenocorticotrophic hormone), insulin and various anabolic agents. The following discussion will be confined to mainstream treatments and in particular the use of insulin which is mentioned because of its importance and relevance to diabetes mellitus, discussed later in this section.

Tube feeding

Many clinicians advocate the use of tube feeding for anorectics only in resistive cases (Bhanji and Mattingly, 1988). However, Williams (1958) suggested that inpatient treatment of anorexia nervosa was ineffective except in those patients who had been intubated. He reported on the progress of 53 female anorectics admitted to the London Hospital between 1897 and 1957. His recommendation that tube feeding be more freely adopted aroused much criticism and was not widely followed. A survey carried out among physicians in the United Kingdom showed that very few used this form of treatment (Bhanji, 1979) and that intravenous nutrition was only used with severe metabolic disturbances when the patient was uncooperative and emaciated (Bhanji and Mattingly, 1988).

Total parenteral nutrition

The usefulness of intravenous nutrition for the treatment of anorexia nervosa has been supported on a number of occasions where intravenous via subclavian vein catheterization proved life-saving (Finkelstein, 1972; Silk, 1983). Four less complicated cases in whom parenteral feeding succeeded in increasing both the patients' weights and their willingness to cooperate with psychotherapy were documented by Maloney and Farrell (1980). However, Pertschuk et al. (1981) drew attention to the potential hazards of this method of feeding and detailed the cases of 11 patients who had developed peripheral weakness and numbness followed by pneumonia after total parenteral nutrition. A transient elevation of serum transaminase levels occurred in five of the cases, one died as a result of hypophosphataemia (depletion of phosphates in the blood) and one patient suffered a pneumothorax (collection of fluid in the lung or lungs usually as a result of infection). Clearly, this method of intervention is fraught with possible medical complications.

Pharmacotherapy

Reviews from several authors suggest that three main factors play a part in the decision to use any particular drug (Johnson, Stuckey and Mitchell, 1983; Crisp, 1984; Russell, 1985; Treasure, 1988). The first is that the chosen drug has been shown to produce weight gain in other conditions. The weight-sustaining effect of insulin in the diabetic and the hunger which may result from hypoglycaemia are well recognized (Nathan *et al.*, 1984), but it is not clear how other drugs may cause weight gain. The neuroleptics may do so by reducing activity, producing water retention, altering carbohydrate metabolism or blocking the actions of hypothalamic dopaminergic neurones. The antidepressants appear to induce a craving for carbohydrates and cyproheptadine was found to increase the appetites of young asthmatics (Bhanji and Mattingly, 1988). Manic depressives on lithium may also gain weight; and delta-tetrahydrocannabinol has been shown to enhance the appetites of those suffering from late stages of cancer but it does not appear to be of any value in anorexia nervosa (Gross *et al.*, 1981).

The second factor in the use of a particular drug for the treatment of anorexia nervosa may result from the fact that certain disturbances have been found in the neurotransmitter of patients with eating disorders. For example, Barry and Klawans (1976) have argued that the disorder is caused by an increase in hypothalamic dopaminergic activity. Hence the dopamine antagonists, such as the neuroleptics, may be effective. If their view that the excess dopaminergic activity results from a defective feedback mechanism is correct, L-dopa should also be effective. An alternative theory is that anorexia nervosa results from a deficiency of hypothalamic catecholamines, especially dopamine (Mawson, 1974). Studies of the effects of

both L-dopa and the dopamine agonist bromocriptine in anorexia nervosa have disappointingly produced inconclusive
findings (Johanson and Knorr, 1977; Harrower *et al.*, 1977).
Redmond, Swann and Heninger (1976) did find that anorectics
gained weight when the alpha-adrenergic blocker phenoxybenzamine was administered rather than the beta-adrenergic
blocker propranolol (a drug often used by public speakers to
'calm their nerves' prior to speaking publicly).

The third factor is that anorexia nervosa is a variant of
some other disorder, such as depressive illness, and as such
may respond to antidepressants. Similarly, anticonvulsants
have been used because of the association with epilepsy as a
substantial proportion of anorectics have abnormal electro-
encephalograms ('brain waves'). However, the association between anorexia nervosa and other disorders such as depressive
illness has often been questioned (e.g. Altschuler and Weiner,
1985).

Evidence for pharmacotherapy

Neuroleptics

Insulin and the neuroleptic chlorpromazine (in daily doses of
up to 1000 mg) were found to reduce anorectics' resistance
towards eating and produced a greater increase in weight than
insulin alone (Dally, Oppenheim and Sargant, 1958). However,
the side effects of chlorpromazine, such as epileptic seizures,
far outweighed its benefits (Dally, 1981; Crisp, 1984). The view
that anorexia nervosa stems from hyperactivity of hypothalamic
dopaminergic neurones led to the use of other neuroleptics
which, unlike chlorpromazine, were pure dopamine antagonists. Such drugs as pimozide and sulpiride have been found
to promote small signs of weight gain (Plantey, 1977) though
support documented in the 1980s was not statistically significant (Vandereycken and Pierloot, 1982; Vandereycken, 1984).

Antidepressants

Paykel, Mueller and De La Vergne (1973) were the first to carry
out a systematic study of weight gain as a side effect of antidepressant drugs. Harris, Young and Hughes (1986) studied
the effects of seven antidepressant regimens on appetite,
weight and preference for carbohydrates and found that flu-

penthixol, trimipramine (plus phenelzine) and trimipramine (plus isocarboxazid) resulted in the greatest increases.

Dally (1981) and Kennedy, Piran and Garfinkel (1985) considered the effects of monoamine oxidase inhibitors (MAOIs) on weight gain but concluded that they were of little value. However, this was contradicted by Hudson *et al.* (1985) who described a case who was eventually treated with tranylcypromine and L-tryptophan. Likewise, Lacey and Crisp (1980) looked at monoamine re-uptake inhibitors, finding that patients on clomipramine showed increased hunger, appetite and calorie intake and became more active. Biederman *et al.* (1985) found no advantages in taking an antidepressant versus a placebo and finally, Halmi *et al.* (1986) found that the effects on weight gain from using amitriptyline were only a little better than a placebo. In conclusion, the major influences on the outcome of treatment seemed to be the hospital at which the patient was admitted and the weight on admission.

Anticonvulsants

Conflicting reports showed that bingeing anorectics who were administered phenytoin 100 mg thrice daily responded well (Green and Rau, 1974). Using a combination of carbamazepine and lithium, Hudson *et al.* (1985) found similar results of weight gain in an anorectic who frequently binged. Wermuth *et al.* (1977) and Rau, Struve and Green (1979) argued that the main role of anticonvulsants, particularly phenytoin, was in the control of compulsive overeating.

Antiserotonergic drugs

Benady (1970) and Dolecek and Janstova (1985) investigated the effects of cyproheptadine and pizotifen respectively, finding that they were effective in producing weight gain in anorexia nervosa. This is probably due to their antihistamine properties and antagonistic action on serotonin causing vasoconstriction of blood vessels and resulting indirectly in a slowed metabolic rate. However, the latter research has not been confirmed since and Vigersky and Loriaux (1977), Goldberg *et al.* (1979) and Halmi *et al.* (1986) have all suggested that cyproheptadine in particular has few advantages, if any, over placebo.

Opiate antagonists

Treatment of anorexic patients using naloxone has been reported by Moore, Mills and Forster (1981) and, in combination with amitriptyline and anticonvulsants, by Mills and Medlicott (1984). Although relatively successful, the treatment is very expensive and has to be given by continuous intravenous infusion which again poses the problems of infection and other possible medical complications apart from the ones of compliance.

Named drugs

1. **Bethanecol and domperidone**: accelerate gastric emptying but the value of this in anorexia nervosa is undetermined (Dubois, Gross and Ebert, 1980; Russell *et al.*, 1983).
2. **Lithium**: evidence of weight gain was found in anorectics receiving lithium carbonate (Kerry, Liebling and Owen, 1970; Barcai, 1977; Gross *et al.*, 1981) but the side effects of lithium prevented its use for patients who had cardiac complications or who where hypokalaemic.
3. **Metoclopramide**: increases stomach emptying by increasing gastric peristalsis, relaxing the pylorus and duodenum and increasing tonus in the lower end of the oesophagus. It also acts on the medullary vomiting centre to produce an antiemetic effect. It may also block dopaminergic nervous transmission with the hypothalamus. Saleh and Lebwohl (1980) confirmed that food tends to accumulate in the stomach in those suffering from anorexia nervosa and that metoclopramide can help relieve this situation.
4. **Zinc**: absence produces nausea and thus worsens the aversion for food (Safai-Kutti and Kutti, 1984). Results from trials using zinc sulphate showed marked increases in appetite and weight though there is an absence of double-blind trials using this drug with patients suffering from anorexia nervosa (Safai-Kutti and Kutti 1986; Bryce-Smith and Simpson, 1984; Bryce-Smith, 1986).
5. **Insulin**: produces hypoglycaemia (apart from restoring glucose imbalance in diabetes mellitus). The use of insulin in the treatment of anorexia nervosa began soon after its discovery with one of its earliest reports from Andersen (1928). Clow (1932) and McCullagh and Tupper (1940) have also

mentioned how anorectics were highly sensitive to insulin but Bond (1949) noticed that this had no effect on the patient's weight. It would seem that the majority of the literature suggests that the potentially serious consequences of hypoglycaemia resulting from insulin administration in anorectics make it an unviable treatment option. However, the reader is referred to the literature on diabetes mellitus in the presence of anorexia nervosa for details on insulin treatment to produce weight gain in diabetic anorectics, a condition originally thought to be rare before the 1980s (Fairburn and Steel, 1980; Hudson *et al.*, 1985; Szmukler and Russell, 1983; Hillard and Hillard, 1984; Malone and Armstrong, 1985; Rodin *et al.*, 1985; Rosmark *et al.*, 1986; Peveler and Fairburn, 1989). This topic is also addressed in further detail in the research section for anorexia nervosa (Chapter 3).

Family therapy

Much support has been received for family therapy as an alternative to other interventions for the treatment of anorexia nervosa (e.g. Minuchin, Rosman and Baker, 1978). Since the first report by Liebman, Minuchin and Baker (1974) of the results of simultaneous behaviour therapy and family psychotherapy, their approach to the psychiatric management of anorexia nervosa has been supported by several researchers (Bhanji and Mattingly, 1988). After a period of observation, during which the staff join the patient for lunch, it is stipulated that the anorectic will be allowed out of bed only if her weight has increased by 1/4 kg during the previous day. This procedure is repeated with a review by the family and clinician before discharge. After the patient has left hospital the family continue with a behavioural regimen supported by the clinician. Long-term and short-term goals are constantly reviewed with regular meetings with the patient, the family and the clinician. A sample treatment plan is provided by Vandereycken and Meermann (1984b) who describe the process of goal-setting in more detail, and also by Eisler (1988).

Self-help

There is little documentation on the efficacy of self-help programmes for anorectics; but the use of self-help groups is possibly useful if only to give support for sufferers and their families (e.g. Lewis and MacGuire, 1985). This topic is presented by way of research discussion in Chapter 3. The reader is also referred to the Further Reading section at the end of this chapter for information about self-help organizations (Gillie, Price and Robinson, 1982).

OTHER TREATMENT OPTIONS FOR ANOREXIA NERVOSA

A large number of alternative treatments have been tried for anorexic patients with varying degrees of success. So far the mainstream treatments have been detailed and discussed; with the exception of family therapy, the remaining interventions are generally considered to be less successful. These have included:

1. Surgery (leucotomy; pituitary transplants; implantation of calves' hypophysis);
2. Electroconvulsive therapy;
3. Supportive psychotherapy;
4. Dream analysis;
5. Videotape playback therapy;
6. Bedrest;
7. Provision of 'substitute parents' in hospital;
8. Psycho-education;
9. Aversive counter-conditioning;
10. Psychoanalysis.

TREATMENT AS AN INPATIENT

The treatment of anorexia nervosa is interdisciplinary in nature, especially in an inpatient setting such as a hospital. The team will generally involve psychiatry, clinical psychology, internal medicine, nursing, dietetics and physical/physiotherapy. Such treatment should only take place within a unit that specializes in the care of such patients. However, because of the relative rarity of the disorder, there are few units devoted solely to the treatment of anorexia nervosa, such as the Cullen Centre of the Royal Edinburgh Hospital, Edinburgh, Scotland, which treats anorexia nervosa and bulimia patients. One treatment model is a behavioural medicine unit in which psychiatry and medicine share the medical responsibility, while other team members share in the treatment.

Treating anorexia nervosa

Phases of inpatient treatment

These vary slightly between hospitals, but the following plan has been extracted from a mixture of sources, particularly the Maudsley Hospital, London, England and the Cullen Centre of the Royal Edinburgh Hospital, Edinburgh, Scotland:

1. **Setting the goal weight range.** Sometimes it is best to consider setting a weight range of 3–5 lbs rather than an absolute weight. The patient should aim to settle in the middle of this range. Usually the goal weight range is taken from a set of standards such as the Metropolitan Insurance Companies 1983 Tables.
2. **Frame size.** This may be measured from the elbow breadth and compared with standard charts.
3. **Target weight.** It should be a team decision as to whether the patient is informed of their target weight or kept in ignorance. The general policy of the Cullen Centre is to keep the patient as informed as possible about his or her treatment, though some clinicians see difficulties with implementing this policy.
4. **Clothes.** In the past, it has been the preference of the Maudsley Hospital staff to nurse anorexic patients in night clothes from the time of admission until the patient reaches the healthy weight agreed by the team. The rest of the clothes are given to the parents who will be asked to bring clothes to fit at the appropriate time in the treatment phase.
5. **Supervision.** 24-hour supervision is provided and shared by day and night staff. During meal times the nurse should observe very carefully for patients hiding food or throwing it out of a window. Staff should insist on patients finishing their food so that nothing remains on the plate. Typically, during rest periods, two hours after each meal, for one hour the patient should rest on the bed with feet up and then for one hour sitting in the lounge. The nursing staff should be vigilant in seeing that patients do not try to exercise on the bed or spend too long in toilets or bathrooms when they might vomit food eaten or exercise. To reduce this possibility, restrictions are made on times of bathing and duration and frequency of toileting.
6. **Weighing.** Patients are weighed at frequent, regular intervals with their back to the scales and wearing night clothes

only (after emptying the bladder). Patients are not told
their weight in order to lessen fears and preoccupation
with weight, unless they have reached a healthy weight
and are allowed to dress.

7. **Photographs**. On admission, anorectics may be photographed and again on reaching a healthy weight.

8. **Communication**. This is important between staff and
patient. Developing a good rapport with the anorectic is
vital for cooperation and progress in treatment.

9. **Searching lockers**. If patients are suspected of hiding food,
tablets or using laxatives, it is explained to the patient that
a locker search will be made and this is conducted with
two nurses present.

10. **Visitors**. No visitors or telephone calls are allowed in the
first week but this is reviewed weekly and the privilege
increased on reaching a healthy weight.

11. **Food**. This is prescribed as medication in its normal form
with only occasional use of milk-shake types of high calorie
products. Food should be discussed with the patient in
terms of portions or exchanges (i.e. sizes of products with
known calorific values) rather than actual calories. The
initial food intake should be between 1200–1500 calories
per day (i.e. 6–8 portions) according to the patient's admission weight. The diet should be low in fat and lactose;
these enzymes for digesting milk products take time
to build up following prolonged starvation and the body
should not be overwhelmed with these products until
proper inducement of enzymes has occurred. Calories
should be increased by 500–750 calories per week until
a maximum of 3500–5000 calories per day is achieved.
The exact number will depend on the rate of weight
gain, the size of the patient and the presence of discomfort. If too many low calorie foods are permitted in
the diet, the physical quantity occupied by the daily intake
is enormous.

12. **Reassurance**. Patients need to be reassured that they will
not be allowed to eat more than is prescribed for them and
that they will not be allowed to get overweight. Some
patients benefit from small quantities of anti-anxiety agents
about an hour before meals for the first week or two of
treatment or from the use of relaxation training.

13. **Psychiatric examination**. This will be concerned with detection and subsequent treatment of particular associated symptoms such as obsessional symptoms, phobic anxiety, childlike behaviour, domineering parents, etc. Treatment from a variety of options will be carried out: chemotherapy, psychotherapy, family therapy, behaviour modification, cognitive–behavioural therapy.

TREATMENT AS AN OUTPATIENT

The principles involved in treatment are exactly the same as outlined for inpatient care and outpatient follow-up. Assessment should be followed by an agreement that unless weight is gained at a reasonable rate (e.g. 0.1 kg per day determined by measurements at weekly intervals) the patient and family will agree to immediate hospitalization.

Treatment should commence by working out a reinforcement system for weight gain, should it be feasible and appropriate. Such a system will probably only be possible for the younger anorectic living at home, although for the college age patient, return to college at a particular weight level can be reinforcing. Patients may be asked to be active in their treatment by counting the number of bites of food that they eat and to plot the number of 'bite counts' for each meal and for each day on a graph (Agras, 1987). Such a record is useful to the patient because the number of bites taken parallels caloric intake, allowing the patient to better adjust the amount eaten in order to gain the desired amount of weight.

The initial stage of treatment has three primary goals:

1. For the clinician to form an effective therapeutic relationship with the patient and family members;
2. For the clinician to establish initial control over treatment;
3. For the clinician, family and patient to develop, agree upon and implement strategies for reversing the symptoms of anorexia nervosa (Sergent and Liebman, 1984).

In the middle phase of treatment, once the patient is gaining weight steadily, the clinician should begin to shift the focus of sessions to the psychosocial developmental difficulties of the patient and to unresolved conflicts. In the final phase, the clinician carries out individual therapy for the anorectic and this will involve work with other family members such as the parents.

The major problem in outpatient treatment is the complexity of family interactions which may impede progress; difficulty in consuming more than 3000 calories each day, making changes in exercise levels and preventing self-induced vomiting are also important areas which pose problems for the outpatient anorectic. It is difficult to estimate success rates in these patients but often they have more chance of long-term success than inpatients if they can manage a more normal and healthy lifestyle out of the inpatient hospital setting.

OUTCOME OF ANOREXIA NERVOSA

Hilde Bruch (1962) was convinced that unless patients with anorexia nervosa changed their attitudes concerning their body image, their immediate outcome would be unfavourable. Garner *et al.* (1976) confirmed this prediction, finding that those patients who overestimated their own physiques had a poor prognosis. Slade and Russell (1973) also found that patients who continued to overestimate their body size at discharge were the most likely to relapse after leaving hospital.

In 1985, using the repertory grid technique, Button found that patients who responded favourably at outcome were those whose elaboration of self went beyond the concept of weight (see also Crisp 1980a). The clinician may promote the process by gradually helping the patient to:

1. identify and modify weight-related self-schemata;
2. articulate specific beliefs about the meaning of weight;
3. challenge the basis for construing oneself in terms of shape.

Hsu (1980) reviewed research on the outcome of anorexia nervosa between 1954 and 1978 and discussed findings in the areas of mortality, nutritional status, eating difficulties, menstrual function, psychiatric status, psychosexual and psychosocial adjustment and treatment effects. This is one of the most comprehensive reviews on outcome research. Hsu concluded his review with the finding that most of the research seemed to support the view that outcome in a given series (i.e. treatment study) depends largely on the selection of cases that constitute the series and the criteria with which the outcome is assessed. Whether treatment focused on certain predictors or poor outcome, such as disturbed family relationships, can substantially alter the course of the illness still remained unclear at this time. However, Warah (1989) did find overestimation of body size amongst anorectics a predictor of poor prognosis; but at the same time, to make the picture less clear, Warah (1989) also found that body size overestimation was not confined to anorectics and that not all anorectics overestimate their body size. Clearly there is still a need to identify a predictor or predictors for the outcome of anorectic treatment series and the factors which increase the chance of therapeutic success.

FURTHER READING

Assessment

Dally, P., Gomez, J. and Isaacs, A.J. (1979) *Anorexia Nervosa*. Heinemann, London.

Types of treatment

Francis, A. and Clarkin, J.F. (1981) No treatment as the prescription of choice. *Archives of General Psychiatry*, **38**, 542–5.
Larocca, F.E.F. (1984) *The Psychiatric Clinics of North America*. W.B. Saunders, Philadelphia.

Behaviour therapy

Agras, W.S., Barlow, D.H., Chapin, H.N., Abel, G.G. and Leitenberg, H. (1974) Behaviour modification of anorexia nervosa. *Archives of General Psychiatry*, **30**, 279–86.

Cognitive therapy

Blackburn, I.M. and Davidson, K.M. (1990) *Cognitive Therapy for Depression and Anxiety: A Practitioner's Guide*. Blackwell, Oxford.

Cognitive–behavioural therapy

Garner, D.M. and Bemis, K.M. (1982) A cognitive–behavioural approach to anorexia nervosa. *Cognitive Therapy and Research*, **6**, 123–50.

Feeding schedules for people with learning disabilities

Thompson, S.B.N. and Gittins, D.K. (1989a) Finding the right incentive. *Therapy Weekly*, **16**(18), 8.

Thompson, S.B.N. and Gittins, D.K. (1989b) Using a pethna to increase the independence in feeding of a woman with profound mental handicap. *International Journal of Rehabilitation Research*, **12**, 204–7.

Feeding behaviour in anorectics

Uhe, A.M., Szmukler, G.I., Collier, G.R., Hansky, J., O'Shea, K. and Young, G.P. (1992) Potential regulators of feeding behavior in anorexia nervosa. *American Journal of Clinical Nutrition*, **55**(1), 28–32.

Effects of informational feedback on patients

Thompson, S.B.N. and Morgan, M. (1990) *Occupational Therapy for Stroke Rehabilitation*. Chapman & Hall, London and New York.

Misuse of drugs by patients

Mitchell, J.E., Pomeroy, C. and Huber, M. (1988) A clinician's guide to the eating disorders medicine cabinet. *International Journal of Eating Disorders*, **7**(2), 211–23.

Self-help groups

Gillie, O., Price, A. and Robinson, S. (1982) *The Sunday Times Self-Help Directory*. Granada, London.

Hartley, P. (1988) The role of self-help groups in eating disorders, in *Anorexia and Bulimia Nervosa: Practical Approaches*, (ed D. Scott), Croom Helm, London.

Inpatient and outpatient treatment of anorexia nervosa

Pierloot, R., Vandereycken, W. and Verhaest, S. (1982) An inpatient treatment program for anorexia nervosa patients. *Acta Psychiatrica Scandinavica*, **66**, 1–8.

Sergent, J. and Liebman, R. (1984) Outpatient treatment of anorexia nervosa. *Psychiatric Clinics of North America*, **7**(2), 235–45.

Outcome of anorexia nervosa

Hsu, L.K.G. (1980) Outcome of anorexia nervosa. A review of literature (1954 to 1978). *Archives of General Psychiatry*, **37**, 1041–6.

For further information about anorexia nervosa contact:

Anorexia Aid, Priory Centre, 11 Priory Road, High Wycombe, Buckinghamshire.

3

Research into anorexia nervosa

The purpose of this chapter is to present a selection of research topics in anorexia nervosa in order to provide the reader with not only detail of the research undertaken but also the types of methodologies used in such studies.

There have been numerous studies into anorexia nervosa and it would be impossible to summarize here the topics studied. However, it is possible to mention some of the main areas covered: familial alcoholism related to anorexia nervosa; development of pharmacological approaches; sociocultural models of anorexia nervosa; outcome and prognosis; family work; dental characteristics of anorectics; personality disorders; nutritional knowledge; support groups for parents; links with other disorders such as diabetes mellitus; cognitive dysfunction in anorexia nervosa. This list is by no means exhaustive and serves only to represent a 'flavour' of the sort of investigations that have been carried out. The latter four of these areas will now be discussed in greater detail with reference to particular studies; the remainder are referenced at the end of this chapter under the Further Reading section where the reader will find a source of typical studies under each heading.

NUTRITIONAL KNOWLEDGE

People suffering from anorexia nervosa and bulimia present with abnormal eating behaviour and are preoccupied with food, dieting and body weight (Garfinkel and Garner, 1982). Often they collect and read literature relating to food and body function, energy consumption and appear extremely interested in dietary matters. Therefore, it may be expected that they should have a fairly good knowledge of nutrition and that they know what to eat if they could only bring themselves to do so (Russell, 1978). Despite the probable relevance of nutritional knowledge for modification of eating behaviour and eating attitudes, few attempts have been made to investigate the extent of the nutritional knowledge of patients with eating disorders. Beumont *et al.* (1981) found that patients with anorexia nervosa had better nutritional knowledge only with respect to diets, roughage and the caloric content of food. Twenty five percent of the patients possessed less knowledge of nutrition than normal controls.

Laessle *et al.* (1988) developed a questionnaire to measure specific areas of nutritional knowledge and used 56 patients with DSM-III diagnoses of anorexia nervosa, bulimia or atypical eating disorders and 144 normal controls. An analysis of subscales of the questionnaire revealed that patients with anorexia nervosa or bulimia had significantly higher scores for nutritional knowledge than controls on subscales 'macronutrients and roughage' and 'calories', but did not differ from them on the subscale 'micronutrients and vitamins'. Patients with bulimia and patients with anorexia nervosa had equivalent scores; and 15% of these two types of patients scored below the 25th percentile of normal controls.

In the Laessle *et al.* (1988) study, a pool of 119 true–false items were generated for the questionnaire. Selection was governed by curriculum guidelines for the domestic sciences in Germany and by recommendations of the German Nutritional Board (DGE, 1984). The items were categorized into three subscales:

1. **Macronutrients and roughage**, containing questions about food composition with regard to carbohydrates, protein, fat and different types of roughage and the relevance of the latter to a healthy diet.
2. **Micronutrients and vitamins**, containing questions about minerals such as calcium, potassium, iron, etc. and vitamins; minimum requirements of these substances and about the nutrients that contain them.
3. **Calories**, containing questions about the caloric content of food, caloric consumption and energy requirements.

There was a 50% probability of answering true–false items correctly by chance. To correct for mere guessing (Grosse and

Wright, 1985), each item response (1: correct, 0: incorrect) was weighted by an additional rating of certainty about correctness of response (1: sure, 0: unsure). If an item was answered correctly but the respondent had stated that s/he was unsure about the response, it was assumed that s/he had guessed and the item was not marked as correct. Scores for the total scale and each subscale were tallied by adding up the correct answers after weighting (Laessle *et al.*, 1988).

Psychometric quality of the revised form of the Nutritional Knowledge Questionnaire in the Laessle *et al.* (1988) study seemed satisfactory, but the authors advised that it should be tested again in an independent sample. In addition to content validity, which was established by adequate selection of items, criterion validity was indicated by high scores for nutritional 'experts'. As a group, patients with anorexia nervosa or bulimia displayed a relatively thorough knowledge of nutritional matters. They scored higher than normal young adults not only with respect to caloric content of food but also with respect to questions concerning macronutrients and roughage, or micronutrients, minerals and vitamins. Thus, anorexic or bulimic patients generally seem well prepared for a dietary management programme as one component of multidimensional treatment. However, similar to the findings of Beumont *et al.* (1981), about 15% of the patients with anorexia nervosa or bulimia lacked some dietary knowledge.

Long-term normalization of disturbed eating behaviour depends on motivational and ability factors. If motivation to normalize eating behaviour has been established during psychological treatment, this might not be sufficient to maintain a nutritionally adequate diet, if the knowledge and the ability to compose such a diet are lacking. In many cases, patients cannot resort to internal cues to regulate intake, even after months of treatment (Beumont, 1985). They have to go through a 'transition period' of structured and controlled eating (Andersen, Morse and Santmyer, 1984) which requires a high level of nutritional knowledge. Therefore, even patients whose knowledge is relatively good might find additional information useful. A study by Kirkley, Agras and Weiss (1986) illustrates this problem. A large group of patients treated for bulimia with cognitive–behavioural therapy showed nutritional inadequacies after treatment, although binge-eating had stopped. Similar observations were also found in weight-recovered anorectics one year after inpatient treatment (Schweiger, Laessle and Pirke, 1986).

Laessle *et al.* (1988) concluded that the Nutritional Knowledge Questionnaire could be a useful tool for screening patients with poor nutritional knowledge. It could also be applied during a nutritional counselling programme (Beumont, 1985) to motivate and educate patients to improve their knowledge of nutrition, which is clearly an important factor for the improvement of anorexic and bulimic patients.

SUPPORT GROUPS FOR PARENTS

A two-year experience in running a group essentially for parents of children with anorexia nervosa has been described by Lewis and MacGuire (1985). The Anorexic Unit at the Royal Free Hospital, London, is part of a large psychiatric department in which inpatients were treated on a behavioural programme and attended a twice-weekly group. Family therapy or support to parents of either in- or outpatients was offered depending on the inclination and availability of staff.

The group met in the evening for 1½ hours on the first Monday of every month with three to 15 parents attending. The composition of the group varied as follows:

1. Husbands of bulimia patients;
2. Mothers whose husbands had died;
3. Divorced mothers;
4. Only mothers attended; two of these were divorced;
5. Both parents attended, some or most of the time.

From the beginning, the therapists encouraged communication among parents by passing questions directed at them back to other parents. There was an expectation that answers to problems would be given by the therapists. After the initial phase of sharing stories, the group moved to offering support to members. The experiences of those whose children were moving out of the eating disorders phase into what appears to be a depressive obsessional phase were helpful to others. At this time, there was resistance to interpretations offering insight. It was as though parents were seeking reassurance about their parenting ability and answers to the illness, before wanting to look at the family dynamics that might contribute to the illness.

The next phase was that of critical examination of the service offered by the unit. However, this was interpreted, on one level, as their difficulty in allowing others to care for their child, although the unit was in the process of policy change and improvement. Finally, questionnaires were sent out to all parents/husbands who had attended the group. A different but similar questionnaire was sent to their daughters/wives. They were asked to reply anonymously. Fifteen questionnaires were sent out; ten of the parents'/husbands' were completed and returned, but only six of the anorectics' questionnaires were completed (Lewis and MacGuire, 1985).

Some of the main themes that had emerged in the groups were as follows:

1. The difficulty in accepting the change in their childrens' behaviour and the anger or helplessness this engendered.
2. Closeness between mothers and daughters. Parents frequently presented with a special link between mother and daughter. The group would be told how some daughters would climb like a toddler into their mother's arms for a cuddle. It was difficult for parents to accept that this served to keep mothers in the mothering role.
3. Negative attitudes towards fathers, sometimes to the extent that the patient would not be in the same room with him.
4. The change in the family's eating pattern in their attempt to keep the anorectic 'normal'.
5. Concern was expressed as to the effect of the patient's illness on the rest of the family, particularly the siblings.
6. Particular difficulties parents experienced when patients were discharged from the unit – their lack of confidence in their parenting ability and their need for extra support from the treatment unit at this time.
7. The deepening of the depression and dependency the girls developed as they relinquished their symptoms of anorexia nervosa.
8. The girls' acknowledgement of their lack of feeling of self, e.g. 'I have to dress in this striking way. As I am no longer anorexic, I need something to make me different'.
9. Marital problems among the parents.

Husbands' replies to the questionnaires about the group were positive; parents' replies were generally critical towards the professionals involved in the treatment, wanting more positive suggestions and advice, but said that they had obtained mutual support and reassurance. It was felt that the group met some of the parents' needs for information and support but therapists were generally cautious in looking at family dynamics and their effects. Indeed, Boszormenyi-Nagy and Spark (1973) have found that the direct challenge of rigid and implicit family beliefs is likely to have the paradoxical effect of strengthening these beliefs.

The authors concluded that the group appeared to offer a safe setting for parents to unburden themselves and to gain guidance and advice from both other parents and the therapists. It would appear that a group of this type is of positive, though limited, value in helping parents to adjust to their child's illness; however, as Lewis and MacGuire (1985) suggest, it may be a useful adjunct in the overall treatment of anorexia nervosa.

DIABETES MELLITUS AND ANOREXIA NERVOSA

There are many case reports of patients with eating disorders (anorexia nervosa and bulimia in particular) and diabetes mellitus. The first case report was by Bruch (1973) followed by a study reported by Fairburn and Steel (1980). It was initially believed that such cases were rare, but the number of case reports has continued to grow. Dietary restraint, such as that required for satisfactory management of diabetes mellitus, may predispose patients to develop an eating disorder and the findings of some uncontrolled studies suggest that the prevalence of eating disorders may be higher among diabetic patients than among the general population (Hudson *et al.*, 1985; Rodin *et al.*, 1985; Rosmark *et al.*, 1986).

Early reports commented that the combination of eating disorders and diabetes mellitus presented a formidable therapeutic challenge (Fairburn and Steel, 1980; Szmukler and Russell, 1983). However, Peveler and Fairburn (1989) reported on a case of anorexia nervosa in a 22 year old woman with diabetes mellitus who was successfully treated using cognitive–behavioural techniques; the author described the modifications to the standard cognitive–behavioural treatment approaches (Garner and Bemis, 1985; Fairburn, 1985; Fairburn and Cooper, 1988) necessary for patients in whom these disorders co-exist.

The subject of the Peveler and Fairburn (1989) study was a 22 year old female laboratory worker who developed diabetes mellitus at the age of ten years. Her diabetes was described as always being 'difficult to control' in spite of regular clinical attendance and apparently good compliance with medical advice. The patient developed hypothyroidism at the age of 14 years with marked weight gain at the time of onset, settling after the commencement of thyroid hormone replacement therapy.

The presenting problem was a deterioration in metabolic control over a period of three months with frequent episodes of severe hypoglycaemia necessitating hospital admission. It emerged that this was associated with marked self-induced weight loss (Peveler and Fairburn, 1989).

At assessment, the patient was clearly underweight and distressed. She complained of depressed mood, lethargy, impaired concentration, episodes of depersonalization and extreme sensitivity to cold. Although she did not admit that her weight was low, she also had an intense fear of gaining any weight and admitted to powerful feelings of guilt after eating anything.

A baseline period of assessment and self-monitoring was instituted before treatment commenced. Measures used to monitor progress included weight, daily insulin dose, frequency of episodes of hypoglycaemia and glycosylated haemoglobin (HbAlc) (Nathan *et al.*, 1984). General psychological symptomatology was assessed using the Symptom Checklist (SCL-90R) (Peveler and Fairburn, 1989). Specific eating disorder symptomatology was assessed with the Eating Attitudes Test (EAT) (Garner and Garfinkel, 1979) and the Eating Disorders Inventory (EDI) (Garner, Olmsted and Polivy, 1983). These latter instruments provide valid and reliable indices of eating disorder psychopathology in non-diabetic populations, although the validity of some items (e.g. 'avoids food with sugar in them') is in question when the instruments are used with patients with diabetes mellitus.

The patient agreed to an initial treatment plan of 24 weekly outpatient appointments and was taught to monitor her behaviour and related thoughts. She was also asked to keep a detailed record of all food eaten, insulin injected, episodes of hypoglycaemia and the results of blood tests. Written information about the psychological and physiological effects of starvation was provided. The primary goal of treatment at this point was to engage the patient in a potentially therapeutic collaborative relationship and to encourage her to embark upon gradual weight gain (Peveler and Fairburn, 1989).

At the first stage of treatment, the patient's weight continued to fall, reaching a low point of 45 kg after four weeks. As she was continuing to weigh herself frequently, it was decided that she should be weighed at each weekly hospital visit and should not weigh herself in between. This instruction provoked considerable anxiety.

Dietary advice, agreed with the physicians responsible for routine diabetic care, centred on increasing the total amount of food consumed at each meal or snack time and the inclusion of more calorific foods in the diet. At each interview, the effects of changes in eating habits on glycaemic control were noted and appropriate adjustments in the insulin dose discussed. Increases in food intake were praised. Changes in eating were related to events in the patient's life and the effects of personal relationships upon eating and mood were also discussed when appropriate. Advice was directed towards abandoning extreme restraint and including 'banned' foods in the diet in moderate amounts (Peveler and Fairburn, 1989).

Subsequent treatment sessions diminished fears about anticipated weight gain and permitted increased eating for a week or two, but then observation of real weight gain would lead to a resurgence of anxiety and reduction of food intake. One of the patient's greatest fears concerned the return of her normal appetite. She reported that before the onset of anorexia nervosa she had felt constantly hungry and was not satisfied by the diabetic diet. Since achieving a low weight, her appetite had largely subsided.

Towards the end of the weekly appointments, weight gain was proceeding satisfactorily and the patient was adjusting her insulin dose as required. The next phase of treatment consisted of fortnightly appointments and more intensive use was made of cognitive techniques (Beck, 1976; Garner and Bemis, 1985). These were used to elicit and examine specific thoughts associated with weight and shape and with diabetes mellitus. Examples of diabetes-related thoughts included the following:

'How dare you eat if your sugar level isn't perfect?'
'This "hypo" serves you right for not managing your diabetes
properly.'

The patient's attributions for certain events were also examined, e.g. episodes of hypoglycaemia were regarded as a consequence of taking excess insulin, rather than as a consequence of undereating. The patient's perfectionistic approach to self-care contributed to the high frequency of hypoglycaemic attacks because she aimed to keep her blood glucose levels within unrealistically narrow limits and overcompensated for small deviations. She was able to accept a slightly wider range of glucose levels once she recognized the self-defeating nature of her unrealistic goals.

Soon after the shift to fortnightly appointments a target weight range of 55–58 kg was agreed. After almost one year of treatment, comprising 24 weekly and 14 fortnightly sessions, the target weight range was attained. The patient's attitudes to shape and weight were less distorted as may be seen by the fall in both the total EAT score (from 52 to 21) and the 'Drive for Thinness' (DT) subscale of the EDI (from 18 to 6). General psychological distress was also diminished as indicated by the fall in the score on the SCL-90R, from 133 to 50. Glycaemic control, as shown by the glycosylated haemoglobin level, remained satisfactory throughout and the frequency and severity of episodes of hypoglycaemia were markedly reduced.

The patient was seen for three months after the completion of treatment. The gains made in treatment had been well maintained, with no significant weight loss or continuing low levels of psychological disturbance as assessed by self-report and at interview; and there was a persisting change in attitudes to shape and weight. The patient had also made considerable progress in dealing with other problem areas, such as her career development. Regular menstruation had not resumed, however.

Peveler and Fairburn (1989) concluded that a cognitive–behavioural approach can succeed in selected patients who have co-existing anorexia nervosa and diabetes mellitus. Flexible multiple injection insulin regimens appear to facilitate the treatment of patients with eating disorders and the establishment of adequate glycaemic control. However, the treatment may be most effective if the therapist takes responsibility for the management of both eating disorder and diabetes. Therefore, the therapist requires a sound knowledge of the principles of treatment of both conditions. Finally, a close liaison between medical (i.e. hospital medic, general practitioner, general nurse, etc.) and psychiatric teams (i.e. clinical psychologist, psychiatrist, psychiatric nurse, etc.) is essential.

COGNITIVE DYSFUNCTION IN ANOREXIA NERVOSA

Apart from physical symptoms there are often psychiatric overlays with anorexia nervosa. Obsessional and phobic anxiety symptoms are occasionally so prominent that the features of anorexia nervosa are missed. Depression of mood, disturbance of sleep and other symptoms and signs which can accompany depression are by no means rare. Suicidal gestures are common among those who binge (Bruch, 1978) but suicide itself occurs in 2% of patients with long-standing anorexia nervosa (Dally, Gomez and Isaacs, 1979), from despair and eventual loss of hope of recovery. Carrier (1939) considered depression to underlie many of his cases of anorexia nervosa and like Dally, Gomez and Isaacs (1979), recommended that eating disorders associated with obvious depressive illness should not be termed anorexia nervosa.

Several writers, including Kraepelin (1920), have tried to equate anorexia nervosa with manic depressive illness. Decourt (1951) argued that some of his patients were depressed and described cyclothymic swings in one patient. Carrier (1939), too, quoted a case of a girl who had repeated episodes of anorexia nervosa between the ages of 18 and 32 years; from 28 years onwards she developed mania which alternated with depression. Manic depressive illness has been seen to occur in association with anorexia nervosa-like behaviour (Dally, Gomez and Isaacs, 1979); but patients with such a combination should not be diagnosed as suffering from anorexia nervosa.

It has also been suggested in the past that schizophrenia can be related to anorexia nervosa (Dubois, 1913); Nicolle (1938) also supported this view. Using Bliss and Hardin Branch's (1960) very broad diagnostic criteria for anorexia nervosa, it can be seen that schizophrenia could be related; however, these views are very much in the minority amongst clinicians who generally accept that anorexia nervosa may be distinguished as a disorder in its own right as defined by the DSM-III-R criteria.

Some theories have implicated disturbed cognitions in the aetiology and perpetuation of anorexia nervosa. However, the specific nature of these disturbances has received only limited empirical attention (e.g. Strauss and Ryan, 1988). Over 20 years ago, Bruch noted the primacy of perceptual and conceptual disturbances in anorexia nervosa (Bruch, 1962; 1973). Her clinical descriptions spawned a host of studies examining body image distortions and faulty satiety cues. Current theories continue to emphasize cognitive factors in the aetiology and perpetuation of anorexia nervosa though focus has now shifted to logical errors, cognitive slippage and conceptual complexity (e.g. Swift and Letven, 1984; Fairburn, 1985; Garner, 1986).

Garner and Bemis (1982; 1985) and Garner (1986) have stressed the significance of logical errors in the development and maintenance of anorexia nervosa. Akin to Beck's (1967; 1976) theory of depression, this approach to eating pathology centres on the identification and correction of cognitive distortions, such as overgeneralization, selective abstraction, catastrophizing and personalization. Despite the clinical descriptions of these specific types of faulty thinking in eating disorders, to date there has been only one empirical investigation of these phenomena (e.g. Strauss and Ryan, 1988). These authors examined logical and conceptual thinking in anorectics and controls but did not consider subjects' abilities to maintain a cognitive set or to shift a perceptual set. However, a study by Thompson (1991b) was different in that it included measures of all of these capabilities. A small number of studies have attempted to establish whether neurobiological factors implicated in this disorder include specific cognitive deficits. It has been suggested that a distorted body image may be a consequence of impairment in right hemisphere function, resulting in visuospatial deficits. Preliminary findings support this hypothesis (Fox, 1981; Hamsher, Halmi and Benton, 1981). Small (1984) also found evidence for both conceptual laxity and poor reality testing in anorectics' Rorschach protocols. However, in his review of psychodiagnostic literature, he noted serious methodological flaws in the surveyed research.

Other cognitive features often associated with anorexia nervosa involve more purely intellectual capabilities. Although the anorectic tends to demonstrate above-average abilities on intelligence tests (Bemis, 1978; Hamsher, Halmi and Benton, 1981), some theorists point out that anorectics do not develop formal operational thinking or mature conceptual complexity (Garfinkel and Garner, 1982). One investigation, using the Loevinger Sentence Completion Test (Loevinger and Wessler, 1970), failed to confirm this speculation (Swift *et al.*, 1984) but awaits replication.

Motor restlessness and/or hyperactivity, decreased food efficiency and anxiety have been found to be indicative of a high level of arousal and found to be present in sufferers of anorexia nervosa. These symptoms also appear to be associated with a relatively poor performance on tasks which assess automatic information processing or incidental learning (Fox, 1981; Strupp *et al.*, 1986). However, processing of information requiring concentration and cognitive effort is not impaired in anorectic subjects (Strupp *et al.*, 1986). This finding is consistent with theories which propose a link between heightened arousal and a narrowing of attentional focus (Bacon, 1974; Eysenck, 1979). Various studies which have employed the Stroop Test as an objective measure of anorectics' preoccupation with food-related stimuli have demonstrated that these individuals selectively attend to such stimuli. When compared with controls, patients were significantly more distracted by high-threat words, such as 'cake, cream, butter, sugar' (Channon, Helmsley and de Silva, 1988; Ben Tovim *et al.*, 1989). Such results suggest that anorectics have reduced information processing capacity because they are constantly monitoring input for food-related cues.

Cognitive impairment in anorectics has received scant empirical attention despite its prominence in contemporary theories of anorexia nervosa. The few investigations using patients with anorexia nervosa (as compared with bulimia) describe conflicting findings and seem to suffer from inadequate research designs (e.g. dependence on a single dependent variable or failure to distinguish between restricting and bulimic subtypes). There have been exceptions to this in which cognitive deficits have been reported under sound methodological conditions. For instance, Hamsher, Halmi and Benton (1981) reported a range of cognitive deficits in a group of 20 anorectics, including slowed reaction time, poor short-term visual memory and impaired information retrieval. Of particular interest is their finding that patients who still demonstrated cognitive impairment after refeeding had lost weight again at one year follow-up when compared with those whose cognitive function improved with weight gain. However, again this study lacks comprehensiveness in its measures of cognitive function such as problem-solving abilities and ability to shift perceptual and cognitive sets which the Thompson (1991b) study was careful to include. Further research into cognitive function in anorexia nervosa will enable researchers to determine whether neuropsychological abnormalities in this group are transient features associated with the disorder and/or its treatment. Alternatively, it may be that abnormalities in cognitive function predispose some anorectics towards an eating disorder and limit their progress.

A possible organic origin?

The major methodological flaws of existent studies of neuropsychological performance in anorectics derive from their reliance on inappropriate control groups and inadequate investigation and/or reporting of concomitant psychopathology in the patient groups. Both depression and obsessionality frequently co-exist with anorexia nervosa (Kasvikis *et al.*, 1986; Holden, 1990) and are likely to influence performance on psychometric tests. A well designed study must incorporate screening for these disorders in both the patient and the control groups.

Obsessive–compulsive disorder (OCD) is an illness in which recurrent and persistent thoughts, ideas, impulses or images may give rise to repetitive intentional behaviours. Obsessions and compulsions are recognized by the patient as unrealistic, excessive and unwanted, but often become overwhelming and can cause disruption of occupational and social functioning (American Psychiatric Association, 1987). Since obsessionality and compulsivity are common among anorectics, it may follow that their neuropsychological performances on psychometric tests, which assess cognitive function, are similar.

Several studies have shown neuropsychological deficits in OCD patients (Flor-Henry, Yeudall and Koles, 1979; Insel, Donnelly and Lalakea, 1983; Behar, Rapoport and Berg, 1984).

These are thought to be mainly frontal lobe in nature. The selective response to psychopharmacological agents and operative interventions, together with a possible increased concordance rate for OCD amongst monozygotic twins, has been cited as evidence for a biological rather than a psychoanalytical basis for OCD. Several lines of evidence have converged to implicate the caudate nucleus in OCD pathophysiology with several cases having been reported in which typical OCD symptoms followed acquired striated damage (Wilbom, 1960; Weilburg, Mesula and Weintraub, 1989). Luxemberg *et al.* (1987) showed significantly smaller caudate volumes in ten male OCD sufferers compared to controls. Baxter, Phelps and Mazziotta (1987) concluded that there were significantly increased metabolic rates in both caudate nuclei and the left orbitofrontal gyrus in 14 OCD patients. However, five of the subjects were on psychotropic medication and the others had only been drugfree for two weeks. As both these studies involved only small numbers, or an atypical patient group (only males or childhoodonset cases), the applicability for all OCD sufferers is unclear.

It is also possible that anorectics have different pathophysiologies compared with controls and that these might be responsible for any difference in cognitive function as reflected by their performance on psychometric tests. As Snaith (1981) suggests, anorexia nervosa is the complex interaction between psychogenic factors, reduced food intake and weight loss. The possibility remains of an organic predisposition among anorectics rather than a unitary psychiatric disorder. Since the neuropsychological features of anorexia nervosa are poorly understood, it is important that future studies employ comprehensive test batteries to assess a range of cognitive functions as well as providing additional data on visuospatial deficit and selective attention. The Thompson (1991b,c) study discussed here employed a test battery which was appropriately comprehensive and includes tests which were chosen for their sensitivity and efficacy in different clinical settings. Therefore, it is possible to investigate these hypotheses, that is, of an organic origin to the disorder by way of examining the neuropsychological performances of anorectics.

The psychometric components of the test battery also formed part of a battery of tests being used by another researcher at the Cullen Centre, Royal Edinburgh Hospital, to assess cognitive impairment in OCD patients. These tests were well known and have been widely used elsewhere. Details and rationale of the battery will now be discussed.

Rating scales

1. Yale-Brown Obsessive and Compulsive Scale (Y-BOCS)
2. Eating Attitudes Test-40 (EAT-40)
3. Montgomery-Asberg Depression Rating Scale (MADRS)
4. Morgan-Russell Scale (MRS)
5. Detailed interview

Psychometric tests

6. Trail Making Test A and B (TMT)
7. Wechsler Adult Intelligence Scale – Revised (WAIS-R)
8. Rey-Osterreith Complex Figure Test (CFT)
9. Auditory Verbal Learning Test (AVLT)
10. Paced Auditory Serial Addition Test (PASAT)
11. Wisconsin Card Sorting Test (WCST)
12. Controlled Oral Word Association Test (COWAT)
13. National Adult Reading Test (NART)
14. Stroop Test

Description and rationale of the test battery

1. Y-BOCS

A two-part checklist determining the frequency of a number of obsessions and/or compulsions that the patient performs (Goodman, 1989; DeVeaugh *et al.*, 1990). The first part requires the patient or therapist to place a tick against any current or past obsessions or compulsions including aggressive obsessions, contamination obsessions, somatic obsessions, cleaning/washing compulsions, counting compulsions, etc. A target symptom list can then be established. The second part consists of ten items each with a 0–4 scale (none, mild, moderate, severe, extreme) at which the therapist rates, for example, time spent on obsessions, control over obsessions, distress from compulsions, etc. from an interview with the patient. Scores are derived from summing items 1–5 (obsession subtotal), 6–10 (compulsion subtotal) and Y-BOCS total (sum of items 1–10).

2. EAT-40

A 40-item questionnaire to be completed by the patient. Statements are related to food and enable the clinician to distinguish between responses made by anorectics or bulimic subtypes (Garner and Garfinkel, 1979; Garner *et al.*, 1982). A scale allows the patient to mark an 'X' under the column which best applies to each statement: Always, Very Often, Often, Sometimes, Rarely, Never. A score of 0–3 is assigned to each response and totalled to give an overall score. Example statement: 'Feel bloated after meals'.

3. MADRS

A 10-item depression rating scale which rates each item on a subscale 0–6. For example, item 1 'Apparent Sadness': representing despondency, gloom and despair (more than just ordinary transient low spirits), reflected in speech, facial expression and posture. Rate by depth and inability to brighten up: 0 – no sadness; 2 – looks dispirited but does brighten up without difficulty; 4 – appears sad and unhappy most of the time; 6 – looks miserable all the time, extremely despondent (Montgomery, 1979; Montgomery and Asberg, 1979; Peyre *et al.*, 1989). Intermediary scales (1,3,5) allow the rater intermediate positions on the rating scale where appropriate. The rating is based on a clinical interview moving from broadly phrased questions about symptoms to more detailed ones which allow a precise rating of severity. The rater must decide whether the rating lies on the defined scale steps (0,2,4,6) or between them (1,3,5).

4. MRS

A 14-item questionnaire used as a guided interview exploring the clinical features regarded as central to the syndrome of anorexia nervosa (Morgan and Russell, 1975; Morgan and Haywood, 1988). Five scales (A–E) cover food intake, menstrual state, psychosexual state and socio-economic state. With the exception of subscale D3, 'overt sexual behaviour' (which has three scores: 0,6,12), each scale has four nominal scores: 0,4,8,12. Example statement: 'Attitude to menstruation (if it has returned)' – Active Dislike (0); Variable: dislike or disinterest (4); Disinterest (8); Pleased that it has returned (12).

5. Detailed interview

Salient points were noted in the patient's family history: genetic susceptibility to an eating disorder, history of obesity, anorexia nervosa, bulimia, social pressures, etc. Birth history: caesarean/ normal, meningitis, head injuries, accidents. Milestones: age talked, walked, etc. Also, number of years of continuous education from nursery through schooling and on to further education, secretarial or apprenticeships. Personal details (marital status, date of birth) and weight details were also recorded: present weight and height; highest and lowest past weight (excluding pregnancy) and for how long; how long ago; patient's view of her ideal weight; age at which problems began; present occupation; mother's and father's occupation. These data were considered important in order to (a) check on previous diagnoses; (b) screen for a possible eating disorder among controls; (c) establish baselines of body weight for potential follow-ups in future research. This was also in keeping with data collected in previous studies on eating disorders (e.g. Garner and Garfinkel, 1979; Garner *et al.*, 1982; Thompson and Muir, 1993).

6. TMT

Test measures visual–conceptual and visuomotor tracking ability. Motor speed and attention are also required (Army Individual Test Battery, 1944; Reitan, 1958). The test is given in two parts (A and B) and the patient must first draw lines to connect consecutively numbered circles on one work sheet (Part A) and then connect consecutively numbered and lettered circles on another work sheet by alternating between the two sequences (Part B). The patient is urged to connect the circles 'as fast as you can' without lifting the pencil from the paper. Both parts are timed. Reitan and Tarshes (1959) suggested that patients who perform very much better on Part A than B are likely to have left-sided lesions; however, this has been both supported (Wheeler and Reitan, 1963) and refuted (Korman and Blumberg, 1963).

7. WAIS-R

Seven subtests of the WAIS-R were used: Digit Symbol, Information, Similarities, Block Design, Object Assembly, Digit Span and Comprehension. The reader is referred to the following sources for a description of this well-known and widely used test: Wechsler, 1944; 1955; 1981. For most adults, the Digit Symbol is a test of psychomotor performance that is relatively unaffected by intellectual prowess, memory or learning (Murstein and Lcipold, 1961; Glosser, Butters and Kaplan, 1977; Erber, Botwinick and Storandt, 1981). Estes (1974) points out that skill in encoding the symbols verbally also appears to contribute to success on this test and may account for a consistently observed feminine superiority on symbol substitution tasks (Wechsler, 1958; Smith, 1967).

Information subtest claims to measure 'general ability': mental alertness, speed and efficiency. It also tests verbal skills, breadth of knowledge and, particularly in older populations, remote memory (Lezak, 1983). Information tends to reflect formal education and motivation for academic achievement (Saunders, 1960). It is one of the few subtests in the WAIS-R that can give spuriously high ability estimates for overachievers or fall below the patient's general ability level because of early lack of academic opportunity or interest and contains ten items that are not equally difficult for men and women, the difference favouring men to a significant degree (Lezak, 1983). Information performance can be a fairly good predictor of the hemispheric side of a suspected brain lesion (Reitan, 1955; Spreen and Benton, 1965; Smith, 1966).

Similarities is a test of verbal concept formation and tends to be more sensitive to the effects of brain injury regardless of localization than the other verbal subtests (Hirschenfang, 1960). Its vulnerability to brain conditions that affect verbal functions compounds its vulnerability to impaired concept formation, so that a relatively depressed Similarities score tends to be associated with left temporal and frontal involvement (Newcombe, 1969; McFie, 1975) and is one of the best predictors of left hemisphere disease in the WAIS-R battery. Rzechorzek (1979) found that patients with left frontal lobe lesions had significantly lower Similarities scores than did those with anterior lesions on the right, whose Similarities scores tended to be unaffected (Bogen et al., 1972; McFie, 1975). Lower Similarities scores are also associated with bilateral frontal lesions (Sheer, 1956).

Block Design is generally recognized as the best measure of visuospatial organization in the Wechsler scales. It reflects general ability to a moderate extent so that intellectually capable but academically or culturally limited persons frequently obtain their highest score on this test (Lezak, 1983). Block Design scores tend to be lower in the presence of any kind of brain injury. They are likely to be least affected when the lesion is confined to the left hemisphere, except when the left parietal lobe is involved (McFie, 1975). They tend to be moderately depressed by diffuse or bilateral brain lesions such as those resulting from traumatic injuries or diffuse degenerative processes that do not primarily involve cortical tissue. Patients with severe damage to prefrontal cortex or extensive right hemisphere damage that includes the parietal lobe are likely to perform very poorly (Luria, 1973) and left parietal lesion patients tend to show confusion, simplification and concrete handling of the design. However, their approach is likely to be orderly, they typically work from left to right as do intact subjects and their construction usually preserves the square shape of the design. Their greatest difficulty is likely to be in placing the last block, which will typically be on their right (McFie, 1975).

Object Assembly has the lowest association with general intellectual ability of all the Performance Scale subtests but the speed component renders it relatively vulnerable to brain damage generally. Since it tests constructional ability, it tends to be sensitive to posterior lesions, more so to those on the right than the left (Black and Strub, 1976; Long and Brown, 1979).

Digit Span tends to be more vulnerable to left hemisphere involvement than to either right hemisphere or diffuse damage (Newcombe, 1969; Weinberg *et al.*, 1972). What Digits Forward (of the Digit Span subtest) measures is more closely related to the efficiency of attention than to what is commonly thought of as memory (Spitz, 1972). Also, anxiety tends to reduce the number of digits recalled (Pyke and Agnew, 1963). The Digits Backward requirement of storing a few data bits briefly while juggling them around mentally is an effortful activity that calls upon the working memory, as distinct from the more passive span of apprehension measured by Digits Forward (Vernon, 1979; Hayslip and Kennelly, 1980).

Comprehension is only a fair test of general ability, but the verbal factor is influential. Six items have a sex bias with an overall tendency (at the 5% level of significance) for men to make slightly higher scores (Lezak, 1979a). However, as Lezak (1983) points out, it is important to distinguish between the capacity to give reasonable-sounding responses to these structured questions dealing with single, delimited issues and the judgement needed to handle complex, multidimensional real-life situations. Thus, as demonstrated most vividly by many patients with right hemisphere lesions, high scores on Comprehension are no guarantee of practical common sense or reasonable behaviour.

8. CFT

A 'complex figure' was devised by Rey (1941) to investigate both perceptual organization and visual memory in brain injured patients. Osterreith (1944) standardized Rey's procedure, obtaining normative data from the performance of 230 normal children of ages ranging from 4–15 years and 60 adults in the 16–60 age range. In addition to two groups of children with learning and adjustment problems, he studied a small number of behaviourally disturbed adults, 43 who had sustained traumatic brain injury and a few patients with endogenous brain disease. The test material consists of Rey's complex figure, blank A4 size paper and six coloured pens. The patient is first instructed to copy the figure which has been so set out that its length runs along the patient's horizontal plane. The examiner watches the patient's performance closely. Each time the patient completes a section of the drawing, the examiner hands him or her a different coloured pen and notes the order of the colours. For most clinical purposes, switching colours generally affords an adequate representation of the patient's overall approach.

By analysing how patients draw the structural elements of the Rey–Osterreith figure, Binder (1982) obtained three scores: configural units, fragmented units and missing units. Visser (1973) suggests that a fragmented or piecemeal approach to copying the complex figure is characteristic of brain damaged persons and reflects their inability to process as much information at a time as do normals. Thus, brain damaged persons tend to deal with smaller visual units, building the figure by accretion. Many ultimately produce a reasonably accurate reproduction in this manner, although the piecemeal approach increases the likelihood of size and relationship errors (Messerli, Seron and Tissot, 1979).

Giving the patient six different coloured pens may be substituted by just a single colour to avoid disruption; what is more important is the analysis of the completed drawings which is achieved by obtaining scores for properly placed lines and completed segments, etc. An 'immediate recall' of the drawing may be obtained by removing the complex figure and asking the patient to draw it from memory. A 'delayed recall' can also be obtained after a lapse of about 30 minutes.

9. AVLT

A 15-word list is read aloud to the patient who then must recall as many of the words as possible in any order. However, the order of their recall and any confabulations or associations is also recorded. This is repeated for four more presentations after which a second different list of 15 words is presented demanding the same task of the patient. The patient is then asked to recall the first list of words and, after a 30-minute lapse, is asked to recall the first list yet again for the final occasion (Taylor, 1959; Rey, 1964).

Most brain damaged patients show a learning curve over the five trials. The appearance of a curve, even at a low level (3 to 4 words on trial I to 8 or 9 on trial V), demonstrates some ability to learn if some of the gain is maintained on the delayed recall trial VI. Craik (1977) suggests that on supraspan learning tasks such as this, both short-term retention and learning capacities (i.e. primary and secondary memory in Craik's terminology) of intact subjects are engaged. Many brain damaged patients do as well as normal subjects on the initial trial, but have less learned carry-over on subsequent trials (Lezak, 1979a,b). (See McKenzie *et al.*, 1991; Thompson *et al.*, 1991; Thompson, 1992b, for effects of rehearsal on memory and self-help tips.)

10. PASAT

This sensitive test simply requires that the patient adds 60 pairs of randomized digits so that each is added to the digit immediately preceding it (Gronwall and Sampson, 1974; Gronwall and Wrightson, 1974; Gronwall, 1977). For example, if the examiner reads the numbers '2-8-6-1-9', the subject's correct responses, beginning as soon as the examiner says '8', are

'10-14-7-10'. The digits are presented at four rates of speed, each differing by 0.4 seconds and ranging from one every 1.2 seconds to one every 2.4 seconds. (For the present study, digits were presented at 4 second intervals in trial I and at 2 second intervals in trial II.)

Postconcussion patients consistently perform well below control group averages immediately after injury or return to consciousness. The overwhelming tendency is for their scores to return to normal within 30 to 60 days. Based on an evaluation of how the PASAT performance was associated with performances on memory and attention tasks, Gronwall and Wrightson (1981) concluded that the PASAT is very sensitive to deficits in information processing ability. By using the PASAT performance as an indicator of the efficiency of information processing following concussion, the examiner can determine when a patient is able to return to a normal level of social and vocational activity without experiencing undue stress, or when a modified activity schedule would be best (Gronwall, 1977).

11. WCST

This widely used test was devised to study 'abstract behaviour' and 'shift of set'. The reader is referred to the following sources for details of test description and administration: Berg, 1948; Grant and Berg, 1948; Lezak, 1983. A poor performance of this test can result from different kinds of intellectual deficits. The patient may have difficulty sorting according to category, which suggests an impaired ability to form concepts. This problem occurs most often in patients with frontal lobe (particularly left frontal lobe) damage involving the medial area (Drewe, 1974). Difficulty in shifting when the category changes, i.e. perseveration, was also a common error made by Drewe's brain injured patients regardless of the side of the lesion.

Taylor (1959) associated perseverative errors with dorsolateral lesions of the frontal lobes, but reported that more patients with left-sided lesions displayed permanent impairment on this task after lobectomy. Robinson *et al.* (1980) found that both frontal lobe patients and those with diffuse brain damage were highly susceptible to making perseverative errors. Perseveration also characterizes the performance of long-term alcoholics (Tarter and Parsons, 1971; Parsons, 1975).

12. COWAT

Benton and Hamsher (1976) and Benton *et al.* (1983) have systematically studied the oral production of spoken words beginning with a designated letter. The 1976 version was developed as part of Benton and Hamsher's Multilingual Aphasia Examination and provides norms for two sets of letters, CFL and PRW. These letters were selected on the basis of the frequency of English words beginning with these letters. In each set, words beginning with the first letter of these two sets have a relatively high frequency, the second letter has a somewhat lower frequency and the third letter has a still lower frequency.

The examiner asks the patient to say as many words as s/he can think of that begin with the given letter of the alphabet, excluding proper nouns, numbers and the same word with a different suffix. The score, which is the sum of all acceptable words produced in the three one-minute trials, is adjusted for age, sex and education. Word fluency has proven to be a sensitive indicator of brain dysfunction. Frontal lesions, regardless of side, tend to depress fluency scores, with left frontal lesions resulting in lower word production than right frontal ones (Ramier and Hécaen, 1970; Perret, 1974; Miceli *et al.*, 1981). Benton (1968) found that not only did patients with left frontal lesions produce on the average almost one-third fewer words than patients with right frontal lesions, but bilateral lesions tended to lower verbal productivity even more. Reduced capacity to generate words has also been associated with Alzheimer's-type disease (Miller and Hague, 1975). In contrast, verbal fluency holds up when symptoms of depression mimic organic deterioration (Kronfol *et al.*, 1978).

13. NART

To better estimate the actual premorbid vocabulary of patients with dementing conditions, Nelson and O'Connell (1978) recommended using phonetically irregular words that can only be read correctly by someone who has prior familiarity with them.

The NART list comprises 50 phonetically irregular words. Patients with cortical atrophy made many more errors reading the NART list than a list of regularly formed words. A control group made as many errors as did the patients on the irregular list but fewer errors on the list of phonetically regular words.

NART's increased sensitivity to premorbid vocabulary level appears to permit more accurate prediction of premorbid ability for patients who had been of high average or better intelligence than do other reading vocabulary tests.

14. Stroop Test

Measures the ease with which the patient can shift perceptual set to conform to changing demands (Stroop, 1935; Lezak, 1983). Talland (1965) used the Stroop Test to examine the effects of perceptual interference and incidentally found that it provided data on reading fluency. Dodrill (1978) included it in his Neurological Battery for Epilepsy as a test of concentration which, if impaired, may contribute to problems in shifting responsively.

Ten female outpatients (one in full-time employment, nine unemployed) diagnosed as suffering from anorexia nervosa, in a new phase of treatment at the Cullen Centre, Royal Edinburgh Hospital, were used in the study together with ten healthy females (eight in full-time employment, two in full-time education) from the Edinburgh area. The two groups were matched, as closely as possible, for age, number of years of continuous education, premorbid intelligence quotient and social class. In addition, in order to check that the diagnosis of anorexia nervosa only applied to the anorectic group, all subjects were asked to complete the Morgan-Russell Scale (MRS) and the Eating Attitudes Test (EAT-40). The anorectic group had a mean age of 25.8 years; mean number of years of continuous education of 15.8 years; and mean premorbid IQ of 115.4. Subjects in this group satisfied the diagnostic criteria for anorexia nervosa for both the MRS (poor/intermediate outcome categories) and the EAT-40. The control group had a mean age of 23.2 years; mean number of years of continuous education of 16.7 years; and a mean IQ of 119.7. All subjects were willing volunteers and had responded to verbal requests for participation from the researcher. It was explained to patient-subjects that participation would not in any way constitute or interfere with their treatment and all subjects were given an information sheet at least 24 hours before them signing a consent form for participation.

All subjects were presented with the same test battery which was administered on two separate occasions at the Cullen Centre, Edinburgh.

The results revealed that 16 out of the 40 neuropsychological test scores and rating scales scores were found to be significantly different between the anorectic group and the control group. Of these scores, the following were found to be highly correlated with depression (as represented by a high MADRS score): Auditory Verbal Learning Test-Trial B (AVLT-B); Rey-Osterreith Complex Figure Test-Copy Trial (CFT-Copy); Trail Making Test-Trial A (TMT-A); Yale-Brown Obsessive and Compulsive Scale (Y-BOCS-O and Y-BOCS-C).

The question asked is whether or not the subjects' test performances had been affected by depression or obsessionality/compulsivity, or by combinations of these factors. Or in fact, whether the scores were attributable only to the effects of anorexia nervosa. In other words, could the scores be attributed to the variables being partialled out in an analysis of covariance? To answer this, the effect of partialling out the MADRS score across all subjects was examined; this revealed only five test scores to be significantly different between the two groups of subjects: AVLT-III; TMT-B; Wechsler Adult Intelligence Scale-Revised (WAIS-R)-Information subtest; Y-BOCS-O; and Y-BOCS-C. All other variables were not significantly different between groups after controlling for depression. There are at least two possible reasons for the above results: (1) the test scores and rating scores were significantly different between the groups because four out of ten of the anorectics were suffering from depression (which may have affected their test scores) thus producing an abnormal difference between the groups; (2) those scores that were not significantly different between the groups were 'masked' by the effects of depression on four out of ten of the anorectics' data (i.e. in the absence of depression, these scores would be higher or lower).

These reasons seem plausible and are consistent with the findings of past studies. For example, Strauss and Ryan (1988) found that in all of their eating disordered groups, dysphoria and depression were prominent features which may have significantly affected subjects' cognitive functioning and subsequent performance on tests. Evidence for depression was also found in the eating disordered patients of the Abbey *et al.* (1990) study.

It also seems possible that the scores of the WAIS-R-Information subtest may have been masked by the presence of depression since they were not significant before the MADRS score was partialled out but were significant ($p < 0.05$) after controlling for depression. The scores for the Y-BOCS-O and Y-BOCS-C may also have been affected by the partialling out; but in this case, there was a greater significant difference between groups ($p < 0.01$ for both scales) in the presence of depression than after controlling for depression ($p < 0.05$ for both scales). This might have been because obsessionality and compulsivity were both highly correlated with depression ($p < 0.01$ and $p < 0.05$, respectively). This finding is consistent with the knowledge that depression and obsessionality (and compulsivity) are often found together, especially among sufferers of obsessive–compulsive disorder (OCD) and anorexia nervosa (Holden, 1990). The AVLT-III, however, seemed unaffected by partialling out depression, remaining significant between groups both in the presence ($p < 0.05$) and in the absence ($p < 0.05$) of depression. Perhaps the effects of rehearsal were greater on subjects' ability to store auditory material in short-term memory than were the effects of depression on these processes.

The effects of partialling out the EAT-40 score were also examined; for example, there was a difference between the groups in the TMT-B when the EAT-40 was partialled out. The difference in scores on the WAIS-R-Similarities subtest was also significant after partialling out (but not beforehand); thus suggesting that the difference in scores between groups may possibly be attributable to the effects of anorexia nervosa. Although not directly confirmed by other studies, past research has indicated that cognitive dysfunction, exhibited by poor neuropsychological performance, is present in anorexia nervosa (Fox, 1981). Other studies have also suggested differences in information processing among anorectics (e.g. Strupp *et al.*, 1986) though this has not always been convincingly evidenced.

Combinations of variables were also partialled out to see if they affected the significance of other scores between the two groups. Results of this covariance indicated that a significant difference between groups on the TMT-B and AVLT-V had possibly been masked by the presence of obsessive and compulsive symptoms and depression as there was a significant difference (p < 0.05) after, but not before, partialling out. On the CFT-Delayed Recall trial, there was a significant difference before and after partialling out Y-BOCS-O and Y-BOCS-C (p < 0.05), but not when EAT-40 or MADRS was partialled out. Hence, this score may be attributable to the diagnostic differences between the two groups and/or to the effects of depression. For the EAT-40, there was a change in the level of significance between groups (p < 0.01 to p < 0.05) following partialling out of the Y-BOCS-O, thus indicating the possible effects of obsessionality on the EAT-40 score. Therefore, there is additional strong evidence to support the finding that obsessional symptoms co-exist with anorexia nervosa (Solyom, Freeman and Miles, 1982; Rothenberg, 1990).

Finally, a comparison between test scores on their significance before and after partialling out depression, obsessionality, compulsivity and symptoms of anorexia nervosa revealed that the AVLT-III, CFT-Copy and CFT-Delayed Recall trials may possibly be attributable to the diagnostic differences between the two groups. Of these variables, only the CFT-Delayed Recall was found to be highly correlated with the EAT-40; and the CFT-Copy was highly correlated with depression. These results suggest that some forms of memory failure (as tested by AVLT-III) and poor visuospatial ability (tested by CFT) may be present in anorexia nervosa. These deficits, when applied to victims of head injury, imply impairment of the right hemisphere, part of which is considered to be responsible for visuospatial coordination (Fox, 1981). Furthermore, Hamsher, Halmi and Benton (1981) have suggested that it is because of a poor visuospatial ability that anorectics tend to distort their body image. Evidence to suggest that anorectics process information less well than non-anorectics might also be implied from poor performances on the AVLT trials.

It does seem likely that obsessionality co-exists with anorexia nervosa; however, it is also likely that not all anorectics exhibit compulsive symptoms or suffer depression, as supported by Dally, Gomez and Isaacs (1979). The effects of depression and obsessionality/compulsivity, though, seem to affect subjects' performances on neuropsychological tests which, singularly or in combination, do tend to confound results. What this study does provide is strong evidence to suggest that there were differences between the controls and the anorectics on some tests and, therefore, there is strong evidence to suggest cognitive impairment.

The study is not conclusive, on the other hand, in providing irrefutable evidence to suggest that anorexia nervosa has an organic origin. This is mainly because of insubstantial evidence on some tests. But results of poor performance on neuropsychological tests do tend to implicate anatomical structures in the brain. If obsessionality is to be associated with the function of the caudate nucleus as with OCD (Weilburg *et al.*, 1989; Richfield *et al.*, 1987; Luxemberg *et al.*, 1987), then it is possible that this anatomical site may be responsible for the obsessionality found in anorectics.

The exact function of the caudate nucleus is unresolved; it is known that pyramidal and extrapyramidal motor systems are responsible for the central control of somatic motor activities (Munn, 1956). The former, which is well developed in mammals, governs the initiation of movements and fine motor control; the phylogenetically older extrapyramidal system regulates gross bodily movements and motor programmes (Eysenck, Arnold and Meili, 1975). Extrapyramidal motor disorders include Parkinson's disease and Huntington's chorea. The caudate nucleus, contained within the corpus striatum, is therefore likely to play a role in motor system control. The corollary of this would imply that disruption or damage to the caudate nucleus is likely to affect motor control. It is proposed that obsessionality also results from damage to this area and is perpetuated by a misperception during motor activities (i.e. it may stem from inadequate or incomplete proprioception or 'internal body awareness').

Clearly, further research into anorexia nervosa is indicated. Future studies should focus on visuospatial deficits and problems with memory (e.g. Weingartner *et al.*, 1983); tests which identify these deficits should be used, perhaps in association with single photon emission tomography (SPET) or, if possible, with the more expensive PET which has the advantage of enabling radioactive isotopes of shorter half-lives (than for the SPET) to be administered in order to monitor cerebral activity during, for example, neuropsychological testing.

It would also be interesting to see if there is any change in anorectics' test performances as weight is gained during treatment. Perhaps this would increase the chances of resolving the debate over the origin of anorexia nervosa: whether organic or psychological.

FURTHER READING

Familial alcoholism

Halmi, K.A. and Loney, J. (1973) Familial alcoholism in anorexia nervosa. *British Journal of Psychiatry*, **123**(572), 53–4.

Pharmacotherapy

Morley, J.E. (1989) An approach to the development of drugs for appetite disorders. *Neuropsychobiology*, **21**(1), 22–30.

Sociocultural models

Engel, K. and Hohne, D. (1989) An interaction model of anorexia nervosa. *Psychotherapy and Psychosomatics*, **51**(2), 57–61.

Outcome and prognosis

Rosenvinge, J.E. and Mouland, S.O. (1990) Outcome and prognosis of anorexia nervosa. A retrospective study of 41 subjects. *British Journal of Psychiatry*, **156**, 92–7.

Family work

Engel, K. and Wigland, G. (1989) Empirical coverage of psychodynamic configurations of anorexia nervosa. *Psychotherapy and Psychosomatics*, **51**(1), 1–10.

Lunt, P., Carosella, N. and Yager, J. (1989) Daughters whose mothers have anorexia nervosa: A pilot study of three adolescents. *Psychiatric Medicine*, **7**(3), 101–10.

Slagerman, M. and Yager, J. (1989) Multiple family group treatment for eating disorders: A short-term program. *Psychiatric Medicine*, **7**(4), 269–83.

Dental characteristics of anorectics

Altshuler, B.D. (1990) Eating disorder patients. Recognition and intervention. *Journal of Dental Hygiene*, **64**(3), 119–25.

Personality disorders

Kennedy, S.H., McVey, G. and Katz, R. (1990) Personality disorders in anorexia nervosa and bulimia nervosa. *Journal of Psychiatric Research*, **24**(3), 259–69.

Torem, M.S. (1990) Covert multiple personality underlying eating disorders. *American Journal of Psychotherapy*, **44**(3), 357–68.

Nutritional knowledge of anorectics

Beumont, P.J.V., Chambers, T.L., Rouse, L. and Abraham, S.F. (1981) The diet composition and nutritional knowledge of patients with anorexia nervosa. *Journal of Human Nutrition*, **35**, 265–73.

Support groups for parents

Rose, J. and Garfinkel, P.E. (1980) A parents' group in the management of anorexia nervosa. *Canadian Journal of Psychiatry*, **25**, 228–33.

Yager, R. (1982) Group parent training versus individual family therapy: An outcome study. *Journal of Behavioural Therapy and Psychiatry*, **13**, 119–22.

Diabetes mellitus and anorexia nervosa

Fairburn, C.G. and Steel, J.M. (1980) Anorexia nervosa in diabetes mellitus. *British Medical Journal*, **280**, 1167–8.

Hillard, J.R. and Hillard, P.J.A. (1984) Bulimia, anorexia nervosa and diabetes – deadly combinations. *Psychiatric Clinics of North America*, **7**, 367–79.

Rosmark, B., Berne, C., Holmgren, S., Lago, C., Renholm, G. and Sohlberg, S. (1986) Eating disorders in patients with insulin-dependent diabetes. *Journal of Clinical Psychiatry*, **47**, 547–50.

Cognitive dysfunction in anorexia nervosa

McKenzie, K., Thompson, S.B.N. and Weeks, D.J. (1991) *Your Memory Manual: A Self-Help Guide to Help People Overcome Everyday Memory Difficulties*. Lothian Health Board, Edinburgh.

Thompson, S.B.N. (1991c) Distorted image. *Therapy Weekly*, **18**(18), 8.

Thompson, S.B.N., McKenzie, K. and Weeks, D.J. (1991) Aide-mémoire. *Therapy Weekly*, **18**(20), 7.

Thompson, S.B.N. (1992a) Implications from neuropsychological test results of women in a new phase of anorexia nervosa. *Eating Disorders Review*, (in press).

Thompson, S.B.N. (1993a) *Anorexia Nervosa: An Organic Origin?* Paper presented at XXV International Congress of Psychology at Brussels International Conference Centre, Brussels, Belgium, 19–24 July 1992, in *Le Journal des Psychologues*, (in press).

Obsessive–compulsive disorder and anorexia nervosa

Pigott, T.A., Altemus, M., Rubenstein, C.S. *et al.* (1991) Symptoms of eating disorders in patients with obsessive–compulsive disorder. *American Journal of Psychiatry*, **148**, 1552–7.

4

Epidemiology of bulimia

DEFINITION OF BULIMIA

The clinical picture of bulimia is distinctive (Beumont, George and Smart, 1976; Russell, 1979; Huon and Brown, 1984). Bulimic patients report that they are constantly preoccupied with thoughts of food. This preoccupation is a reaction to their long-continued restricted eating patterns. Their eating pattern is characterized by dieting or starvation on the one hand and episodes of gorging or unrestricted eating on the other (Fairburn, 1982; Fairburn and Cooper, 1982). The dieting behaviour comes first and is motivated by the extreme importance the patients attribute to being slender, or at least to not being plump. Self-induced vomiting and purgation usually occur after the gorging behaviour has become established and patients often recall their delight at discovering how to induce vomiting, as they believed they would be able to eat as much as they liked without gaining weight.

An increase in the incidence of bulimic behaviour in young adult women has generated a substantial demand for treatment and curiosity about the disorder. One of the earliest accounts of bulimic behaviour can be found from records of Ancient Rome where *vomitaria* were commonly employed in order to allow the rich and gluttonous the opportunity to eat compulsively for many hours on end without ever becoming or feeling satisfied (Skidmore, 1985). In a historical review of the symptoms of bulimia, Casper (1983) found that although clinical descriptions of bulimia date back to the 1900s, it was not until the 1940s that more detailed accounts of bulimic behaviour began to emerge in the literature. In these early reports, however, the symptomatic behaviour was always referred to as a symptom of anorexia nervosa. Bulimia among individuals who did not have histories of weight disorders, such as anorexia nervosa and obesity, was first observed in 1976 by Marlene Boskind-White who coined the term 'bulimarexia' to describe this category of patients (Boskind-White, 1984; Johnson, Lewis and Hagman, 1984). Shortly afterwards various labels emerged describing the population that included bulimia nervosa (Russell, 1979), dietary chaos syndrome (Palmer, 1979) and abnormal weight control syndrome (Crisp, 1981). Bulimia emerged as a distinct diagnostic entity in 1980 with the publication of the third edition of the *Diagnostic and Statistical Manual of Mental Disorders* (American Psychiatric Association, 1980) which was revised in 1987 – DSM-III-R (American Psychiatric Association, 1987). (For a discussion of differences in DSM-III criteria and use of them in research, see Gartner *et al.* (1989) and Yager, Landsverk and Edelstein (1989a) respectively.)

The DSM-III-R criteria for the diagnosis of bulimia are:

1. Recurrent episodes of binge-eating (rapid consumption of a large amount of food in a discrete period of time).
2. At least three of the following:
   (a) consumption of high-caloric, easily ingested food during a binge;
   (b) inconspicuous eating during a binge;
   (c) termination of such eating episodes by abdominal pain, sleep, social interruption or self-induced vomiting;
   (d) repeated attempts to lose weight by severely restricted diets, self-induced vomiting or the use of cathartics or diuretics;
   (e) frequent weight fluctuations due to alternating binges and fasts.
3. Awareness that the eating pattern is abnormal and fear of not being able to stop eating voluntarily.
4. Depressed mood and self-deprecating thoughts following eating binges.

In bulimia (without anorexia nervosa) weight loss may be substantial, but the weight does not fall below a minimal normal weight (Russell, 1979; Casper *et al.*, 1980). This is one of the distinctions bulimia *per se* has from anorexia nervosa.

The dietary chaos syndrome

Palmer (1979; 1982) coined the term 'dietary chaos syndrome' to describe some individuals who come to have a body weight in the normal range for perhaps many months or years, even though this is achieved in spite of a highly eccentric and disordered style of eating. A few young women seem to arrive at this same position without ever having been in a state of primary anorexia nervosa. It is difficult to be certain of the implications and prognosis of such a state, although the individual herself often feels very upset and distressed by her own lack of control. She may feel her state to be worse than her former anorexia nervosa. Her concern with eating is predominant and can be seen as loaded with neurotic meaning. However, the force about weight may be relatively less strong because the biological regression which is present in an anorectic at low weight may be inoperative at a more normal weight. As Beumont, Burrows and Casper (1987) have pointed out, essentially, Palmer's description corresponds to the DSM-III-R criteria for bulimia, except that the latter also specifies the presence of depressive moods and self-deprecating thoughts following episodes of binge-eating.

AETIOLOGY AND PREVALENCE

Some patients with eating disorders develop reactive episodes of hyperphagia (bulimia) about which they feel exceedingly guilty (Beumont, Burrows and Casper, 1987). Once the patient has learnt to induce vomiting or abuse laxatives so as to rid herself of the unwanted calories, the bulimic episodes serve to reduce tension and hence are difficult to relinquish. Thus the syndrome of bulimia is established. Not all bulimic patients have passed through a phase of prior anorexia nervosa, but the development of the condition appears essentially similar even in those who have not. Persistent dietary restraint is eventually interrupted by reactive hyperphagia; vomiting and/or purgation are used to counteract the unwanted ingestion of high calorie foods and the behavioural disturbance becomes the focus of intense guilt feelings, but is nevertheless experienced as anxiety reducing.

It has been suggested that the number of bulimic patients seeking treatment probably represents only a small proportion of those suffering from the disorder (Strangler and Printz, 1980; Larocca, 1984; Schliessener-Stropp, 1985; Agras, 1987; Beumont, Burrows and Casper, 1987). Although these figures are inconsistent and although the samples surveyed were certainly not representative of the general population, there can be little doubt that the condition is very widespread among young women and adolescent girls in most developed Western societies.

Part of the difficulty in collecting data on the incidence of bulimia is due to the fact that patients are initially very secretive about their bulimic episodes. It is not infrequent that overeating and self-induced vomiting have occurred for many years without family members being aware of its presence. However, once others do become aware of it, patients will sometimes overeat in the company of family or friends.

Numerous factors have been identified as precipitants of binge-eating. These include dysphoric mood states such as anxiety and tension or boredom, preoccupation with thoughts of food, drinking alcohol, going out with members of the opposite sex or returning home from school or work. It is worth noting that only a small proportion of patients admit that hunger is a precipitant of bulimia.

Approximately 50% of bulimics regularly induce vomiting (Halmi, Falk and Schwartz, 1981; Fairburn and Cooper, 1982) and the temptation to do so is usually greatest at home. The reason is to ensure that this behaviour remains concealed from others. The preferred method of inducing vomiting is to induce a gag reflex by inserting the fingers into the mouth and throat. Some individuals are able to induce vomiting at will by contracting their thoracic and abdominal muscles. Others simply chew their food and spit it out afterwards. Most individuals feel relieved after they have induced vomiting. They no longer experience abdominal discomfort and are aware that they will not gain weight as a result of their binge. Patients frequently take purgatives immediately after their bulimic episode; the dosage is often excessive and it is not uncommon for a patient to take up to 20 times the recommended amount (Touyz and Beumont, 1985).

Psychological theories

Several researchers have suggested that over the last three decades the sociocultural milieu for adolescent and young adult women has become progressively unstable; this has precipitated identity confusion among this age group (Bardwick, 1971; Bruch, 1973; Selvini Palazzoli, 1974; Garner, Garfinkel and Olmsted, 1983). Changing role expectations in women have included accommodating more traditional feminine expectations such as physical attractiveness and domesticity, incorporating more modern standards for vocational and personal achievement and taking advantage of increased opportunity for self-definition and autonomy. Garner, Garfinkel and Olmsted (1983) suggested that 'while the wider range of choices available to contemporary women may provide personal freedom for those who are psychologically robust, it may be overwhelming for the field-dependent adolescent who lacks internal structure'.

Personality, precipitating factors and bulimia

On reviewing the data regarding personality traits of bulimics, two major factors emerge as being generally characteristic. Firstly, there is substantial evidence to indicate that bulimics as a group experience significant instability that is manifested in fluctuating mood states, impulsive behaviour, low frustration tolerance and high anxiety (Johnson, Lewis and Hagman, 1984). Secondly, that they experience significant difficulties with self-esteem that is expressed through feelings of inadequacy, helplessness, ineffectiveness, guilt, self-criticism and feelings of being undifferentiated (Larocca, 1984). Individuals who do experience affective instability are at substantial risk for having difficulties with self-esteem because the fluctuating feeling states can give them the experience of being out of control and helpless. Taken together, these two character factors suggest that bulimic patients would have significant and repeated difficulty with self-regulation when exposed to events that trigger dysphoric feelings (Goodsitt, 1983).

Loro and Orleans' (1981) review and findings on binge eaters showed these individuals to evidence deficits in interpersonal, self-esteem and stress management areas (Mehrabian, 1987). The exception was a study by Johnson et al. (1982) in which clinically diagnosed bulimics were found to be relatively symptom-free according to standard indicators of psychiatric symptoms. This latter review of findings on the common characteristic of clinically diagnosed bulimics and binge eaters suggests that individuals exhibiting these problems are more likely to evidence other signs of psychological maladjustment than of adjustment (Mehrabian, Nahum and Duke, 1986; Mehrabian and Riccioni, 1986; Mehrabian, 1987).

On considering the personality traits of sufferers of bulimia, a pattern of premorbid characteristics emerges, as well as a sociocultural context that could shape the specific choice of symptomatic behaviour. The biological factors suggest that bulimic patients would be at risk for experiencing affective instability. Given an adequately structured family environment, this vulnerability may be overcome. Unfortunately, the data indicate that the families of bulimics appear to be poorly structured and disorganized (Larocca, 1984). With a biological vulnerability to affective instability and a disorganized and conflicted family structure that generally has high achievement expectations (Johnson, Lewis and Hagman, 1984), we can presume that an individual would emerge who is faced with dysphoric and variable mood states; not being exposed to sufficient environmental structure does not allow him or her to develop adequate coping strategies for such situations that may evoke dysphoric feelings. Thus, as the developmental demands for identity formation and developing mechanisms for self-regulation are of highest priority, adolescent women in particular begin restrictive dieting in the pursuit of thinness which has become equivalent to the pursuit of self-control and self-esteem. Prolonged calorie restriction (dieting) and weight loss, however, exacerbate affective instability and render the individual tense, anxious, hyperactive, hypervigilant and preoccupied with food (Keys, Brozek and Henschel, 1950) which then interferes with the social relations they desire. Paradoxically, the initial efforts to etablish self-control through dieting and weight loss place them at more risk for losing control because of the heightened vulnerability to affective instability.

Given these predisposing factors, the stage is set for the emergence of binge-eating symptoms. Research has indicated that the onset of bulimic symptomatology often follows a period of restrictive dieting. In their clinical sample, Pyle, Mitchell and

Eckert (1981) found that 30 out of the 34 patients they inter-viewed indicated that the onset of their bulimic behaviour occurred during such a period of restrictive dieting and 34% of the Johnson, Stuckey and Lewis (1982) sample reported the same relationship between restrictive dieting and the onset of bingeing.

Traumatic events such as loss or separation from a signifi-cant person in their lives were recalled by 30 patients of Pyle, Mitchell and Eckert (1981) as being associated with onset of bulimic behaviour. Also frequently mentioned in association with the emergence of bulimic behaviour were arguments and conflictual feelings about sexuality. Difficulty in handling specific emotions was reported by 40% of the respondents questioned by Johnson, Stuckey and Lewis (1982) as the cause for the initial bingeing behaviour. Emotions most frequently reported as precipitants to bingeing included depression, lone-liness, boredom and anger. Other factors cited as precipitors included interpersonal conflict such as stressful job situations, parental and marital conflicts, unfulfilling relationships and loss or separation from friends, family or work. The pattern thus emerges that being called upon to handle difficult emo-tions in situations, often during the time of extended food de-privation and dieting, increases the possibility of binge-eating and the onset of a bulimic pattern for these women.

CHARACTERISTICS OF THE BULIMIC PATIENT

Overall, it is probably true to say that bulimics tend to appear more normal than anorectics in terms of current ideas of what constitutes an acceptable body shape. Classic anorectics are always obviously thin (Lambley and Scott, 1988). However, it is the bingeing episodes that have led some researchers to draw a distinction between bulimia and anorexia nervosa. Bulimic episodes are sometimes planned. Binge foods are selected because they are easy to swallow or to regurgitate, e.g. ice cream, yoghurt, etc. Most patients include foods they do not allow themselves to eat at other times and refer to these taboo items as 'junk foods'. It is not uncommon for individuals to throw away food they have recently purchased to avoid eating it, despite the expense involved.

Beumont, Burrows and Casper (1987) noted large individual differences in the quantity of food consumed during a binge and some patients may consume as much as 20 to 30 times the recommended daily allowance of calories in one episode. Although it is widely believed that patients gorge predominantly on foods high in carbohydrates, an analysis of their food records reveal that large amounts of fat and protein are consumed as well. There is a tendency to eat very rapidly early on in the disorder but once it has become well established, patients tend to eat slowly, especially if there is little risk of being discovered. Some patients report 'picking' behaviour (Beumont, Burrows and Casper, 1987). They move around the kitchen eating very small quantities of food, e.g. a teaspoon of jelly or yoghurt, a slice of apple or a portion of cheese. They often continue to do so for hours at a time so as to ingest thousands of calories.

There are currently no long term outcome studies on bulimia but it is known that medical complications may arise from recurrent binge-eating and purging. Pyle, Mitchell and Eckert (1981) reported that 44 of 85 bulimic patients they studied had abnormal electrolyte balances. Common abnormalities were metabolic alkalosis, hypochloraemia (low blood levels of chloride) and hypokalaemia (low blood levels of potassium). The depletion of chloride and potassium is associated with fatigue, muscle weakness, constipation and dysphoria, all of which mimic depression. Also reported are oedema and possible kidney dysfunction and a predisposition to cardiac arrhythmias (Johnson, Lewis and Hagman, 1984). Furthermore, laxative abuse has been associated with damage to submucosal nerve fibres in the intestines. Gastric dilation has also been reported by Saul, Dekker and Watson (1981) with one case resulting in death due to rupture of the intestines. Other associated medical problems are parotid gland enlargement from vomiting and poor diet (Ahola, 1982; Hasler, 1982) and dental caries and erosion of enamel from frequent exposure to hydrochloric acid from vomiting (Gallo and Randel, 1981).

FURTHER READING

General

Beumont, P.J.V., Burrows, G.D. and Casper, R.C. (1987) *Handbook of Eating Disorders. Part 1: Anorexia Nervosa and Bulimia Nervosa.* Elsevier, Amsterdam.

Charnock, D.J.K. (1989) A comment on the role of dietary restraint in the development of bulimia nervosa. *British Journal of Clinical Psychology*, **28**, 329–40.

Dennis, A.B. (1992) Divergent forms of purging behavior in bulimia nervosa patients. *International Journal of Eating Disorders*, **11**(1), 17–24.

Lawrence, M. and Dana, M. (1990) *Fighting Food: Coping with Eating Disorders*. Penguin, London.

Wilson, C.P., Hogan, C.C. and Mintz, I.L. (1983) *Fear of Being Fat: The Treatment of Anorexia Nervosa and Bulimia Nervosa*. Jason Aronson, New York.

Epidemiology of bulimia

Rand, C.S.W. and Kuldau, J.M. (1992) Epidemiology of bulimia and symptoms in a general population – sex, age, race and socioeconomic status. *International Journal of Eating Disorders*, **11**(1), 37–44.

Personality traits

Strien, T.V. (1986) *Eating Behaviour, Personality Traits and Body Mass*. Swets and Zeitlinger, Lisse.

Prevalence of bulimia

Pope, H.G., Hudson, J.I., Vurgelen-Todd, D. and Hudson, M.S. (1984) Prevalence of anorexia nervosa and bulimia in three student populations. *International Journal of Eating Disorders*, **3**, 45–51.

Whitehouse, A.M., Cooper, P.J., Vize, C.V., Hill, C. and Vogel, L. (1992) Prevalence of eating disorders in three Cambridge general practices: Hidden and conspicuous morbidity. *British Journal of General Practice*, **42**(355), 57–60.

5

Assessment, treatment and outcome of bulimia

HOW TO ASSESS

Fichter (1990) claims that we have no satisfying explanation for the impressive persistence of bulimia in many individuals despite their recognition of its malicious effect on their lives. It is true to say that, although effective treatments have been developed, it remains difficult to 'match' the patient to the correct therapy and as Fichter (1990) reminds us, we cannot predict with any confidence who will do well and who poorly. It is therefore with some caution that an outline of assessment is presented for bulimics. Basically, the assessment of bulimic patients is not dissimilar to that of anorectics in that there are generally three phases: screening (usually the administration of screening questionnaires); an initial diagnostic interview (where psychological well-being is also assessed, notably focusing on depression of mood, lack of confidence, lack of assertiveness, etc.); and finally self-monitoring (using charts and food diaries). However, with bulimic patients there is almost always an element of secrecy attached to their bingeing behaviour which hinders the assessment process. Therefore, a thorough diagnostic interview is of paramount importance and the following information will be important to collect:

1. Patient's lifestyle;
2. Any complications, such as physical illness (e.g. diabetes);
3. Presence of depression;
4. Extent to which the patient is underweight or overweight;
5. Pattern of binge-eating and purging (and severity);
6. Patient's degree of dissatisfaction with their body.

Patient's name .... Date ....

1. Do you have a regular day to day eating pattern?   Yes/No
2. Are you a strict dieter?   Yes/No
3. Do you feel a failure if you break your diet once?   Yes/No
4. Do you count the calories of everything you eat, even when not on a diet?   Yes/No
5. Do you ever fast for a whole day?   Yes/No
6. If yes, how often is this?

   Every second day – 5   2–3 times a week – 4
   Once a week   – 3   Now and then   – 2   Have once – 1

7. Do you do any of the following to help you lose weight? (Circle number)

	Never	Occasionally	Once/ wk	2–3/ wk	Daily	2–3/ wk	5+/ wk
Take diet pills	0	2	3	4	5	6	7
Take diuretics	0	2	3	4	5	6	7
Take laxatives	0	2	3	4	5	6	7
Make yourself vomit	0	2	3	4	5	6	7

8. Does your pattern of eating disrupt your life?   Yes/No
9. Would you say that food dominated your life?   Yes/No
10. Do you ever eat and eat until you are stopped by physical discomfort?   Yes/No
11. Are there times when all you can think about is food?   Yes/No
12. Do you eat sensibly in front of others and make up in private?   Yes/No
13. Can you always stop eating when you want to?   Yes/No
14. Do you ever experience *overpowering* urges to eat and eat and eat?   Yes/No
15. When you are feeling anxious do you tend to eat a lot?   Yes/No
16. Does the thought of becoming fat *terrify* you?   Yes/No
17. Do you ever eat largish amounts of food rapidly (not a meal)?   Yes/No
18. Are you ashamed of your eating habits?   Yes/No
19. Do you worry that you have no control over how much you eat?   Yes/No
20. Do you turn to food for comfort?   Yes/No
21. Are you able to leave food on the plate at the end of a meal?   Yes/No
22. Do you deceive other people about how much you eat?   Yes/No
23. Does how hungry you feel determine how much you eat?   Yes/No

Figure 5.1 Bulimic Investigatory Test, Edinburgh (BITE; Henderson and Freeman, 1987).

24. Do you ever binge on large amounts of food?   Yes/No

25. If yes, do such binges leave you feeling miserable?   Yes/No

26. If you do binge, is this only when you are alone?   Yes/No

27. If you do binge, how often is this?

Hardly ever...............	1	Once a month	2
Once a week	3	2–3 times a week	4
Daily	5	2–3 times a day	6

28. Would you go to great lengths to satisfy an urge to binge?   Yes/No

29. If you overeat do you feel *very* guilty?   Yes/No

30. Do you ever eat in secret?   Yes/No

31. Are your eating habits what you would consider to be normal?   Yes/No

32. Would you consider yourself to be a compulsive eater?   Yes/No

33. Does your weight fluctuate by more than 5 lbs in a week?   Yes/No

Figure 5.1 *Continued*

Screening questionnaires

The caloric intake of bulimic individuals varies markedly. Some patients consume as many as 15 000 calories a day, others less than 1000 calories (Agras, 1987). Some binges, then, may consist of eating a small amount of food that the patient's 'food rules' permit. Once the food rule is broken, some patients immediately purge, whereas others go on to consume large amounts of food. Almost all bulimics demonstrate a restricted pattern of caloric intake, eating little breakfast and lunch and tending to binge in the afternoons and evenings. It is important to gather as much of this sort of information as possible and this can be achieved by asking the patient to complete, truthfully, a screening questionnaire such as the Bulimic Investigatory Test, Edinburgh (BITE), as used with bulimic patients at the Cullen Centre, Royal Edinburgh Hospital, Edinburgh (Figure 5.1). It should be emphasized that unless the patient is truthful in the way she completes the questionnaire, it is impossible for any therapeutic intervention to be successful and is therefore a waste of the clinician's time.

The diagnostic interview

Interviewing the bulimic patient is perhaps the most important stage of the assessment phase. By careful probing into the patient's life history a pattern of eating and purging behaviour is found, often revealing elaborate ways in which the patient has kept secret aspects of their behaviour such as bingeing and vomiting. The clinician should ask the patient to describe his or her food intake for a typical day in some detail, both for so-called normal meals and for binges. Alcohol intake, drug use and abuse and stealing of either food or other goods (see Casper *et al.* (1980) on kleptomania in bulimic patients) should be investigated during the interview as these types of behaviour have been found in some bulimic patients.

Once the pattern of eating has been clarified, the methods used in purging should be examined. The clinician should help the patient disclose the nature of the problem by asking how vomiting is induced (use of fingers, automatic vomiting, use of purgative like ipecacuanha, etc.); when and where it is induced; the use of rituals such as cleaning up afterwards; and methods used to hide the behaviour. The use of diuretics, laxatives, fasting alternating with binges and strenuous exercise should also be covered in detail, even if the patient has answered 'no' to the screening questionnaire questions or to initial questions in the interview.

Other important areas to discuss in the interview are the patient's dissatisfaction with body size and shape – the precise dissatisfaction should be discerned and the patient's degree of rigidity of these beliefs. Such questions as 'How do you think you would feel if you put on 3 lbs?' etc. can help to gather this necessary information and thus the patient's erroneous beliefs about food, weight and body shape can often be explicated by the clinician.

It has been found that most bulimics are slightly underweight by 5–15% (Agras, 1987), some are of normal weight and a few are overweight. The therapeutic approach taken may be different depending upon the patient's current weight. Should weight loss be in the 20–25% range, the restoration of normal body weight becomes the first task, with treatment of binge-eating and purging as a secondary concern. The Body Mass Index (BMI), below which mortality rates are elevated above those for persons of normal weight, is 18 for women and 20 for men, values that are below the tenth percentile of the population (Agras, 1987). For the overweight bulimic, attention must be directed not only towards the binge-eating and purging, but also towards the accompanying obesity. Here the paradox is that by increasing the number of meals eaten during the day, total caloric intake is reduced as binge-eating ceases.

Self-monitoring

This is perhaps the most difficult stage of the assessment for the bulimic. It is not only about self-admission of the problem but it is also about allowing others to become aware of it – a part of the syndrome which is not readily exposed by the bulimic individual. However, the daily food diary (Figure 5.2) can be an important part of information collation and should be encouraged by the clinician. It is useful to compile a small booklet so that the patient can keep a week's log of her eating pattern and binges, and so build up a picture of her eating behaviour to be reviewed at subsequent interviews.

HOW TO TREAT

The causal factors in bulimia are still not completely understood; most bulimic patients report a history of dieting prior to developing their bulimic symptoms. As Martin (1990) comments, society is now obsessed with dieting, weight and food. This can be seen not only in the media but also on the supermarket shelves. Indeed, such products as 'Lean Cuisine' and 'Lite' food ranges were not in evidence before the 1980s.

Increase in the incidence of bulimia (Halmi, Falk and Schwartz, 1981; Wardle and Beinart, 1981; Pyle *et al.*, 1983) has generated significant demands on treatment. A number of treatment interventions have been attempted including behavioural (Thornton and DeBlassie, 1989), exposure plus response prevention (Johnson *et al.*, 1984), cognitive–behavioural (Bossert, Schnabel and Krieg, 1989; Laessle *et al.*, 1990), pharmacotherapy (Mitchell *et al.*, 1990; Stevenson and Solyom, 1990), family therapy (Willard, Swain and Winstead, 1989), self-help (Johnson and Connors, 1987), progressive relaxation (Chaitow, 1983), counselling (Hornak, 1983) and imaginal

Date ....   Day ....

	Vomit	Laxative	Other
Breakfast			
Lunch			
Evening meal			
Totals :	:	:	:

Comments:

1. The desire to starve myself today has been:

Not at all   As strong as it
possibly could be

2. Today, the urge to overeat has been:

Not at all   As strong as it
possibly could be

3. Today, in general I have felt:

Not at all   Extremely
emotionally   emotionally
upset   upset

Figure 5.2 Food diary for bulimia patients.

desensitization (McConaghy and Blaszczynski, 1988). Yet, as Fichter (1990) comments, there is still difficulty in reliably matching patients to the 'right' treatment and the predictability of outcome remains uncertain. Techniques used for assessing therapeutic progress in anorexia nervosa have been commonly adopted for bulimics, e.g. image marking, visual size estimation and distorting video techniques (Whitehouse, Freeman and Annandale, 1988; Bowden et al., 1989). Putting aside for one moment the debates concerning any similarities between anorexia nervosa and bulimia, it would appear that techniques first used with anorectics are continually tried out with bulimics.

Behaviour therapy

A behavioural approach in the treatment of bulimia focuses on increasing control over eating, eliminating food avoidance and changing maladaptive attitudes. This is done by positive reinforcement of abstinence from bulimic symptoms or, indirectly, by modifying one or more of the proposed reinforcers (Martin, 1990).

The first report on the effectiveness of a specific treatment programme for bulimia was by Boskind-Lodahl (1978). The treatment involved Gestalt-type experiential work coupled with behavioural techniques such as self-monitoring and goal setting within a feminist perspective. White and Boskind-White (1981) continued to use this treatment concept in a group format. In an uncontrolled study involving 14 bulimics they ran group meetings five hours a day for five days. Postgroup frequency of binge/purge episodes was not reported, but at six months follow-up the authors reported three out of 14 patients (21%) were totally remitted, seven out of 14 (50%) reported significant reduction and four out of 14 (28%) had little or no improvement.

A number of successful interventions using behaviour therapy have been reported. For example, Cooper and Cooper (1989) reported on a study of eight bulimic patients using purely behavioural techniques and without explicit cognitive procedures. All subjects had been systematically assessed before and after treatment while seven had been re-assessed at a one-year follow-up. The authors reported that, as a group, they showed 'substantial improvement in terms of eating habits, a global index of specific psychopathology and mental state'. These results are comparable to those reported by the authors in an earlier study using a cognitive–behavioural approach. Results of the 1989 study, according to the authors, question the need for cognitive procedures in order to produce change in bulimic patients.

Exposure and response prevention

Rosen and Leitenberg (1982) hypothesized that the driving force behind bulimia may be vomiting rather than bingeing. They suggested that the anxiety-reducing function of the vomiting may be similar to that in compulsions such as hand-washing in obsessive–compulsive disorders. Once the bulimic has learned that vomiting reduces the anxiety concerning weight gain, there are fewer inhibitions to overeating and the vomiting response has been reinforced (Johnson and Larson, 1982). Thus, their treatment addressed the vomiting component of bulimia, rather than the bingeing. Their 1982 study employed a multiple baseline involving exposure to preferred binge foods and prevention of the vomiting response. In the treatment sessions the bulimic subject was encouraged to eat as much of these foods as possible and then refrain from vomiting. After eating she was encouraged to focus on her feelings of discomfort and anxiety until the urge to vomit vanished. Three phases of supervised exposure and response prevention were conducted. Following this, the subject was instructed to decrease vomiting gradually over the next several weeks. The results indicated that over the successive treatment phases the subject was able to increase the amount of food eaten and both her anxiety and frequency of vomiting decreased.

These promising results led to several other studies investigating the efficacy of exposure and response prevention (e.g. Hoage, 1989). Leitenberg *et al.* (1984) treated five subjects meeting criteria for bulimia. After a five-week baseline period subjects received between 12 and 18 individual sessions. Sessions were divided into two-week phases in which subjects were exposed to various foods according to their self-rated degree of difficulty with them. Subjects were instructed to eat until they felt a strong urge to vomit and then would deal with the anxiety-provoking cognitions together with the clinician. Generally the subjects ate more and reported less anxiety over time. At the end of the treatment 40% had ceased vomiting entirely, 40% had reduced by more than half and 20% had not changed. At a 3- to 6-month follow-up these results were maintained. Recording psychological functioning, positive changes were reported on the BDI (Beck Depression Inventory), EAT (Eating Attitudes Test), Rosenberg Self-Esteem Scale (Rosenberg, 1979) and the Lawson Self-Esteem Scale (Lawson, Marshall and McGrath, 1979), although no statistical analysis was performed. (The reader is referred to Chapter 2 where the BDI and EAT questionnaires have been presented in full.)

Behaviour therapy is particularly helpful as an approach when it is part of a treatment programme. Its success is possibly attributable to the fact that it addresses the vicious bingeing and purging cycles so commonly seen in bulimic patients. As with any approach, there are some disadvantages: it places minimal emphasis on the patients' body image (Martin, 1989a,b), low self-esteem, feelings of helplessness and the loneliness and shame felt as a result of their maladaptive behaviour. Therefore, it is most usefully conducted within the framework of additional supportive therapy.

Cognitive–behavioural therapy

The main therapeutic procedures used in cognitive–behavioural therapy, as first described by Fairburn (1981), are aimed at interrupting the revolving cycle of dietary restriction, binge eating and purging by reinstating normal dietary habits while challenging the distorted beliefs that accompany the disorder. In brief, the first step is to enhance social control by urging the patient to disclose the full nature of the problem to significant others. Following this, the restricted dietary pattern, which is identified through the use of self-monitoring, is tackled by gradually shaping the patient's eating behaviour towards a balanced diet of three meals a day. Exposure to binge foods is then accomplished by introducing small amounts of such foods into the diet. This process is usually made problematic by the patient's distorted cognitions concerning food and body image. Such cognitions are identified and modified by challenge and the application of logic, thus clearing a way for the patient to try out the necessary behaviour changes. Typical automatic thoughts include: 'I mustn't eat today because I binged yesterday. I feel very depressed'; 'I'll never be able to stop bingeing; food is the only thing that gives me pleasure nowadays'. In the final phase of therapy, procedures to reduce the chance of relapse are used, including re-establishing self-monitoring, problem-solving, coping with high-risk situations and obtaining help from friends.

It is also important to offer advice to the bulimic patient concerning other aspects of health, e.g. to check with their general practitioner whether or not they need iron or potassium supplements; to take exercise in moderation; to drink alcohol only in moderation or else give it up completely; and finally, brushing teeth after vomiting serves only to scrub acid into the tooth enamel, so it is better to brush teeth several hours following vomiting so that teeth are protected.

Several researchers have advocated the use of cognitive–behavioural therapy for bulimics (e.g. Kirkley *et al.*, 1985) but of 15 non-single case studies reviewed involving such an approach, only five had some sort of control, i.e. multiple baseline, two-group comparison, or waiting list control (Beumont, Burrows and Casper, 1987). Many of these studies were uncontrolled pilot programmes with small samples and were thus flawed in design; follow-ups were lacking, many studies omitted measures of psychological functioning as well as binge/purge behaviour and a number of studies did not specify their results clearly. Nonetheless, as a group these studies suggest that cognitive and behavioural interventions are relatively effective in their impact upon binge/purge behaviour and psychological functioning. However, this has not been supported in later studies, such as that by Freeman *et al.* (1988) who concluded that bulimia is amenable to treatment by once-weekly psychotherapy in either individual or group form.

Group treatment programmes using this approach seem also to have had some degree of success (e.g. Ordman and Kirschenbaum, 1985; Schneider and Agras, 1985). Using an adaptation of Fairburn's (1981) cognitive–behavioural approach, Schneider and Agras reported a 91% improvement in symptoms. Similarly, Hsu and Holder (1986) have used the approach to treat 56 bulimic patients and continued to follow them for at least one year after completion or dropping out of the treatment. Their approach followed the lines of similar studies, e.g. Fairburn, 1981; Long and Cordle, 1982; Boskind-Lodahl, 1976; 1978; and Lacey, 1983. Emphasis was placed on dietary intake and recognizing the antecedents to bingeing. Alternative coping strategies were taught and the responsibility for change was shifted onto the patients themselves. Indeed, this is probably the main advantage of this approach: the responsibility for regulating food intake becomes the patient's instead of the therapist's. The disadvantage, however, is that regular input is required from the clinical psychologist and the paramedical professionals such as dietitians and occupational therapists.

Pharmacotherapy

Over the years, many researchers have suggested that bulimic patients often present with symptoms that are characteristic of unipolar or bipolar affective psychoses (i.e. depressive illnesses). This has been supported by Hudson, Laffer and Pope (1982), Johnson and Larson (1982) and Walsh, Roose and Glassman (1983). A high incidence of major affective disorder among first- and second-degree relatives has also been found (Strober, 1981; Hudson, Laffer and Pope, 1982; Pope *et al.*, 1983; Strober *et al.*, 1982; Gwirtsman *et al.*, 1983; Brotman, Herzog and Woods, 1984; Herzog, 1984; Mitchell *et al.*, 1984; Stewart *et al.*, 1984). It is for these reasons that tricyclic medication (e.g. imipramine) has been tried with bulimics. Likewise, open trial investigation of the use of lithium with character-disordered bulimics has been reported (e.g. Hsu, 1984); and because of a suggested link between bulimia and certain neuropsychological disorders, phenytoin has also been prescribed to bulimics under controlled conditions (e.g. Green and Rau, 1974; Wermuth *et al.*, 1977).

In reviewing the medication literature, it appears that pharmacological interventions are promising. Many bulimic patients have affect regulation difficulties and for some, a biological vulnerability plays a predominant role in the aetiology of the disorder. It is unclear, however, which bulimics are responsive to medication as some bulimics with significant depressive symptoms are poor responders. Other confusions arise over results presented from using small sample sizes, a lack of monitoring serum levels in patients and inadequate long term follow-up data. A placebo-controlled, double-blind trial carried out by Mitchell and Groat (1984) also acted on the association between bulimia and affective disorders. Using amitriptyline hydrochloride as the drug of choice, 32 female outpatients with bulimia were treated and monitored at frequent intervals. The authors reported that these patients had fewer days each week when they binged, spent fewer hours binge-eating each week and had a lower number of vomiting episodes each week.

Such methods of treatment have been used with other antidepressants, including tricyclic imipramine and the monoamine oxidase inhibitor (MAOI) phenelzine (Strober, 1981; Hudson, Laffer and Pope, 1982; Sabine *et al.*, 1983; Kennedy, Piran and Garfinkel, 1985; Kronig, 1986). However, some clinicians argue that tricyclics can produce a carbohydrate craving which exacerbates the symptoms of bulimia (Paykel *et al.*, 1973). Therefore, alternatives have been tried, such as naltrexone, a long-acting opiate antagonist (Jonas and Gold, 1987) and fenfluramine (Robinson, Checkley and Russell, 1985).

It is an interesting fact that some bulimic patients respond to pharmacotherapy irrespective of exhibiting symptoms of depression or other affective disorders. While some studies have shown that antidepressants can have beneficial effects in treating bulimia, none has systematically examined the maintenance of patients' improvement or the effects of drug discontinuation, side effects, poor compliance or suicide risks. Until further research is conducted using a variety of medications versus placebo under controlled conditions, this situation remains inconclusive.

Family therapy

While there have been a number of reports on the use of family therapy with patients suffering from anorexia nervosa (e.g. Minuchin, Rosman and Baker, 1978), very few data based reports have appeared concerning family therapy for patients with bulimia. Exceptions to this have included Schwartz's (1982) single case study and Schwartz, Barrett and Saba's (1984) larger scale study of family therapy. In the latter study, 30 bulimic patients and their families were seen for an average of 33 sessions over nine months. At the close of treatment, 66%

were having less than one binge/purge episode per month and feeling nearly always in control; 10% were having two episodes per month to once per week but feeling usually in control; 10% were having between two and four episodes weekly and 14% were binge/purging more than five times per week and feeling out of control. While these outcome figures are positive, it is clear that further work needs to be carried out before this approach to the treatment of bulimia is anywhere near conclusive.

Group (psychodynamic) therapy

Group therapy is a form of treatment in which people are seen to grow and change through various mechanisms (Martin, 1990). Psychodynamic theories on bulimia see a basic deficit in self-regulation in which the patient uses his or her bingeing, vomiting and dietary restrictions to help internal tension regulation and self-definition (Stern, 1986). Schwartz (1982) argues that food is viewed as the semi-symbolic equivalent of the oral mother and that, for the bulimic individual, the bingeing–vomiting syndrome is a 'concrete expression of the introjection–projection struggles of early infancy'.

Boskind-Lodahl (1976, 1978) reported on this form of approach as one of the earliest treatments for bulimia, using a feminist perspective. The author reported a reduction in bingeing and purging by the end of the treatment, with group members also reporting improvements in social competence, self-esteem and emotional stability. Given the intensity of group treatment, results are slow to show improvement. However, the maintenance of these results over a longer period is more impressive.

Group treatment approaches are particularly useful when working with bulimic patients because of the secrecy and isolation surrounding the condition. It is possible for group members to confront each other in sessions on how to use their dependency on diet. Shisslak *et al.* (1986) see interactional group therapy as an ideal format for tackling the four distortions common to the beliefs of bulimic patients: appearance is the sole criterion by which others evaluate them; they will be abandoned if they do not devote themselves to fulfilling the desires of others; the expression of emotion is unacceptable; and they are unlovable unless they achieve perfection.

Other researchers (e.g. Sykes, Currie and Gross, 1987) emphasized the importance of goal setting with their patients at the outset of treatment. These goals included control of symptoms; improved social family and/or marital relationships; normalized eating patterns and weight; goals pertinent to the developmental stage of the group and the individual patient; and individual goals as determined by the patient. The authors felt that this approach examined both the behavioural and the psychodynamic aspects of the condition.

As with all treatment approaches, there is always a tendency for drop-out or non-attendance of patients. Some therapies seem to have higher rates of drop-out than others; therefore, it is a consideration to be borne in mind when establishing any therapeutic programme. The reader is referred to the Further Reading section where a source of references on this subject may be found.

Self-help

Huon (1984) detailed the success of a self-help programme by mail in Australia. Subjects were 90 DSM-III bulimic females who responded to an invitation in a magazine to participate in a study. The self-help components consisted of task-orientated suggestions for change sent to each individual monthly over seven months. The majority of participants in all experimental groups improved; 19% were symptom-free at the end of seven months, while 68% improved to the point where they were binge/purging less than once per week. At a 6-month follow-up, 32% were symptom-free and 45% reported 'significant improvement'.

The authors noted that those willing to self-monitor tended to remain in the programme, while those unwilling to comply with this request dropped out. It is interesting that providing bulimics with psycho-educational materials can also be effective in the absence of therapeutic contact.

Progressive relaxation

Connors, Johnson and Stuckey (1984) have reported on the use of progressive relaxation as a component in several treatment programmes, but there are few studies which have employed it as a primary intervention (e.g. Mizes and Lohr, 1983; Mizes and Fleece, 1984). Whilst progressive muscle relaxation in particular has been beneficial to patients in other settings (Thompson, 1990b), many patients attempting this relaxation procedure under the urge of the stress to binge find it impossible and hence need a variety of alternative activities to consider when having the desire to binge.

Counselling

A number of counselling approaches have been used with bulimic patients. For example, Hornak (1983) used structured group counselling while Leclair and Berkowitz (1983) utilized a personal insight approach. Loganbill and Koch (1983) and also Weber and Gillingham (1984) de-emphasized topics which centred around food and eating patterns while Neuman and Halvorsen (1983) reported on counselling groups which focused on nutritional advice, peer self-help groups, psychoanalytically oriented psychotherapy, cognitive–behavioural therapy and assertiveness training. The reader is referred to the original sources (cited in the Further Reading section) for detailed accounts of these practices.

Imaginal desensitization

In a study by McConaghy and Blaszczynski (1988), a 33 year old bulimic woman was taught a relaxation procedure which she was encouraged to carry out prior to visualizing the first behaviour of a scene, such as 'driving to a particular shop to buy cream cakes'. The dramatic results reported by the authors seem most promising as this technique could be carried out simply and with little rehearsal.

TREATMENT AS AN INPATIENT OR AN OUTPATIENT

Many clinicians and researchers still consider hospitalization essential for the treatment of bulimia (e.g. Russell, 1979; Garfinkel and Garner, 1982; Levitt, 1986). Indeed, Garfinkel and Garner (1982) see the external controls imposed by the hospital setting as 'necessary to break an unending cycle of starvation and vomiting in non-emaciated patients'. Russell

(1979) sees hospital admission as necessary in order 'to interrupt the vicious cycle of over-eating, self-induced vomiting (or purging) and weight loss'. He also sees hospitalization as essential if there is a risk of suicide or if medical complications prevail.

Garfinkel and Garner (1982) have recommended that two to three weeks' hospitalization is necessary in order to reduce the urge to vomit. This should comprise total bedrest with denied self-access to lavatories for two hours after meals. According to the authors, patients should be encouraged to talk to staff instead of vomiting.

Martin (1990) asserts that providing inpatient care for a patient with bulimia is often crucial in breaking the long-standing and life-threatening patterns of behaviour associated with the condition. The purpose of hospitalization of bulimic patients is seen by Levitt (1986) to include the following: interrupting uncontrolled habits which are associated with the condition, such as bingeing and purging; assessing the patient's current medical and psychosocial status; initiating a therapeutic process; initiating psychosocial treatment; and developing a long term plan following discharge.

There are others, however, that advocate outpatient treatment for bulimia (Schliessener-Stropp, 1985). It has been argued that a day hospital treatment plan is more cost-effective and successful in the long term for treating bulimic patients who can continue to face the problems they encounter in everyday life which are often avoided during periods of sustained inpatient treatment. Clearly, there is room for both views and it is important, as stated earlier, to fit the best treatment to the patient.

OUTCOME OF BULIMIA

It is still sometimes difficult to determine which set of patients will respond to which particular treatment interventions. It may well be that a subgroup of patients with a true biological vulnerability will respond to nothing but medication, while another group will respond to a larger variety of interventions. The fact that variable outcome results have been obtained with similar methods of intervention raises the question of patient vulnerability. Researchers have suggested several different patient variables which they found to be associated with poorer treatment outcome: anorexic tendencies (Stevens and Salisbury, 1984); higher EAT (Eating Attitudes Test) and EDI (Eating Disorders Inventory) scores (Leitenberg *et al.*, 1984); level of personality disorder (Brotman, Herzog and Woods, 1984); borderline personality organization (Johnson and Larson, 1982); major depression (Mitchell and Groat, 1984); and continuing to live at home throughout treatment (Schwartz, Barrett and Saba, 1984).

The general level of psychopathology is also thought to influence outcome and also the degree to which patients comply with the demands of a particular treatment programme. In a psycho-educational group study, Johnson and Connors (1987) found the best predictor of improvement was compliance with the different aspects of the treatment programme. This was supported by Connors, Johnson and Stuckey (1984). Pyle *et al.* (1984) argued that patients entering a programme where abstinence is demanded from the first night are likely to be a relatively healthy group with high motivation and little ambivalence about relinquishing their usual behaviour. Hence, the outcome is likely to be favourable.

In conclusion, it remains difficult to generalize across groups of individuals as to the best predictors of treatment outcome. However, as research becomes more stringent in both criteria for the selection of patients and in their methodology and reporting, comparison between different research is made more feasible. Then, there is a greater possibility of knowing reliable predictors of treatment outcome for bulimic patients.

FURTHER READING

Screening questionnaires

Agras, W.S. (1987) *Eating Disorders: Management of Obesity, Bulimia and Anorexia Nervosa*. Pergamon, New York.

Diagnostic interview and self-monitoring

Garfinkel, P.E., Moldofsky, H. and Garner, D.M. (1980) The heterogeneity of anorexia nervosa: Bulimia as a distinct subgroup. *Archives of General Psychiatry*, **37**, 1036–40.

Russell, G. (1979) Bulimia nervosa: An ominous variant of anorexia nervosa. *Psychological Medicine*, **9**, 429–48.

Treasure, J. (1989) Bulimia nervosa and anorexia nervosa. *Practitioner*, **233**(1479), 1525–7.

Types of treatment

Freeman, C.P.L., Barry, F., Dunkeld-Turnbull, J. and Henderson, A. (1988) Controlled trial of psychotherapy for bulimia nervosa. *British Medical Journal*, **296**, 521–4.

Long, C.G. and Cordle, C.J. (1982) Psychological treatment of binge eating and self-induced vomiting. *British Journal of Medical Psychology*, **55**, 139–45.

Turnbull, J., Freeman, C.P.L., Barry, F. and Henderson, A. (1989) The clinical characteristics of bulimic women. *International Journal of Eating Disorders*, **8**(4), 399–409.

Behaviour therapy

Cooper, P. and Cooper, Z. (1989) Behavioural treatment of bulimia nervosa. *International Journal of Eating Disorders*, **8**, 87–92.

Linden, W. (1980) Multicomponent behaviour therapy in a case of compulsive binge eating followed by vomiting. *Journal of Behavioural Therapy and Experimental Psychiatry*, **11**, 297–300.

Wolf, E.M. and Crowther, J.H. (1992) An evaluation of behavioral and cognitive-behavioral group interventions for the treatment of bulimia nervosa in women. *International Journal of Eating Disorders*, **11**(1), 3–16.

Cognitive–behavioural therapy

Fairburn, C.G. (1981) A cognitive–behavioral approach to the treatment of bulimia. *Psychological Medicine*, **11**, 707–11.

Fox Kales, E. (1991) Cognitive factors in eating behavior in bulimia. *Appetite*, **17**(3), 241.

Freeman, C.P.L., Barry, F., Dunkeld-Turnbull, J. and Henderson, A. (1988) Controlled trial of psychotherapy for bulimia nervosa. *British Medical Journal*, **296**, 521–4.

Pharmacotherapy

Kennedy, S., Piran, N. and Garfinkel, P.E. (1985) Monoamine oxidase inhibitor therapy for anorexia nervosa and bulimia: A preliminary trial of isocarboxazid. *Journal of Clinical Psychopharmacology*, **5**, 279–85.

Mitchell, J. and Groat, R. (1984) A placebo-controlled double-blind trial of amitriptyline in bulimia. *Journal of Clinical Psychopharmacology*, **4**, 186–93.

Walsh, B.T., Roose, S.P. and Glassman, A.H. (1983) *Depression and Eating Disorders*. Paper presented at the Annual Meeting of the American Psychiatric Association, Washington DC.

Family therapy

Schwartz, R.C. (1982) Bulimia and family therapy. A case study. *International Journal of Eating Disorders*, **2**, 75–82.

Self-help

Ernst, S. and Goodison, L. (1981) *In Our Hands*. The Women's Press, London.

Group (psychodynamic) therapy

Cox, G. and Merkel, W. (1989) A qualitative review of psychosocial treatment for bulimia. *Journal of Nervous and Mental Disorders*, **177**, 77–84.

Roy-Byrne, P., Lee Benner, K. and Yager, J. (1984) Group therapy for bulimia: A year's experience. *International Journal of Eating Disorders*, **3**, 97–116.

Progressive relaxation

Mizes, J.S. and Fleece, E.L. (1984) *On the Use of Progressive Relaxation in the Treatment of Bulimia: A Replication and Extension*. Paper presented at the Annual Meeting of the Society of Behavioral Medicine, Philadelphia.

Counselling

Hornak, N. (1983) Group treatment for bulimia: Bulimics Anonymous. *Journal of the College of Studies in Personnel*, **24**, 461–3.

Hsu, L.K.G., Holben, B. and West, S. (1992) Nutritional counseling in bulimia nervosa. *International Journal of Eating Disorders*, **11**(1), 55–62.

Leclair, N. and Berkowitz, B. (1983) Counselling concerns for the individual with bulimia. *Personnel Guidance Journal*, **2**, 352–5.

Loganbill, C. and Koch, M. (1983) Eating disorder group. *Journal of the College of Studies in Personnel*, **24**, 174–275.

Neuman, P. and Halvorsen, P. (1983) *Anorexia Nervosa and Bulimia: A Handbook for Counsellors and Therapists*. Van Nostrand Reinhold, New York.

Weber, K. and Gillingham, W. (1984) Group counselling for anorexic and bulimic students. *Journal of the College of Studies in Personnel*, **25**, 276.

Imaginal desensitization

McConaghy, M. and Blaszcynski, A. (1988) Imaginal desensitization: A cost-effective treatment in two shoplifters and a binge-eater resistant to previous therapy. *Australian and New Zealand Journal of Psychiatry*, **2**, 78–82.

Inpatient and outpatient treatment of bulimia

Levitt, J. (1986) Treating adults with eating disorders by using an inpatient approach. *Health and Social Work*, **11**, 133–40.

Schliessener-Stropp, B. (1984) Bulimia: A review of the literature. *Psychological Bulletin*, **95**, 247–57.

Outcome of bulimia

Luborsky, L., Auerback, A., Chandler, M. and Cohen, M. (1971) Factors influencing the outcome of psychotherapy: A review of quantitative research. *Psychological Bulletin*, **75**, 145–85.

Stevens, E.V. and Salisbury, J.D. (1984) Group therapy for

bulimic adults. *American Journal of Orthopsychiatry*, **54**, 156–61.

Wooley, S.C. and Kearney-Cooke, A. (1986) Intensive treatment of bulimia and body image disturbance, in *Handbook of Eating Disorders*, (eds K.D. Brownell and J.P. Foreyt), Basic Books, New York, pp. 476–502.

Wooley, S.C. and Wooley, O.W. (1985) Intensive residential and outpatient treatment of bulimia, in *Handbook of Treatment for Anorexia Nervosa and Bulimia*, (eds D. Garner and P.E. Garfinkel), Guildford Press, New York, pp. 391–430.

Drop-outs in treatment

Bakeland, F. and Lundwall, L. (1975) Dropping out of treatment: A critical review. *Psychological Bulletin*, **82**, 738–83.

Margittae, K., Blouin, A. and Perez, E. (1986) A study of drop-out and psychopharmacological research with bulimics. *International Journal of Psychiatry and Medicine*, **16**, 297–303.

Merrill, C., Mines, R. and Starkey, R. (1987) The premature dropout in the group treatment of bulimia. *International Journal of Eating Disorders*, **6**, 293–300.

Mushlin, A. and Appel, A. (1977) Diagnosing potential non-compliance. Physician's ability in a behavioural dimension of medical care. *Archives of Internal Medicine*, **137**, 318–21.

For further information about bulimia (or anorexia nervosa) contact:

Eating Disorders Association, Sackville Place, 44–48 Magdelin Street, Norwich, Norfolk NR3 1JE.

6

Research into bulimia

A selection of research topics in bulimia is presented in this chapter. Detail is given to the individual research undertaken with particular reference to the methodologies adopted. As it is not possible to cover all of the research areas investigated, the reader is directed to the Further Reading section at the end of this chapter for additional information.

There have been few long term outcome studies into bulimia, but one notable exception is the study by Hsu and Sobkiewicz (1989) in which 45 female bulimic patients were followed over a six year period. Such studies face many practical difficulties such as the tendency of bulimics towards extreme secrecy in their bingeing behaviour. Nevertheless several centres have been active in eating disorders research (e.g. Cullen Centre, Edinburgh, Scotland; Addenbrooke's Hospital, Cambridge, England) and short term studies continue to yield interesting results and have covered a remarkable variety of topics, e.g. experiential aspects of bulimia and effects of cognitive therapy; perception of weight; teaching psychological techniques to other health care staff such as dietitians; heat pain threshold in bulimics; prevalence of bulimia; serotonin levels in bulimics; bulimia as a variant of anorexia nervosa; bulimia as a distinct subgroup of anorexia nervosa; efficacy of eating disorder questionnaires in male bulimics; binge-eating behaviour *per se*; and educational approaches. The last four in this list will be discussed here in greater detail.

BULIMIA AS A DISTINCT SUBGROUP OF ANOREXIA NERVOSA

Some researchers consider bulimia to be a subgroup of anorexia nervosa; those who do generally believe it is a poor prognostic sign in anorexia nervosa (e.g. Garfinkel, Moldofsky and Garner, 1980). However, one question that has often been raised is whether bulimia represents an 'end stage' of chronic anorexia nervosa or whether bulimic patients are a distinct subgroup. In a study by Garfinkel, Moldofsky and Garner (1980), patients were seen between 1970 and 1978 and detailed histories were taken for each of them. Of these patients, 68 experienced bulimia and 73 did not (restricters). Those that satisfied modified criteria of Feighner *et al.* (1972) (criteria often used for psychiatric research) were included in the study.

All subjects seen by the authors personally between 1970 and 1978 were included in the study provided they met modified criteria of Feighner *et al.* (1972). Although the Feighner *et al.* (1972) criteria were generally used (which incidentally is not advised for clinical work since they are believed to be too vague – DSM-III-R criteria are preferred), the authors disagreed with three of their points:

1. The age of onset (some patients in the study were older than the specified 25 years);
2. The need for 'anorexia' (many patients did not have loss of appetite);
3. The degree of weight loss being greater than 25% of original body weight (if someone was relatively thin at the onset or still growing and lost only 20% of their weight it would not negate the diagnosis).

Bulimia was defined as an abnormal increase in one's desire to eat, with episodes of excessive ingestion of large quantities of food that the patient viewed as 'ego-alien' and beyond her control (Garfinkel, Moldofsky and Garner, 1980). Of the 141 patients seen, 68 patients experienced bulimia at the time of initial consultation and 73 did not. In 14 patients, these data were not clear and they were omitted from analyses. Of the bulimic patients, 25 experienced episodes of excessive ingestion of food at least on a daily basis; 28, one to five times per week, and 15, one to three times per month. Patients who clearly did not display bulimia and only curtailed dietary intake were placed into the 'restricting' group. Patients were seen, when referred by other physicians, during various phases of their illness and with varying degrees of chronicity. Bulimic patients, however, were not ill for a substantially longer period than restricters.

Both groups of patients showed similar social characteristics, with the upper and middle social classes being over-represented in comparison with the general population. Of importance, there were no differences between the bulimic and restricter groups in age of onset or duration of illness, arguing against bulimia simply representing a manifestation of chronicity (Garfinkel, Moldofsky and Garner, 1980).

Of patients in whom bulimia developed, the onset of bulimic episodes occurred at varying phases of the disorder. In six patients, it preceded or was coincidental with the weight loss. For those patients on whom these data were available (71%), bulimia developed 19.2 ± 8.0 months after the onset of dieting. There were major differences between the bulimic and restricting groups: bulimic patients had a history of weighing more and in fact 32% were obese premorbidly; by contrast, obesity was rare in the restricters. Similarly, bulimic patients weighed significantly more at the time of initial contact and at their minimum weights. They also vomited and misused laxatives and displayed a variety of impulsive behaviour, including use of alcohol and street drugs, stealing, suicide attempts and self-mutilation. With regard to family history, the high frequency of obesity in the mother of bulimic patients was noteworthy. In conclusion, the authors found that the two groups shared features common to primary anorexia nervosa. However, these results suggested a different group of women who were pre-disposed to have anorexia nervosa develop with bulimia.

EFFICACY OF EATING DISORDER QUESTIONNAIRES IN MALE BULIMICS

In the past, there has been debate concerning the reliability of eating disorder questionnaires in identifying people with an eating disorder. In an unusual study, because of its use of only male subjects, Turnbull *et al.* (1987) collected the case histories of five men who met DSM-III criteria for bulimia. Various eating disorder questionnaires were administered and the results indicated that most of these instruments would not have identified the men as suffering from an eating disorder.

All the subjects were assessed over a period of two or three weeks to check that they met DSM-III criteria for bulimia and to see whether or not they also met Russell's (1979) criteria for 'bulimia nervosa'. They were weighed and their heights noted. A full personal history and history of weight and eating patterns were taken. The BITE (Henderson and Freeman, 1987), EAT-40 and EAT-26 (Garner and Garfinkel, 1979; Garner *et al.*, 1982) and EDI (Garner, Olmsted and Polivy, 1983) were administered. The BITE (which has already been mentioned in Chapter 2 and Chapter 5) is a self-rating 33-item questionnaire designed to detect subjects with bulimia or binge-eating. It has two scales, a symptom scale and a severity scale, which allow for the measurement of the degree of symptoms present and an index of the severity of bingeing and purging behaviours. The EDI, EAT-40 and EAT-26 are standard instruments which assess the attitudes and objective features of eating disorders.

Subjects were asked to keep a diary of everything they ate and drank and of how often they binged, vomited and abused laxatives. They were asked to note the occasions and quantities of other drugs taken and how often they engaged in exercise designed to counter the effects of bingeing (Turnbull *et al.*, 1987).

Zinkland, Cadoret and Widmes (1984) noted a tendency for bulimic men to be taller and heavier than men without eating disorders, but Herzog *et al.* (1984) found them to be lighter. The bulimic men described in this study were taller and lighter than average. The thinner subjects' ideal weights were close to their present weights, whilst the two heavier subjects, while of perfectly normal weight, wanted to be much thinner. Herzog *et al.* (1984) found a mean age of onset in bulimic men of 18.6 years, while in this sample the mean age of onset was higher (22.4 years).

The scores the subjects obtained on the EDI and EAT would not have identified these men as having eating problems (Turnbull *et al.*, 1987). Subjects' scores on the subscales of the EDI were more similar to those of normal than bulimic women. The cut-off scores on the EAT-40 and EAT-26 are 30 and 20 respectively; the subjects' scores were below these values. Inspection seemed to indicate that the men's scores on the EAT and subscales of the EAT were between those of normal and bulimic women. Turnbull *et al.* (1987) commented that these subjects had scores for bulimia which were well elevated above those of normal men and women on both the EDI and EAT scales. It was on the less objective scales and more on those indicating attitude that they failed to show large differences from normals. However, it is clear that the subjects' scores would have identified them as being bulimic using the BITE; the cut-off is 25 for the total score. The subjects' scores were much more similar to those of bulimic than to those of normal women.

Finally, Turnbull *et al.* (1987) concluded that bulimia may be more common in men than has previously been supposed. Button and Whitehouse (1981) and Clarke and Palmer (1983) found no evidence of eating disorder in the groups of men they surveyed using the EAT. In view of the results of Turnbull *et al.*'s (1987) study, it would seem that caution must be used in the administration of test instruments derived from and derived for women, as the pattern for men does not seem to be as clear-cut. Most of the subjects described would have been missed if the most widely used instruments (i.e. the EDI and EAT) had been used for screening yet all subjects had clinically significant and distressing pathology.

BINGE-EATING BEHAVIOUR

Towards the end of the 1970s there was an increased interest in the condition known as the 'binge-eating syndrome' (later termed 'bulimia nervosa' and a decade later, 'bulimia'). Indeed, much of this interest arose out of the apparent connection of the binge-eating syndrome with anorexia nervosa. Several investigators found that nearly half of their anorectic patient population had exhibited symptoms of bulimia (Hsu, Crisp and Harding, 1979; Casper *et al.*, 1980; Pyle, Mitchell and Eckert, 1981). Another investigator found that anorexia nervosa patients developed bulimia after they had regained a normal weight (Russell, 1979).

It also became evident that binge-eating and vomiting behaviour occurred in normal weight and even overweight people (Boskind-Lodahl, 1978; Boskind-White, 1984; Strangler and Printz, 1980; White and Boskind-White, 1981). This information led to the classification of bulimia as a distinct disorder from anorexia nervosa in the third edition of the *Diagnostic and Stat-*

istical Manual of the American Psychiatric Association (DSM-III) (American Psychiatric Association, 1980).

Because of the apparent increased requests by college students to be treated for this disorder (White and Boskind-White, 1981) and the clinical information that the disorder had become a recognized problem in the teenage and young adult population, Halmi, Falk and Schwartz (1981) decided to conduct a systematic survey of the prevalence of bulimia.

The data were obtained by questionnaire which was distributed to 539 summer session registrants at a suburban liberal arts campus of the State University of New York; 355 students returned the questionnaire completed.

The 23-item questionnaire was distributed to the summer college population with the approval of the college's human rights committee and the approval and cooperation of the college administrators and psychology department. The distribution was performed during the days of registration at the campus registration site. Completion of the questionnaire by the students was strictly voluntary.

The questionnaire was structured to obtain information regarding sex, college major subject and year of study, age and physical stature, including one year weight change and history of highest and lowest weight, use of diet aids and medication and the behavioural symptoms of bulimia according to the diagnostic criteria of the DSM-III.

The respondents' ages ranged from 14 to 67 years old; of the subjects who participated in this study, 33.4% were males and 59.8% were females (with 6.7% not indicating their sex). The respondents' normal weights were computed based on the Metropolitan Life Insurance Company (1959) weight scales which were corrected for sex and height. The respondents' self-report of their present weight was converted to a percentage of the standard weight by the relationship:

$$\text{Percentage of standard weight} = \frac{\text{Present weight}}{\text{Normal weight}} \times 100$$

The respondents were categorized into five weight groupings by both the calculated percentage of the standard weight and their personal opinion of their weight as described in Roberts (1977).

The results of the study indicated that the prevalence of

binge-eating was higher than that previously reported (Wermuth *et al.*, 1977; White and Boskind-White, 1981). Wermuth *et al.* (1977) noted that the frequency of binge-eating had never been estimated and they reported that only one person out of 600 college age men and women seen during a 5-month recruiting period at the Stanford Student Health Service had complained of binge-eating. Strangler and Printz (1980), however, in their study of psychiatric diagnosis in a university patient population, have found the prevalence of bulimia in a sample of 500 student patients to be 3.8% (of which 89.5% were female and 10.5% were male). Strangler and Printz (1980) pointed out that their prevalence finding for bulimia was conservative, since other cases of bulimia were revealed during therapy but were not recorded as such.

Halmi, Falk and Schwartz's (1981) finding for the prevalence of bulimia was 13%, with a ratio of females to males being similar to that found by Strangler and Printz (1980). The work of White and Boskind-White (1981) has also suggested the prevalence of bulimia (at least in college populations) to be higher than that suggested by Wermuth *et al.* (1977). These results indicated that binge-eating may be a much more serious public health problem than was previously thought.

The analysis of the results of this study also add credence to the DSM-III description of bulimia nervosa by detecting strong inter-relationships among the symptoms:

1. Considering oneself a binge-eater;
2. Having an uncontrollable urge to eat;
3. Feelings of guilt and self-deprecating thoughts;
4. Actual bingeing on food;
5. Experiencing a fear of not being able to stop eating.

The results indicated that vomiting may be present in bulimia, but that the presence of vomiting is not a necessary part of bulimia. The condition of vomiting with other symptoms of bulimia in an individual may represent a severe form of bulimia demanding treatment.

It was also interesting to note from this study a significant direct relationship between self-induced vomiting and laxative use. These, appropriately, may be described as purging behaviours. The results also indicated conclusively that the symptoms of bulimia are more likely to appear in those individuals who at some time had been overweight or tended to be heavy within their normal range. Contrary to the results of Beumont, George and Smart (1976) and Beumont (1977), they found no significant relationship between vomiting and weight history. However, these authors had not differentiated the bulimics into vomiters and non-vomiters. Surprisingly, no significant relationships of binge-eating and vomiting history or an abnormally low weight were detected (Halmi, Falk and Schwartz, 1981). This is surprising, since many authors have chosen to consider bulimia as a symptom of anorexia nervosa, if not a subclass within anorexia nervosa (Monti, McCrady and Barlow, 1977; Nogami and Yobana, 1977; Russell, 1979; White and Boskind-White, 1981). The results of Halmi, Falk and Schwartz's (1981) study strongly suggest that bulimia is a distinct disorder. Symptoms of bulimia may occur in conjunction with anorexia nervosa, but the bulimia symptoms are more likely to occur without the presence of anorexia nervosa. In fact, only one person of the 355 examined indicated having had anorexia nervosa.

EDUCATIONAL APPROACHES

Educational group treatment programmes have been reported by a number of researchers including Katzman, Weiss and Wolchik (1986) and Connor-Greene (1987). These will now be discussed.

Study 1

In the Katzman, Weiss and Wolchik (1986) study, treatment programmes were run which consisted of exercises designed to 'help women to feel better about themselves'. Their programme consisted of seven weekly 90-minute group sessions focusing on a particular topic, such as self-esteem, coping strategies, perfectionism, anger, depression, cultural expectations of thinness for women and enhancing body image. Emphasis was placed on the development of new skills rather than on the eating behaviour.

Each person received a treatment package consisting of reading materials, exercises and homework. This package also doubled as a self-help guide at the termination of the programme.

The authors state that by emphasizing building skills, they encourage women to take responsibility for their own behaviour which, in turn, helps to promote change. Unfortunately, there are no statistics reported concerning successes and/or failures as a result of following this methodology.

Study 2

In the Connor-Greene (1987) study, the treatment group ran weekly for six weeks. Each session focused on a particular topic: the psychological and physical effects of bulimia; effects of dieting/caloric deprivation on behaviour; increasing awareness of eating patterns; alternative coping strategies; nutrition awareness; and social pressure for thinness.

Five patients were involved in the pilot study; four of these reported a decrease in binge frequency and four reported a reduction in self-induced vomiting. By the end of the programme, all reported feeling in control of their eating which is in contrast to their feeling of loss of control at the beginning of the programme. The patients also reduced the regularity with which they weighed themselves. These findings tend to support the idea of a short term educational programme in helping to bring the binge-eating behaviour more under the patient's control.

FURTHER READING

Efficacy of cognitive therapy in bulimia

Hsu, L.K. (1990) Experiential aspects of bulimia nervosa. Implications for cognitive therapy. *Behaviour Modification*, **14**(1), 50–65.

Rossiter, E. and Wilson, G. (1985) Cognitive restructuring and response prevention in the treatment of bulimia nervosa. *Behaviour Research and Therapy*, **23**, 349–59.

Schneider, J. and Agras, S. (1985) A cognitive–behavioural group treatment of bulimia. *British Journal of Psychiatry*, **146**, 66–9.

Perception of weight in bulimics

Mitchell, J.E., Pyle, R.L., Eckert, E.D., Hatsukami, D. and Soll, E. (1990) Bulimia nervosa with and without a history of anorexia nervosa. *Comprehensive Psychiatry*, **31**(2), 171–5.

Teaching psychological techniques to health care staff

Biley, F. and Savage, S. (1988) The role of the nurse in eating disorders, in *Anorexia Nervosa: Practical Approaches*, (ed D. Scott), Croom Helm, London.
Kennedy, F. (1987) Teaching dietitians to use psychological techniques with obese clients. *Behavioural Psychotherapy*, **15**, 88–99.

Heat pain threshold

Lautenbacher, S., Pauls, A.M., Strian, F., Pirke, K.M. and Krieg, J.C. (1990) Pain perception in patients with eating disorders. *Psychosomatic Medicine*, **52**(6), 673–82.

Prevalence of bulimia

Bushnell, J.A., Wells, J.E., Hornblow, A.R., Oakley-Browne, M.A. and Joyce, P. (1990) Prevalence of three bulimia syndromes in the general population. *Psychological Medicine*, **20**(3), 671–80.
Hart, K. and Ollendick, T. (1985) Prevalence of bulimia in working and university women. *American Journal of Psychiatry*, **3**, 851–4.
Pyle, R., Halvorsen, P., Neuman, P. and Goff, G. (1983) The incidence of bulimia in freshman college students. *International Journal of Eating Disorders*, **2**, 75–86.

Serotonin and bulimia

Jimerson, D.C., Lesem, M.D., Hegg, A.P. and Brewerton, T.D. (1990) Serotonin in human eating disorders. *Annals of the New York Academy of Science*, **600**, 532–44.
Jimerson, D.C., Lesem, M.D., Kaye, W.H., Hegg, A.P. and Brewerton, T.D. (1990) Eating disorders and depression: Is

there a serotonin connection? *Biological Psychiatry*, **28**(5), 443–54.

Bulimia as a variant of anorexia nervosa

Russell, G. (1979) Bulimia nervosa: An ominous variant of anorexia nervosa. *Psychological Medicine*, **9**, 429–48.

Bulimia as a distinct subgroup of anorexia nervosa

Casper, R.C., Eckert, E.D., Halmi, K.A., Goldberg, S.C. and Davis, J.M. (1980) Bulimia. Its incidence and clinical importance in patients with anorexia nervosa. *Archives of General Psychiatry*, **37**, 1030–5.

Bulimia and eating disorder questionnaires

Walsh, B.T. (1988) *Eating Behaviour in Eating Disorders*. American Psychiatric Press, Washington DC.

Binge-eating

Cooper, P.J. and Fairburn, C.G. (1983) Binge-eating and self-induced vomiting in the community: A preliminary study. *British Journal of Psychiatry*, **142**, 139–44.

Educational approaches

Connor-Greene, P. (1987) An educational group treatment program for bulimia. *Journal of the American College of Health*, **35**, 229–31.

Fernandez, R. (1984) Group treatment of bulimia, in *Current Treatment of Anorexia Nervosa and Bulimia*, (ed P. Powers and Z. Fernandez), Kayer, Basle.

Katzman, M., Weiss, L. and Wolchik, S. (1986) Speak, don't eat! Teaching women to express their feelings. *Women and Therapy*, **5**, 143–57.

Weiss, L. and Katzman, M. (1984) Group treatment for bulimia women. *Arizona Medicine*, **41**, 100–4.

Bulimia and diabetes mellitus

Peveler, R.C. and Fairburn, C.G. (1992) The treatment of bulimia nervosa in patients with diabetes mellitus. *International Journal of Eating Disorders*, **11**(1), 45–54.

7

Epidemiology of obesity

DEFINITION OF OBESITY

It is a fact that some people become fat and others do not. But there can be numerous reasons for those that do become obese. 'Overweight' or 'obesity' occurs more commonly in certain groups than it does in the general population. These groups can be defined in terms of a variety of categories such as sex, age, occupation, race, ethnicity, socio-economic status, level of education, family history of obesity, habitat, dietary habits and smoking and drinking habits. As VanItallie and Woteki (1987) have commented, other features by which one might identify obesity-prone groups are physical attributes such as stature, body frame size and muscle mass. People who regularly take certain drugs, such as phenothiazine derivatives or beta-adrenergic receptor blocking agents (Munro, 1979), can be placed into groups that are defined by the medication used.

Obesity is commonly defined as being a condition characterized by the Body Mass Index (BMI) where weight in kilograms is divided by height in metres squared (VanItallie, 1985). Life insurance companies (e.g. Metropolitan Life Insurance Company, 1959) have tables detailing categories of age, height and weight and recognize ranges for obesity. The following 'grades' are also commonly used to categorize obesity:

Grade I (Cosmetic) – BMI = 25–30 (or 20–30% in excess of the ideal weight)

Grade II (Medical) – BMI = 30–40 (or 30–80% in excess of the ideal weight)

Grade III (Morbid) – BMI > 40 (or >80% in excess of the ideal weight)

AETIOLOGY AND PREVALENCE

Data obtained in the National Health and Nutrition Examination Survey (NHANES II; National Center for Health Statistics, 1981), which was conducted during 1976–80, have also provided interesting information on the prevalence of overweight according to sex, age, race and socio-economic status. Twelve thousand men and women aged 20–74 years were examined and height and weight measurements were made under standardized conditions. In the sample, men were considered to be overweight when the BMI equalled or exceeded 27.8; they were regarded as being medically overweight when the BMI equalled or exceeded 31.1. For American women, these BMI cut-off points were 27.3 and 32.3, respectively. On the basis of these criteria, it was determined that about 34 million American men and women aged 20–74 years were overweight (Bender and Brookes, 1987); of this group almost 12.5 million were morbidly overweight.

Precipitating factors

American women are at increased risk of becoming obese if they are black or if they are in poverty status (VanItallie and Woteki, 1987). For black women who are also poor, it appears that the risk of becoming obese is compounded. As regards the role of race as a determinant of obesity prevalence in women, it is noteworthy that obesity is common among black females in Africa as well as in the USA. For example, Walker and Segal (1980) reported on studies on new black employees and those in employment for at least a year, showing that while obesity in the males was uncommon, over half the females were obese. According to the authors, obesity in black African females develops even while they are on a diet high in fibre and low in animal fat and protein.

Socio-economic status has also been considered as a determinant of obesity with several studies providing possible evidence both from the UK (Silverstone, 1970; Ashwell and Etchell, 1974) and the USA (Goldblatt, Moore and Stunkard, 1965; Orshansky, 1965; Garn et al., 1977). It would seem from these findings that overweight is more common among lower-class women than among upper-class women. However, a similar difference between upper and lower-class men was not demonstrated (Bender and Brookes, 1987).

It has also been conjectured that people who are at the upper end of the scale as regards frame size and/or muscle mass are also at increased risk of becoming obese. People who are overweight but not obese and people who are both overweight and obese have a larger body frame size (inferred from elbow breadth) and a larger musculature (inferred from arm muscle diameter) than do non-overweight individuals of the same height and age (Benn, 1971; Mrosovsky and Powley, 1977; Wirtshafter and Davis, 1977; Bender and Brookes, 1987).

Genetic factors

It is generally considered that there are two ways in which genetic factors manifest themselves in obesity (Bray, 1976a; 1987; Stunkard, 1958; 1991). First, there is a group of rare diseases, known as 'dysmorphic' forms of obesity, in which genetic factors are of prime importance. Second, there is a genetic substrate upon which environmental factors interact in the development of obesity.

The dysmorphic forms of obesity include the Prader–Willi syndrome (Bray, 1983; Apfelbaum, 1987; Thomas, 1981); Bardet –Biedl syndrome, Cohen's syndrome and Carpenter's syndrome (Bray, 1976b; 1987). In most cases, the presenting obesity is moderate. All these forms of obesity are transmitted both by recessive and dominant modes of inheritance. Facial features, hypogonadism, abnormalities in the eye and hypotonia or polydactyly (i.e. having more than the normal number of fingers or toes) run through this group of syndromes. The Prader–Willi syndrome, the most common syndrome in this group, is associated with a translocation or deletion of the chromosome 15 in about half the cases (Bray, 1983).

Bray and York (1971) and Bray (1987) have discussed several studies of genetic versus environmental factors in obesity. The most definitive studies have come from the examination of the relationship between body weight in twins. Since monozygotic twins presumably have identical genetic material and dizygotic twins have the genetic diversity of brothers and/or sisters, evaluation of these two groups of twins should make it possible to separate nature from nurture most clearly. Newman, Freeman and Holzinger (1937) described 50 pairs of monozygotic twins who grew up together and 50 pairs of dizygotic twins who grew up together; then he compared these with 29 pairs of monozygotic twins who grew up in separate households. The monozygotic twins reared together had a mean difference in body weight of 1.9 kg compared to a 4.5 kg difference between the twins raised apart.

Studying the skinfolds at three different sites in monozygotic twins and dizygotic twins, Borjeson (1976) found that variability for each of the three regions measured in monozygotic twins was approximately one-third of that in the dizygotic twins.

Brook, Huntley and Slack (1975) estimated the heritability of skinfold thickness in twin studies and reported that among individuals under ten years of age there was a significant environmental component, but that in twins over ten years of age the estimated heritability was very high. It would seem that single gene transmission is rare in humans, despite some evidence suggesting single and polygenic inheritance involved in the transmission of obesity.

Metabolic causes of obesity

Several authors have shown evidence that obesity in experimental animals is associated with efficiency for energy storage (Bray and York, 1971; 1979). According to Bray (1987), in the majority of forms of experimental obesity, the gain in body energy stores for a given quantity of food intake is higher than in the corresponding lean animals. However, there is some debate about equating findings from animal studies with humans.

At least seven possible mechanisms have been suggested by which internal biochemical pathways might be altered to enhance metabolic efficiency. They are fairly complex explanations and will not be described here in detail. There is also considerable controversial evidence both for and against these proposals, so the reader is referred to a number of interesting authoritative texts for further information on the subject (e.g. DeLuise, Blackburn and Flier, 1980; Thurlby and Trayhurn, 1980; Glick, Teague and Bray, 1981; Nedergaard and Lindberg, 1981; Schwartz and Brunzell, 1981; Golay, Schutz and Meyer,

1982; Simat, Maynard and From, 1983; Charalambous, Webster and Mir, 1984; Shargill *et al.*, 1984).

The first possible mechanism is through changes in 'futile' metabolic cycles in which phosphorylated compounds are made from adenosine triphosphate or ATP (a compound produced and used by cells in the body to store energy) and then broken down. The second is through alterations in protein turnover; the third is through alterations in ionic equilibrium across the cell and the activity of the sodium-pumping enzyme (sodium–potassium ATPase). The fourth mechanism involves alterations in brown adipose tissue; the fifth, increased levels of lipoprotein lipase which may enhance lipid storage; the sixth and seventh mechanisms involve the efficiency of muscular contraction and the metabolic response to diet-induced thermogenesis (i.e. body heat production).

Dietary and endocrinal causes of obesity

As stated earlier, aberrations in the distribution of body fat have been observed with hypogonadism (Bray, 1976b), but a more substantial obesity occurs in Cushing's syndrome with the increased secretion of cortisol (Bray, 1987). Apart from these abnormalities, physical inactivity and the composition of daily diets can play a large part in a person's body fat distribution.

Hypothalamic obesity, though rare as a syndrome in human beings, has been observed under a variety of circumstances (Kissebah *et al.*, 1982; Bray and York, 1979). The major factors producing hypothalamic damage are trauma, malignancy and inflammatory disease. Three groups of findings accompany the syndrome. The first is related to changes in intracranial pressure, such as headache and diminished vision due to papilloedema (i.e. swelling of the optic disc). The second group of symptoms include amenorrhoea, impotence, diabetes insipidus and thyroid adrenal insufficiency. The symptoms of the third group are a variety of neurological and physiological derangements including coma, convulsions, somnolence and hypothermia or hyperthermia.

Endocrine diseases usually have little genetic involvement. The common types of obesity usually have an important genetic component which interacts with the nutrients in the diet. It cannot be denied, however, as with other disorders of eating, that culture also plays a part in influencing how we dress and what we eat. These important cultural differences can sometimes make an acceptable body shape in one culture totally unacceptable in another.

Psychological theories

There has always been considerable prejudice against obesity. This prejudice operates equally in both sexes and in most ethnic groups, having been found in Hispanic Americans as well as native Americans, Australians, Puerto Ricans, Anglo-Americans and Afro-Americans (Harris and Smith, 1983). Intentional efforts to find populations which might show more tolerance of obesity, such as black men, the elderly, and low income groups, have only confirmed the universality of anti-fat attitudes (Maddox, Beck and Liederman, 1968).

Prejudices can have extremely tangible and concrete effects. It has been found that overweight girls are less likely to be admitted to college than lean peers of equal talents and accomplishments (Canning and Mayer, 1966). Overweight acts as a severe handicap in hiring and promotions. Karris (1977) has even found some landlords less likely to rent to the obese. For women, appearance has often been valued over accomplishment and not surprisingly obese women, as a group, have been found to be downwardly socially mobile (Goldblatt, Moore and Stunkard, 1965; Elder, 1969).

Several authors have shown that prejudice against obesity is learned early and has been repeatedly evidenced in children (e.g. Lerner and Gelbert, 1969; Lerner and Korn, 1972; Staffieri, 1967; Harris and Smith, 1983; Lerner, 1973). Fatness has often been associated in the minds of children with cheating, dirtiness, forgetfulness, argumentativeness, laziness, dishonesty, stupidity, sloppiness, meanness, alcoholism and other negative traits (Harris and Smith, 1982). Even in fictional literature we constantly see obese people ostracized from society. For instance, William Golding's portly character 'Piggy', in *Lord of the Flies*, was victimized and eventually killed by his pre-adolescent peers (Golding, 1960).

The existence of prejudice in even very young children suggests that it is learned from parents. In a study of prospective parents enrolled in childbirth education classes, Sherman (1981) found that drawings of thin and average children were rated as more intelligent, likeable, energetic, mature and clean than heavy children. This prejudice does not seem to wane with maturity and the obese often face further prejudice in those to whom they must turn for help. Maddox and Liederman (1969) found that physicians regarded overweight patients as weak-willed, ugly and awkward. Maiman and colleagues (1979) too found prejudice among a group of health professionals, 86% of whom treated obesity. They found that 84% thought the obese to be self-indulgent; 70% assumed they had emotional problems; 88% assumed they ate to compensate for other problems; and 74% assumed they had family problems. It would seem that even a sophisticated understanding of obesity may be insufficient to alleviate prejudice.

On the other hand, it is possible that the obese do have certain personality characteristics or deficits. McReynolds (1982) conducted a study to compare clinical and non-clinical populations. Obese psychiatric patients, a population selected for psychological disturbance, showed a full range of mental disorders. Obese medical patients, selected for physical but not psychological disorders, failed to display a clear association between obesity and psychological disturbance although many appeared to suffer from mental disorders. Non-patient populations, selected only for their obesity, showed few signs of psychological disturbance and contained relatively few instances of diagnosable mental disorders. Therefore, the range of conditions exhibited by obese people, whether or not disturbed psychologically, would seem to be no different from those displayed by lean people.

There does, however, seem to be some evidence to suggest that 'fat' is feared. In 1984, *Glamour* magazine conducted a survey of 33 000 who had responded to a questionnaire about obesity. Of these, 76% regarded themselves as too fat (*Glamour* magazine, 1984). This figure had included 82% of women categorized as normal weight by the Metropolitan Life Insurance Company (1959) tables. Furthermore, it would seem that women have become more obsessed with their weight over the years. In a survey by Berscheid, Walster and Bohrnstedt (1973), numbers of women dissatisfied with their body weight had risen over an 11 year lapse of time between different surveys.

CHARACTERISTICS OF THE OBESE PATIENT

Many clinicians have concluded that the motivation to lose weight exists entirely apart from medical opinion and increasingly, in direct opposition to it. Despite this, there is a cultural force which drives women towards dieting regimens even in the presence of medical factors preventing their success. Obese people, as a group, are universally believed to be intellectually and personally inferior to thin people. This view is held by their parents, their peers, those who regulate access to social opportunities and even by the very people appointed to help them. Fear and hatred of fatness have become an over-riding social force, dominating the lives of many thin as well as fat people and especially those of women.

Many professionals would agree that medical definitions of what is and is not an abnormality warranting treatment have the potential to be widely influential and it may be shortsighted to set such definitions without consideration of all the consequences. Setting a universal goal in treatment not only fails to balance the risks of excess weight (Thompson, 1992c) against the risk of the procedures used to reduce weight, but also ignores altogether the indirect effects of such recommendations on society, which is badly in need of correctives to weight obsession.

From a psychological point of view, obese people generally do not show markedly different attitudes or personality characteristics to thin people except for the feelings of rejection that society imposes. Medically, the condition has a number of different causes, previously discussed, giving rise to a host of characteristics which are essentially associated with the particular abnormality or dysfunction. The physical appearance of an obese person can also vary according to body frame size and musculature which results in differing attitudes from others with regard to the extent of the obese person's 'overweightness'. Obesity is most generally characterized by excess of body fat which sometimes also appears facially. In short, it is a definition including body weight and height that is medically a strict definition (i.e. using the Body Mass Index or BMI – see Garrow, 1988), but culturally, it is dependent on the consensus of the particular culture, the norms of which usually dictate whether or not a person conforms in appearances and/or in body weight range.

FURTHER READING

General

Kolata, G. (1985) Obesity declared a disease. *Science*, **27**, 1019–20.

Lew, E.A. and Garfinkel, P.E. (1979) Variations in mortality by weight among 750 000 men and women. *Journal of Chronic Disorders*, **32**, 226–32.

Sorlie, P., Gordon, D. and Kannel, W.B. (1980) Body build and mortality. The Framingham study. *Journal of the American Medical Association*, **243**, 1828–31.

Epidemiological studies

Hautvast, F.G.A.F. and Deurenberg, P. (1987) The risks associated with obesity: Epidemiological studies, in *Body Weight Control. The Physiology, Clinical Treatment and Prevention of Obesity*, (eds A.E. Bender and L.J. Brookes), Churchill Livingstone, Edinburgh, pp. 65–79.

Characteristics of obesity

Strain, G.W., Hershcopf, R.J. and Zumoff, B. (1992) Food intake of very obese persons: Quantitative and qualitative aspects. *Journal of the American Dietetic Association*, **92**(2), 199–203.

Specific syndromes of obesity

Anavi, Y. and Mintz, S.M. (1990) Prader–Labhart–Willi syndrome. *Annals of Dentistry*, **49**(2), 26–9.

Croft, J.B. and Swift, M. (1990) Obesity, hypertension and renal disease in relatives of Bardet–Biedl syndrome sibs. *American Journal of Medicine and Genetics*, **36**(1), 37–42.

Shelley, D.R. and Dunaif, A. (1990) Polycystic ovary syndrome. *Comprehensive Therapy*, **16**(11), 26–34.

8

Assessment, treatment and outcome of obesity

HOW TO ASSESS

Gross assessment

A determination of whether or not any one individual is too fat is rather simple, from a practical point of view. Without weighing oneself, looking in the mirror often enables a realistic appraisal of the nude body; if this fails to provide a clear answer, then there is the 'pinch test'. This is particularly helpful for adults who are under 50 years old. At least half of the body fat in young individuals is found directly under the skin. At many locations on the body (e.g. back of the upper arm, side of the lower chest, back just below the shoulder blade, etc.), a fold of skin and subcutaneous fat can be lifted between the thumb and forefinger so that it is held free of the underlying soft tissue and bony structure. Jolliffe (1963) reported that in individuals with normal amounts of fat the layer beneath the skin was 6–12 mm thick. The skinfold is usually double thickness, 12–25 mm thick. In most cases, skinfolds thicker than 25 mm are an indication of excessive body fatness (Foreyt, 1977).

A pinch in several places on the body usually indicates whether or not the first skinfold attempted is characteristic of body fatness. There are, however, variations between men and women and it should be noted that this is only a gross measure. Other simple indicators of fatness include the ruler test and circumference test. When lying flat on the back in a relaxed position, the surface of the abdomen between the flare of the ribs and the pubis is normally flat or slightly concave. A ruler placed on the abdomen parallel with the vertical axis should touch both ribs and pubis.

The circumference test is used to compare the circumference of the chest at the level of the nipples with the circumference of the abdomen at the level of the navel. Normally, the circumference of the chest exceeds abdominal circumference by a few centimetres. When abdominal girth approaches, equals or exceeds the girth of the chest, it usually means an excess of abdominal fat.

Specific assessment

Without the aid of sophisticated techniques, it is possible to measure total body fatness only in cadavers. In the living population, data on total body fatness for groups of people have come from densitometry studies, hydrometry studies and, to a limited extent, from measurements of body electrolytes (e.g. Fryer, 1962; Heald *et al.*, 1963; Novak, 1963; Young, 1963). In the late 1950s and early 1960s, information on total body fatness was also reported from measuring the K^{40} (potassium) content through the use of whole body counters (e.g. Anderson and Langham, 1959; Forbes, Gallup and Hursh, 1961). From these scientific techniques, it has been possible to formulate relationships for use in predicting total fatness on the basis of the simpler techniques. Subsequently, tables of skinfold measurements for men and women according to age have been compiled (Seltzer and Mayer, 1965).

Soft-tissue X-ray

This technique allows the measurement of muscle and bone mineralization as well as fat pads that is sometimes difficult to measure using a caliper. The advantage of this technique is that fat is not compressed during measurement, giving rise to greater accuracy. Fairly extensive data on soft-tissue X-ray measurement of fat are available for children by sex and age and more limited data are available on adults (e.g. Young *et al.*, 1961; Heald *et al.*, 1963). The trochanteric pad is the best single predictor of total fat in men and the iliac fat pad in women (Foreyt, 1977) and it was not until the early 1960s that efforts were made to estimate total body fatness by cross-validating measures from using densitometry and hydrometry with those obtained from using soft-tissue X-rays (Young *et al.*, 1963).

Skinfold caliper method

Skinfold measurements appear to be the best single, simple and eminently practical determination of adiposity. Skinfold measurements reflect the amount of subcutaneous fat (Parizkova, 1961; Young *et al.*, 1963; Tanner and Whitehouse, 1962; Young, 1964). Skinfold thickness is measured by pressing a skinfold caliper on certain selected sites on the body; for example, the triceps skinfold is measured midway at the back of the upper right arm flexed at 90°. It is critical that the midway point between the tip of the acromion and the tip of the olecranon be located because of the gradation of subcutaneous fat thickness for the upper arm from elbow to shoulder. A steel tape is useful in locating and marking the midpoint. The arm of the subject should hang freely when the skinfold measurement is made.

The subscapular skinfold is measured just below the angle of the right scapula (shoulder and arm relaxed) with the fold picked up in a line slightly inclined in the natural cleavage of the skin. Precision of the location is less critical in this measurement because subcutaneous fat is fairly uniform in this region of the body.

Standardization of skinfold calipers is a necessary requirement for universal comparability of fatfold measurements and for conversion to total body fat. It is equally important for their application and use to be standardized. The calipers are normally applied to the skinfold about a centimetre below the fingers so that the pressure on the fold at the point measured is exerted by the faces of the calipers and not by the fingers. The handle of the caliper is released to permit the full force of the caliper arm pressure and the dial is read to the nearest half millimetre. When skinfolds are extremely thick, dial readings should be made three seconds after application of the caliper pressure to provide for utmost accuracy.

The triceps skinfold measurement is a single, easy and reasonably precise measure used to gauge an individual's obesity. The upper arm seems to be the most representative single site for estimating the overall deposition of fat in obese individuals, regardless of fat patterning. Seltzer and Mayer (1965) commented that there seems to be no appreciable advantage to using both the triceps and subscapular skin-folds and that the former does not require the patient to undress.

Distorting photograph technique

This technique was developed by Glucksman and Hirsch (1969) to assess total body size perception in a small group of obese patients as well as in a control group. A discussion of this technique together with a description of its application by Garner *et al.* (1976) is presented on p 55.

HOW TO TREAT

Traditional treatments of obesity have included group therapy and psychotherapy (Bruch, 1957), especially behaviour therapy (Epstein and Wing, 1987) and cognitive–behavioural therapy (Fitzgibbon and Kirschenbaum, 1990), therapeutic starvation (Swanson and Dinello, 1969), medication (Penick, 1970; Chen and Silverstone, 1990) and relaxation and imagery (Nagler and Androff, 1990). Several hundred published reports of outpatient treatment for obesity were reviewed by Stunkard and McLaren-Hume (1959). Taken together, the eight studies that met their criteria for acceptable research design indicated that only 25% of the grossly obese were able to lose 9 kg, while fewer than 5% lost 18 kg or more. The discouraging outcomes of traditional treatments have been summarized by Stunkard (1958): 'most obese persons will not remain in treatment. Of those that remain in treatment, most will not lose weight and of those who do lose weight, most will regain it'. Although this comment was made at the end of the 1950s, the situation has changed little.

Towards the middle of the 1970s, attention focused on behavioural approaches to weight reduction (e.g. Abramson, 1973). A variety of behavioural techniques has been applied to the problem of obesity: aversive conditioning, covert sensitization, coverant conditioning, therapist reinforcement of weight loss and self-control of eating.

Aversive conditioning

Moss (1924) provided one of the first examples of aversive conditioning used to modify eating behaviour. After several trials in which a clicking noise was paired with vinegar consumption, the subject rejected orange juice when it was presented with a clicking noise. Following on from this technique, electric shock has been used by several investigators in the treatment of obesity. Wolpe (1954) paired shocks with images of desirable foods, Meyer and Crisp (1964) with approach to temptation foods and Thorpe *et al.* (1964) with verbalizations of a stimulus word: 'overeating'. Three of the four subjects did not remain in treatment, while the fourth exhibited a considerable weight loss which was maintained for at least 20 months.

It is difficult to discern whether or not these studies are successful interventions as the numbers of subjects involved were very small. Studies using larger samples are more convincing, despite their negative findings on some occasions. For instance, Kennedy and Foreyt (1968) paired the smells of desirable foods with the noxious odour of butyric acid. Although subjects lost 13 kg, treatment had the effect of increasing consumption of non-target foods; the reported weight lost was attributed to other techniques (e.g. increased exercise). In an experimental study, Foreyt and Kennedy (1971) compared the effectiveness of this treatment with a control procedure. Experimental subjects averaged a 9 kg weight loss which was significantly greater than the 0.5 kg loss of the control subjects. Although a 48-week follow-up revealed that experimental subjects maintained an average loss of 4 kg, the authors felt that the relationship that developed with the therapist was 'vital in achieving the initial weight loss'.

Stollak (1967) compared the effectiveness of an aversive technique similar to Wolpe's (1954) with two control and three treatment groups. The aversive treatment did not result in significant weight loss after eight weeks of treatment. It would seem, therefore, that aversive techniques are perhaps best used in conjunction with other techniques to help patients lose weight more easily but that aversive techniques alone are relatively unconvincing in terms of success rates of patients' weight loss.

Covert sensitization

Cautela (1966; 1967) has presented the rationale and procedures used in the application of this technique to the treatment of obesity. Typically, the patient is taught to relax and the therapist vividly presents scenes in which the patient approaches forbidden foods, becomes nauseous and vomits. Interdispersed with these scenes are scenes in which the patient approaches the target food, feels nauseous, retreats and immediately feels a sense of relief. Cautela noted that there was no generalization of treatment response to acceptable eating behaviour, which could have otherwise invalidated this treatment approach. In 1972, Cautela outlined a further treatment programme for overeating which added covert reinforcement to the covert sensitization programme.

Other authors (e.g. Boskind-Lodahl, 1978; Strangler and Printz, 1980; White and Boskind-White, 1981) have found evidence of binge-eating and vomiting behaviour amongst overweight individuals. An excessive preoccupation with food in the family has also been linked with obesity (Mintz, 1983). Treatment such as covert sensitization has thus been useful since it addresses the tendency of some obese individuals to binge-eat and vomit. In the first experimental test of covert sensitization, Meynen (1970) compared the effects of eight weekly group sessions with a modified systematic desensitization treatment, a relaxation treatment and a control group. All treatments resulted in significant weight losses, but there were no significant differences between treatments. Negative findings were also reported by Lick and Bootzin (1971).

More encouraging results have been reported by Janda and Rimm (1972) and Manno and Marston (1972). Janda and Rimm compared covert sensitization to a no-treatment control and a placebo treatment. At a six-week follow-up, the covert sensitization group showed a mean loss of 4.6 kg which was significantly greater than the two other groups. Unlike the Lick and Bootzin (1971) study, a significant relationship ($r = 0.53$) between subjective distress and weight loss was found. This might suggest that the covert conditioning, rather than non-specific factors, was responsible for the weight reduction. Manno and Marston found that both covert sensitization and covert reinforcement treatments were significantly more effective than a minimal treatment group, although the two covert treatments produced similar weight losses.

Several researchers have attempted to assess the relative importance of the various factors of covert sensitization. Manno (1972) compared five treatments, including two that made use of covert imagery without aversive scenes. These treatments were significantly more effective than the typical covert sensitization treatments which made use of aversion. Sachs and Ingram (1972) found that backward conditioning (where patients visualized unpleasant scenes first and then the target food) was as effective as forward conditioning; both treatments resulted in significant decrements in consumption of target foods. The results were interpreted as suggesting that motivational factors rather than aversive conditioning are responsible for the effectiveness of covert sensitization.

If covert sensitization is to be viewed as a technique for reducing consumption of specific problematic foods or decreasing eating in specific situations, it would be reasonable to assess its efficacy by measuring consumption of target foods rather than weight loss. It appears unlikely, however, that covert sensitization used exclusively results in the modification of generalized patterns of inappropriate eating in obese individuals.

Coverant conditioning

Coverant conditioning is an extension of the Premack Principle (Premack, 1959) which is discussed in greater detail in Chapter 10 within the context of treating people with a learning disability. Homme (1965) has described the technique and its rationale for coverant control over weight gain. In this technique, low probability thoughts, i.e. thoughts which occur relatively infrequently to the individual (termed 'covert operants' or 'coverants') and which are incompatible with eating, are reinforced by high probability behaviour. However, the utility of such conditioning for the treatment of obesity remains to be demonstrated since studies reported by Tyler and Straughan (1970) and Horan and Johnson (1971) yielded discouraging results.

Therapist reinforcement of weight loss

Ayllon (1963) has described an environmental manipulation which resulted in a significant weight loss of an institutionalized psychotic patient. Treatment consisted of removing the patient from the dining room when she approached tables other than her own or when she picked up unauthorized food. Following the elimination of food stealing (after two weeks) the patient's weight gradually declined to 71 kg, a 17% weight loss from her original weight. Two later case studies demonstrated the treatment of obesity within the context of a token economy (Bernard, 1968; Upper and Newton, 1971). In both studies, patients were placed on a restricted diet and were reinforced for weight loss with tokens and social approval. Similar procedures were used by Moore and Crum (1969) with a schizophrenic patient in a traditional psychiatric institution and by Dinoff, Rickard and Colwick (1972) with a ten year old emotionally disturbed boy attending a summer camp. In all of these case reports, a significant weight loss was achieved.

Harmatz and Lapuc (1968) compared the effectiveness of behaviour modification, group therapy and diet-only treatments using 21 hospitalized schizophrenic male patients. A 4-week follow-up revealed that the behaviour modification group weighed less than the other two groups. However, therapist-controlled reinforcement can present practical problems when applied outside an institutionalized setting. In typical outpatient treatment, the therapist may be able to control reinforcing contingencies for only an hour per week. Tighe and Elliott (1968) described a technique involving threatened loss of money as a method of establishing therapist-controlled reinforcers in the natural environment. Although the authors applied the technique to modifying smoking behaviour, they suggested that it could be used equally well in overeating and other undesirable behaviour.

In 1972, Mann evaluated a programme in which personal possessions (e.g. money and clothes) were surrendered to the researcher to be used as reinforcers. A contract was signed which specified the patient's terminal weight reduction goal as well as the amount to be lost during each two-week period during the study. All eight patients maintained or increased their weight during the baseline period, lost weight during the first phase of treatment, regained weight during the reversal period and finally lost weight during the second treatment period. A second experiment was conducted which revealed that punishing contingencies (i.e. permanently losing personal possessions) were an essential component of treatment. Although treatment was successful, with five patients reaching their goal and the remaining patients achieving reductions in weight ranging from 40% to 70% of their goal, there were several problems encountered. Since the target was weight, rather than actual eating behaviour, a number of patients resorted to extreme measures such as taking laxatives or diuretics to promote rapid weight loss and achieve their goal. There are also several ethical considerations concerning the use of punishment contingencies. No follow-up data were reported and hence the long term effect of treatment was unknown. However, an indication of the long term effects of treatment has been provided by Jeffrey, Christensen and Pappas (1973). Despite the four patients of this study exhibiting a mean weight loss of 10.6 kg by the end of the treatment, at the 6-month follow-up, one patient had returned to his baseline weight, while a second regained 5.5 of the 12.6 kg he had lost.

While the application of therapist reinforcement is relatively straightforward in an institutionalized setting, outpatient treatment may present a number of problems. For instance, unless the therapist is willing to assume the costs of reinforcers, the requirement that patients surrender possessions prior to treatment may have the effect of excluding potential patients lacking the necessary affluence and/or motivation. Another important point is the long term effects of such treatment. Specific eating behaviour is not modified directly in this paradigm and only weight losses are reinforced. For treatment to result in permanent change, patients must devise their own methods for altering eating patterns. If these methods are aversive to the patient, the reinforcers occurring in the natural environment may not be sufficient to maintain the loss after treatment has concluded. The follow-up data reported by Jeffrey, Christensen and Pappas (1973) strongly suggest that for some patients natural reinforcers are inadequate to maintain the reduction in their weight.

Self-control of eating

The first behavioural self-control programme for overeating (i.e. eating beyond nutritional requirements leading to obesity) was described by Ferster, Nurnberger and Levitt (1962). It was theorized that the act of putting food into the mouth is reinforced by its immediate pleasurable consequences, while the negative consequences (such as becoming obese) are postponed to some indefinite time in the future. The goal of treatment was to make the negative consequences more immediate so that they would become more potent as determinants of eating behaviour.

In the Ferster, Nurnberger and Levitt (1962) study, early group sessions were devoted to training the participants to accurately record their food consumption and to reviewing the unpleasant consequences of their obesity. Suggestions were offered for environmental manipulations intended to promote the acquisition of self-control. Although the results of treatment were not reported, Ferster was later quoted by Penick *et al.* (1971) as characterizing the outcome as 'disappointing'.

Other researchers have also presented similar paradigms (e.g. Goldiamond, 1965; Stuart, 1967; Harris, 1969; Stuart and Davis, 1972) and in a controlled study, Wollersheim (1970) compared three group treatments with a no-treatment control. These were: behavioural self-control, positive expectation–social pressure and non-specific therapy. Patients in the behavioural group were taught deep muscle relaxation to be used in situations where tension would have typically resulted in eating and discussed their food consumption records in order to provide a functional analysis of their eating behaviour. This functional analysis included the development of stimulus control of eating, self-reinforcement of control of eating and establishing alternative behaviour incompatible with eating. The positive expectation–social pressure treatment was an attempt to replicate the procedures of weight reduction clubs, such as Weight Watchers, while the non-specific therapy was devoted to the discussion of 'underlying motives' and 'personality make-up' that are related to obesity. Although patients in all three treatment groups lost significantly more weight than controls, *post hoc* comparisons revealed that the behavioural treatment was more effective than the other treatments. In this study, 61% of the behavioural group lost 3.5 kg or more as contrasted with 6% of the controls, 25% of the social pressure group and 40% of the non-specific treatment group. At the 8-week follow-up, 50% of the behavioural patients still met this criterion.

Behaviour therapy and cognitive–behavioural therapy

The procedures involved in both behaviour therapy and cognitive–behavioural therapy for the treatment of anorexia nervosa and bulimia have been discussed elsewhere (Chapters 2 and 5). These are not too dissimilar for the treatment of obesity except for the important fact that the aim of treatment is weight loss and not weight gain. Several authors have discussed these techniques for treating obese patients (for instance, Epstein and Wing (1987) discuss a behaviour therapy technique and Fitzgibbon and Kirschenbaum (1990) discuss a cognitive–behavioural approach). In both of these approaches, it is useful to monitor the eating behaviour itself to establish a baseline 'pattern' of the patient's food intake. The two types of therapy then differ in their approaches to controlling the eating stimulus (e.g. avoiding eating alone or buying foods that should not be eaten in the prescribed diet) and controlling the act of eating (or feeding).

In behaviour therapy, these behaviours may be reward or punishment linked, whereas in cognitive–behavioural therapy, there may also be the facility for replacing certain attitudes towards eating and generally feeling 'obese'. Examples of the cognitive component of the latter therapy might include statements by the patient, such as:

'If I lose weight at this slow rate, I'll always be fat',

replaced by:

'I know it's a slow process, losing weight, but it *is* progressive and I might even stay thin this time'.

Encouraging 'positive' self-statements is useful in maintaining the patient's motivation and in cognitive (–behavioural) therapy, the patient is gradually taught how to replace their often negative interpretations (and attitudes) towards the situation with more objective (and sometimes more positive) interpretations (and attitudes) by using objective self-statements, thus building up a more positive outlook for themselves.

Drug therapy

New drugs are constantly undergoing evaluation for their potential properties as anti-obesity agents. However, there continues to be no evidence that anti-obesity drugs will restore a normal eating habit or have any lasting effect: their anti-obesity properties usually last only for the duration of the treatment. As a rule, once stopped, the patient regains weight. Therefore, they are most useful only as a short term measure, for example, in order to lose weight rapidly for a pending cholecystectomy (i.e. surgical removal of the gall bladder).

Some agents act primarily on the gastrointestinal tract exerting their effect by inhibition of the absorption of either carbohydrate or fat, by inhibition of pancreatic lipase (Munro, 1979). Certain drugs, the amphetamines and amphetamine analogues, e.g. mazindol, diethylpropion and phentermine hydrochloride (Allen, 1977; Campbell *et al.*, 1977; Cooper and Sweeney, 1980), have largely been discredited. Fenfluramine (Ponderax), however, was the most widely used anti-obesity drug in the 1980s and early 1990s and acts on the serotonergic system. It is still used in 'continuous therapy' where the dose is slowly increased to the maximum tolerated and then on withdrawal, slowly decreased in dosage. As with any drug, there are side effects and in this case these can include: lethargy, diarrhoea, depersonalization and withdrawal depression (Stunkard, Rickels and Hesbacher, 1973; Hudson, 1977; Innes *et al.*, 1977; Turner, 1979; Wales, 1979). It is also contra-indicated in epilepsy and may cause pulmonary hypertension. Dextrofenfluramine is an alternative which has fewer adverse effects.

Other drugs used in the treatment of obesity have included 5-hydroxytryptamine (used experimentally – Edwards and Stevens, 1991a,b) and fluoxetine (e.g. Wurtman and Wurtman, 1979; Gaudoin, 1991) which, unlike fenfluramine, is also an effective antidepressant drug. Metformin (glucophage) is less commonly prescribed in obesity and acts primarily as an anorexient drug (Cairns *et al.*, 1977; Clarke and Campbell, 1977). This has many side effects including: nausea, diarrhoea and subclinical B_{12} deficiency following long term treatment. It is contra-indicated in established cardiac or renal failure but is most useful in the treatment of the obese insulin-dependent diabetic.

As technology advances, new drugs will appear on the prescribers' market and will, no doubt, also appear on the prescriptions of specialist clinics. In which case, inevitably, the more vulnerable and desperate may fall victim, on occasions, to the less scrupulous!

TREATMENT AS AN INPATIENT

There are three general aspects to the treatment of obesity: the cause, the complications and the obesity itself. Sometimes obesity leads to depression and in turn, the ensuing depression results in bouts of excessive eating. In these cases, it may be more successful to treat the cause of the depression rather than the obesity. Similarly, treating any associated complications of obesity may be part of the overall management plan. In the obese bronchitic patient, for example, it may be much more important to give up smoking than to lose weight. However, conversely, weight loss is an important aspect of the general management of Type II diabetes or of hypertension. Finally, treating the obesity itself may be the chosen option.

In an inpatient setting, whether a hospital ward or clinic, a number of treatment options are available. Jaw wiring or dental splinting (Garrow and Gardiner, 1981), for example, prevents mastication and the diet given is usually monotonous and consisting of homogenized food. The patient must carry pliers in order to rapidly untie the splints in the event of vomiting, though this would be carefully monitored if the patient was confined to a hospital bed or ward. Weight loss is usually impressive and well maintained though weight gain is common once the splints are removed. This can be avoided either by combining dental splint with gastric plication or sometimes by applying a nylon rope round the abdomen which monitors the girth of the patient.

Other treatments include surgical bypass (Mason, 1981; Greenwood, 1983) which is usually used as a last resort when the patient is reluctant to live with and accept their obesity problem. This is dependent on the availability of surgical expertise and requires the patient's informed consent.

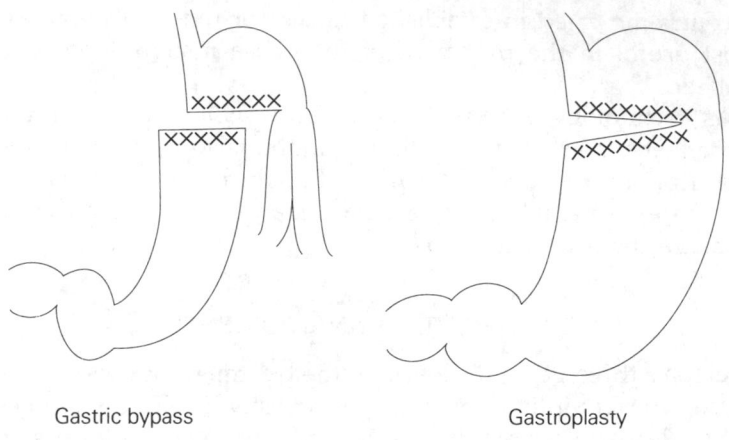

Gastric bypass   Gastroplasty

Figure 8.1 Comparison of gastric bypass with gastroplasty (redrawn from Munro, 1979, p188).

An average reduction of 50% of the excess weight may be expected as a result of a gastric bypass or **jejuno-iliac** bypass, the weight plateauing after 18 months (Hermreck, Jewell and Hardin, 1976; Sorrell and Burcher, 1976; Alden, 1977; Griffen, Young and Stevenson, 1977). The operative mortality for both procedures is usually about 3%, though the morbidity is considerably greater with jejuno-iliac bypass surgery as complications can include liver failure, diarrhoea, vitamin deficiencies, renal stones and gall stones. Lifelong follow-up at a hospital clinic is mandatory for patients with a jejuno-iliac bypass. There is a trend in surgery towards gastric bypass or plication (i.e. 'folding'), especially in the United Kingdom, mainly because of the dangerous complications of a jejuno-iliac bypass. From the late 1980s, there was a tendency to replace the surgical technique known as **'horizontal gastroplasty'** (Printen and Mason, 1973) by another technique termed **'vertical banding gastroplasty'** which may be associated with a reduction in stomal distension and hence weight loss. It is possible that bypass procedures continue to be most valuable in preventing weight regain following substantial non-surgical weight loss (see Figure 8.1 for a comparison of gastric bypass surgery with gastroplasty).

Exclusion and inclusion diets

Exclusion diets are often suitable for the first serious attempt at weight loss. The most frequently prescribed is that of a low carbohydrate, low fat, high fibre regimen. Its efficacy lies in its potential to stimulate satiety satisfactorily and to provide a palatable diet while giving the patient considerable choice of those unrestricted foods. Initial weight loss is dramatic, a feature attributable to a **ketogenic** effect which results in rapid loss of salt and water.

In the inclusion diet regimen, no foodstuff is prohibited but the total daily intake is restricted to a fixed number of calories. Initial weight loss may be more dramatic than with the low carbohydrate diet but is often less sustained. It may prove helpful when previous dietary attempts have failed but requires considerable attention to detail and is most suited to patients with an obsessional personality.

In the normal diet, carbohydrate, fat and protein contribute 5%, 33% and 12% respectively to the total calorie requirements. A calorie intake of between 800 and 1800 calories per day in the majority of people may produce an energy deficit of 1000 kcal per day. Therefore, it is important to set realistic and appropriate energy deficits for the patient with respect to their estimated daily calorie requirements.

TREATMENT AS AN OUTPATIENT

Probably the most important point is to select a target weight that is realistic for the patient. This avoids disappointment in not reaching the target and also helps to maintain the patient's motivation which is of great importance in the outpatient setting where attendance is often voluntary. Material rewards or penalties attached to weight loss can be useful in motivating the patient's maintenance of the treatment programme, but attempts to frighten the patient into losing weight (by, for example, outlining the negative health consequences or the possibility of death) are usually counterproductive to establishing a good rapport between clinician and patient. A realistic rate of weight loss also influences, to a large extent, the success of the treatment. One kilogram of adipose tissue is equivalent to about 7000 kcal. Few patients can maintain a negative energy gap of more than 1000 kcal per day which is about 7000 kcal per week. A realistic weight loss should be targeted at around less than 0.8 kg per week; this would mean a diet comprising 60–100 g of protein with a daily intake of 400 calories. The resultant weight loss would be about 41 kg per year. But it is the permanency of the weight loss that is important. After all, transient loss is of limited value and permanent weight loss demands a permanent change in the patient's eating habits; this is often too great a change for the patient to make or the patient is looking for a quick method of losing weight!

Exercise, although a small part of obesity management, remains an important focus of attention. Indeed, there has been a steady increase in the numbers of people attending aerobic, 'Callanetic' and weight-reducing classes (which might all be loosely termed 'group therapy' for those overweight or obese people that attend). With dietary restriction, three 30-minute training periods each week will reduce the total fat by 40% in one year in the non-obese person but this is much less effective in the obese person and may be a better preventative rather than therapeutic measure. Exercise increases insulin activity, improves glucose tolerance and lowers plasma tri-glycerides. It has also been shown to help lower blood pressure in early hypertension. Simple application for obese patients should be encouraged, such as using stairs in preference to lifts or escalators; walking or cycling to work; avoiding the temptation of 'forbidden' foods by replacing them with gentle exercise, such as a long walk.

Normal daily energy requirements, however, vary with age, sex, occupation, body build and body height. The aim of dietary advice is to provide a regimen deficient in calorie value without lack of essential nutrients. A dietary fibre-rich regimen may be of value by reducing the absorption efficiency of the small intestine, stimulating satiety and possibly reducing the incidence of associated risk factors such as diverticular disease and ischaemic heart disease (see Thompson and Morgan (1990) for a detailed discussion of the latter). Thus a dietary fibre regimen is recommended though there is little to justify the suggestion that it is of therapeutic value in promoting weight loss.

Some therapists and clinicians recommend simple omission diets where minimum knowledge is required of calorific values. These are particularly useful when the dietary origin of obesity is readily identifiable. (Indeed, many people who recognize their weight problem never present to their general practitioner because of the self-use of this technique.) Generally, an omission diet might require avoidance of one or two of the following: crisps, biscuits, sugar, lemonade, alcohol. Any diet, however, requires an adequate fluid electrolyte and vitamin intake and cheap liquid diets, such as 2 pints of skimmed milk per day, may only be effective in short term weight loss. For the majority of people, modifying eating habits still seems to be the only effective long term method of losing weight permanently.

COMMERCIALLY AVAILABLE DIETS

Diets and their definitions

Authors cited in parentheses after the name of the diet are not necessarily the founders nor may they be proponents of the diet; rather, they are intended as citations in which the reader may find further specific information.

1. **Anticellulite Diet** (Ronsard, 1975). Cellulite is described as unevenly distributed lumps of ordinary fat which conventional dieting will not dissolve. Ageing and excessive weight gain are associated with loss of elasticity of the skin which may become dimpled. The diet comprises: raw vegetables, freshly squeezed vegetable juices, 6–8 glasses of water per day.

2. **Beverly Hills Diet** (Mazel, 1981). This diet is nutritionally unsound. It is low in protein and a number of vitamins and minerals, e.g. vitamin B, iron, zinc, calcium and magnesium. For the first ten days, the dieter eats nothing but fruit, all in specific order, i.e. pineapple (day 1); papaya (day 2); papaya and pineapple (day 3). It is also referred to as the 'diarrhoea diet' because it is high in fibre which acts as a laxative and causes flatus.

3. **The Cambridge Diet** (Howard *et al.*, 1978). This is a formula diet sold to the public by 'Cambridge Counsellors' who have used the diet for two weeks but are otherwise untrained. It includes high quality protein, limited fat, vitamins and minerals. For rapid weight loss, the dieter is instructed to drink

three servings of the diet formula daily for a total of 330 calories (33 g of protein; 40 g of carbohydrate; 3 g of fat). Unfortunately, as it is a variant of a modified fast, it is too drastic to be used without medical supervision since the risks can be significant and are similar to those of any very low calorie diet (Blonz and Stern, 1981).

4. **Drinking Man's Diet** (Gardner and Williams, 1974). This diet limits the carbohydrate intake to 60 g per day and includes diet meals such as 'filet mignon with Bearnaise, wine, followed by brandy'. It is nutritionally unsound since dietary choices become limited as alcohol is substituted for food. As with all low carbohydrate, high protein diets, problems can ensue, e.g. fatigue, postural hypotension, hyperlipidaemia, electrolyte imbalance and even cardiac arrhythmias.

5. **Enzyme Catalyst Diet** (Wade, 1976). Weight loss on this diet is due to caloric restriction only. The author proposes dubious suggestions such as eating 'gentle raw enzyme foods' like bananas, raw wheat germ, celery or raw nuts before consuming any high calorie foods (such as desserts or any food with sugar).

6. **I Love New York Diet** (Myerson and Adler, 1982). A variation of the high protein diet, in the form of a rigid menu plan, is proposed which does not specify portion size. Daily totals for the first week are approximately 700 calories per day rising to 1500 calories per day in the second week.

7. **Kempner's Rice Diet** (Kempner, 1949; Kempner *et al.*, 1975). The diet consists mainly of rice and fruit. Blood pressure is reduced, producing postural hypotension in some individuals. Protein intake is inadequate and vitamin and mineral supplements are required because the regimen is low in vitamin A, riboflavin, calcium and iron.

8. **Macrobiotics** (Sakurazawa, 1965). This is a system of diets relying primarily on wholegrain cereal, fish and selected vegetables. Regimen 7 consists of 100% brown rice. However, strict adherence to brown rice will result in nutritional deficiencies (e.g. vitamins A, C and D, calcium and protein) which could lead to scurvy.

9. **Pritikin Program** (Pritikin and McGrady, 1979). Primarily wholegrains, vegetables and fruits, the diet is high in carbohy-

drate (up to 80% of calories) and low in fat (no more than 10% calories). This can result in rough, dry skin. Caffeine, salt, cholesterol, saturated fats and artificial sweeteners are all outlawed. High quality protein intake can be low, as only about 2.5 kg of lean fish or meat is allowed per week. Likewise, the diet is low on calcium since dairy products are also limited. As the diet is particularly high in fibre, a decreased absorption of nutrients may result together with gastric distress and flatulence.

10. **Protein-Sparing Modified Fasts – PSMF** (Linn and Stuart, 1977). This is a modification of the total starvation diet except that the individual consumes 15 g of liquid predigested protein three times per day (approximately 180 kcal) to minimize loss of lean body mass. According to Blonz and Stern (1981), commercial preparations of predigested liquid protein are poor quality proteins which contain a low percentage of essential amino acids relative to non-essential amino acids. Despite an improvement in nitrogen balance, it is not known whether this dietary protein will 'spare' protein in tissues from being used for fuel during fasting; and a number of deaths due to heart failure have been reported (Stern, 1983), having also been attributed to these liquid protein diets. A vitamin and mineral supplement is recommended with this diet together with close medical supervision.

11. **The Scarsdale Diet** (Tarnower and Baker, 1978). One of five variations of menu plans may be chosen which are low in carbohydrate and high in protein. Rapid weight loss in the first week is due partly to the restriction of carbohydrate resulting in water loss. Quantities of food are not specified which may mean that heavy eaters could be eating excess calories. Dairy products are permitted only twice a week which indicates an inadequate supply of calcium, vitamins A and D and probably vitamin B_2.

12. **The Southampton Diet** (Berger and Cohen, 1982). Based on the concept of 'happy' foods (that 'truly satisfy your hunger', such as milk, beef and wholegrains) and 'sad' foods (such as egg yolks, chocolate and lentils) which 'make you feel depressed and more hungry', the diet provides a two-week meal plan that should be followed rigidly. Berger claims that 'happy' foods contain the amino acid tryptophan which is con-

verted in the brain to the neurotransmitter serotonin. Basically, the diet is nutritionally sound despite the dubious 'scientific' explanations.

13. **Starvation Diet** (Silverstone, Stark and Buckle, 1966). Some starvation diets permit fruit juices but usually the regimen is simply not to eat or drink anything except water. Up to 2.5 kg per day can be lost in this way though long term results are discouraging and weight regain is common. Close medical supervision is advisable since total fasting results in a negative nitrogen balance and a loss of lean body mass. More dangerous are a host of other possible complications, including: loss of minerals, ketosis, dehydration, elevated uric acid levels, nausea, dizziness, fatigue and adverse effects on renal and hepatic function. Sudden death has also been reported.

14. **Vegetarian Diets**. If the diet excludes cheese and eggs, it should include vegetables with high quality protein, such as soybeans and foods with complementary protein (e.g. beans and rice). These diets are usually nutritionally sound but are usually high in fibre (which might lead to some gastric distress) and are generally low in cholesterol. They have the advantage of usually costing less than diets that include meats and some feel that they help to support campaigns against inhumane animal farming.

15. **Weight Watchers Diet Plan** (Nidetch and Heilman, 1972). This is a nutritionally sound approach that includes three basic programmes: reducing, levelling and maintenance. Meals can include unlimited amounts of certain vegetables, such as lettuce, but only moderate amounts of others, such as green beans. Techniques to modify eating behaviour and increase exercise are also incorporated into the programme, making the plan a combination of group ('behaviour') therapy and dieting.

OUTCOME OF OBESITY

The outcome of longstanding obesity in an individual is dependent on many factors: the age of the individual; lifestyle; any associated medical complications; how long the individual has been obese, etc. (VanItallie, 1979). The outcome of treatment, therefore, also depends on these factors in addition to those directly related to the particular treatment undertaken (e.g. Kingsley and Wilson, 1977). Certain treatment approaches seem to improve outcome when used in conjunction with others. For example, Levitz and Stunkard (1974) found that behaviour therapy increased the effectiveness of a self-help programme called 'Take Off Pounds Sensibly' (TOPS): fewer TOPS members dropped out of the two behavioural interventions than out of a nutrition and a control group. The behavioural programmes also produced significantly greater losses than the control treatments.

Behaviour therapy does appear to be the only intervention that has been extensively evaluated and it seems to be more effective than rival therapies. Self-help groups also have a good track record of successes possibly because of the commitment of their members. However, such groups as Weight Watchers also incorporate a behavioural approach as a key element of their programme (Nidetch and Heilman, 1972).

In addition to the direct physiological benefits derived from some approaches, such as dieting and exercise, there is the feeling of well-being. Motivation can play an important part in influencing the success or failure of a chosen treatment approach. Psychological and physiological explanations come together when considering the biological mechanisms involved during exercise. In one study, 20 minutes of treadmill running was associated with elevations in plasma concentrations of beta-endorphins (Gambert, Garthwaite and Pontzer, 1981). This may be a partial explanation for the euphoria anecdotally associated with exercise. In individuals who were distressed, anxious or physically unfit, exercise training was associated with improvements of mood (Folkins and Sime, 1981). Collingwood and Willett (1971) found that exercise improved the self-concept of obese adolescent boys; and when combined with a weight reduction programme, exercise has also been associated with a shift towards a more internal locus of control or feelings of self-control over one's life. This may have implications for weight maintenance since Cohen *et al.* (1980) reported that children who maintained lost weight reported more self-regulation than children who regained weight. In terms of weight maintenance, there is strong evidence to suggest that individuals who are successful in maintaining a reduced body weight are those who incorporate physical activity into a daily routine (Grinker, Most and Hirsch, 1980).

Successful weight loss from surgical interventions is less clear. What is known is that weight reduction amounts to approximately one-third of maximum body weight or 50% to 60% of excess weight or overweight. The patient thus remains obese. Greenwood (1983) comments that patient satisfaction is universally high, even in the face of prevalent complications in the order of 30% irrespective of operation. But the malignant abuse of some of these operations, as suggested in Joffe (1981), may well result in discreditation of the surgical approach to morbid obesity. With all these factors taken into account, the best maintenance of reduced weight (as compared with the best immediate success of weight loss) still remains with behavioural approaches when the patient learns to modify his or her eating habits and then, in addition, adheres to this altered style of eating.

FURTHER READING

Assessment

Davis, C. (1990) Body image and weight preoccupation: A comparison between exercising and non-exercising women. *Appetite*, **15**(1), 13–21.

Heald, F.P., Hunt, E.D. Jr., Schwartz, R., Cook, C.D., Elliot, O. and Vajda, B. (1963) Measures of body fat and hydration in adolescent boys. *Pediatrics*, **31**, 226–39.

Young, C.M. (1963) Body composition studies of 'older' women, thirty to seventy years of age. *Annals of the New York Academy of Science*, **110**, 589–607.

Types of treatment

Abramson, E.E. (1973) A review of behavioural approaches to weight control. *Behaviour Research and Therapy*, **11**, 547–56.

Kirschenbaum, D.S., Johnston, W.G. and Stalonas, P.M. Jr. (1987) *Treating Childhood and Adolescent Obesity*. Pergamon Press, Oxford.

Wolf, M.C., Cohen, K.R. and Rosenfeld, J.G. (1985) School-based interventions for obesity: Current approaches and future prospects. *Psychology in the Schools*, **22**(2), 187–200.

Aversive conditioning

Foreyt, J.P. and Kennedy, W.A. (1971) Treatment of over-weight by aversion therapy. *Behavior Research and Therapy*, **9**, 29–34.

Meyer, V. and Crisp, A.H. (1964) Aversion therapy in two cases of obesity. *Behavior Research and Therapy*, **2**, 143–7.

Morganstern, K.P. (1974) Cigarette smoke as a noxious stimulus in self-managed aversion therapy for compulsive eating: Technique and case illustration. *Behavior Therapy*, **5**, 255–60.

Wijesinghe, B. (1973) Massed electrical aversion treatment of compulsive eating. *Journal of Behavior Therapy and Experimental Psychiatry*, **4**, 133–5.

Covert sensitization

Cautela, J.R. (1972) The treatment of over-eating by covert conditioning. *Psychotherapy: Theory, Research and Practice*, **9**, 211–16.

Diament, C. and Wilson, G.T. (1975) An experimental investigation of the effects of covert sensitisation in an analogue eating situation. *Behavior Therapy*, **6**, 499–509.

Foreyt, J.P. and Hagen, R.L. (1973) Covert sensitisation: Conditioning or suggestion? *Journal of Abnormal Psychology*, **82**, 17–23.

Janda, L.H. and Rimm, D.C. (1972) Covert sensitisation in the treatment of obesity. *Journal of Abnormal Psychology*, **80**, 37–42.

Maletzky, B.M. (1973) 'Assisted' covert sensitisation: A preliminary report. *Behavior Therapy*, **4**, 117–19.

Manno, B. and Marston, A.R. (1972) Weight reduction as a function of negative covert reinforcement (sensitisation) versus positive covert reinforcement. *Behavior Research and Therapy*, **10**, 201–7.

Murray, D.C. and Harrington, L.G. (1972) Covert aversive sensitisation in the treatment of obesity. *Psychological Reports*, **30**, 560.

Sachs, L.B. (1972) Covert sensitisation as a treatment for weight control. *Psychological Reports*, **30**, 971–4.

Coverant conditioning

Horan, J.J. (1971) Coverant conditioning through a self-management application of the Premack Principle: Its effect on weight reduction. *Journal of Behavior Therapy and Experimental Psychiatry*, **2**, 243–9.

Horan, J.J., Baker, S.B., Hoffman, A.M. and Shute, R.E. (1975) Weight loss through variations in the coverant control paradigm. *Journal of Consulting and Clinical Psychology*, **43**, 68–72.

Therapist reinforcement of weight loss

Dinoff, M., Rickard, H.C. and Colwick, J. (1972) Weight reduction through successive contracts. *American Journal of Orthopsychiatry*, **42**, 110–13.

Jeffrey, D.B., Christensen, E.R. and Pappas, J.P. (1973) Developing a behavioral program and therapist manual for the treatment of obesity. *Journal of the American College of Health Association*, **21**, 455–9.

Mann, R.A. (1972) The behavior-therapeutic use of contingency contracting to control an adult behavior problem: Weight control. *Journal of Applied Behavior Analysis*, **5**, 99–109.

Self-control of eating

Hagen, R.L. (1974) Group therapy versus bibliotherapy in weight reduction. *Behavior Therapy*, **5**, 222–34.

Harris, M.B. and Hallbauer, E.S. (1973) Self-directed weight control through eating and exercise. *Behavior Research and Therapy*, **11**, 523–9.

Jeffrey, D.B. (1974) A comparison of the effects of external control and self-control on the modification and maintenance of weight. *Journal of Abnormal Psychology*, **83**, 404–10.

Levitz, L.S. and Stunkard, A.J. (1974) A therapeutic coalition for obesity: Behavior modification and patient self-help. *American Journal of Psychiatry*, **131**, 423–7.

Mahoney, M.J. (1974) Self-reward and self-monitoring techniques for weight control. *Behavior Therapy*, **5**, 48–57.

Ogden, J. (1992) *Fat Chance! The Myth of Dieting Explained*. Routledge, London.

Penick, S.B., Filion, R., Fox, S. and Stunkard, A.J. (1971) Behavior modification in the treatment of obesity. *Psychosomatic Medicine*, **33**, 49–55.

Behaviour therapy

Epstein, L.H. and Wing, R.R. (1987) Behavioral treatment of childhood obesity. *Psychological Bulletin*, **101**(3), 331–42.

Hall, S.M. (1973) Behavioral treatment of obesity: A two-year follow-up. *Behavior Research and Therapy*, **11**, 647–8.

Romanczyk, R.G., Tracey, D.A., Wilson, T. and Thorpe, G.L. (1973) Behavioral techniques in the treatment of obesity: A comparative analysis. *Behavior Research and Therapy*, **11**, 629–40.

Cognitive–behavioural therapy

Fitzgibbon, M.L. and Kirschenbaum, D.S. (1990) Heterogeneity of clinical presentation among obese individuals seeking treatment. *Addictive Behavior*, **15**(3), 291–5.

Relaxation and imagery

Nagler, W. and Androff, A. (1990) Investigating the impact of deconditioning anxiety on weight loss. *Psychological Reports*, **66**(2), 595–600.

Drug therapy

Chen, Y. and Silverstone, T. (1990) Lithium and weight gain. *International Clinical Psychopharmacology*, **5**(3), 217–25.

Greenwood, M.R.C. (1983) *Obesity*. Churchill Livingstone, New York.

Guy-Grand, B. (1992) Clinical studies with d-fenfluramine. *American Journal of Clinical Nutrition (Supplement)*, **55**(1), 173S–6S.

Matthews, P.A. (1975) Diethylpropion in the treatment of obese patients seen in general practice. *Current Therapy and Research*, **17**, 340.

Moe, J.F. (1977) Phentermine hydrochloride therapy for

exogenous obesity: An evaluation of interrupted therapy. *Current Therapy and Research*, **22**, 666.

Munro, J.F. (1979) Clinical use of anti-obesity agents, in *The Treatment of Obesity*, (ed J.F. Munro), MTP Press, Lancaster, pp. 85–121.

Wise, S.D. (1992) Clinical studies with fluoxetine in obesity. *American Journal of Clinical Nutrition (Supplement)*, **55**(1), 181S–4S.

Inpatient and outpatient treatment of obesity

Brownell, K.D., Kelman, J.H. and Stunkard, A.J. (1983) Treatment of obese children with and without their mothers: Changes in weight and blood pressure. *Paediatrics*, **71**, 515–25.

Foreyt, J.P. (1977) *Behavioural Treatments of Obesity*. Pergamon Press, Oxford.

Gomez, C. (1981) Gastroplasty in intractable obesity. *International Journal of Obesity*, **5**, 413.

Joffe, S.N. (1981) Surgical management of morbid obesity. *Gut*, **22**, 248.

Mason, E.E. (1981) Surgical treatment of obesity. *Major Problems in Clinical Surgery*, **26**, 1–493.

Outcome of obesity

Beneke, W.M., Paulson, B. and McReynolds, W.T. (1978) Long-term results of two behavior modification weight loss programs using nutritionists as therapists. *Behavior Therapy*, **9**, 501–7.

DeWind, L.T. and Payne, J.H. (1976) Intestinal bypass surgery for morbid obesity: Long-term results. *Journal of the American Medical Association*, **236**, 2298–301.

Epstein, L.H., Thompson, J.K. and Wing, R.R. (1980) The effects of contract and lottery procedures on attendance and fitness in aerobics exercise. *Behaviour Modification*, **4**, 465–80.

Fremouw, W.J. and Zitter, R.E. (1980) Individual and couple behavioral contracting for weight reduction and maintenance. *Behavior Therapy*, **3**, 15–16.

Lee, J., Cornelissen, E. and McCargar, L. (1991) Criteria for evaluating the success of weight loss programs. *Canadian Home Economics Journal*, **41**(4), 168–70.

Sanders, T.A.B. and Manning, J. (1992) The growth and development of vegan children. *Journal of Human Nutrition and Dietetics*, 5(1), 11–21.

Sjöström, L. (1981) Can the relapsing patient be identified? in *Recent Advances in Obesity Research: III*, (eds P. Björntorp, M. Cairella and A.N. Howard), John Libbey, London, p. 85.

Wilson, G.T. and Brownell, K.D. (1980) Behavior therapy for obesity: An evaluation of treatment outcome. *Advances in Behavior Research and Therapy*, 3, 49–86.

For further information about obesity contact:

The British Dietetic Association, 7th Floor, Elizabeth House, 22 Suffolk Street, Queensway, Birmingham B1 1LS.

For further information about the Prader–Willi syndrome contact:

The Prader–Willi Association (UK), 37 Jasmine Close, Goldsmith Park, Woking, Surrey GU21 3RQ.

For further information about diabetes contact:

The British Diabetic Association, 10 Queen Anne Street, London W1M 0BD.

9

Research into obesity

A considerable amount of research has focused on obesity as a medical condition with much debate arising over how best to treat the condition either pharmacologically or by surgical intervention. Traditional dietary interventions have brought little success and are often interrupted by bouts of weight regain and remissions. Sometimes the focus on dietary restraint has even led to complications and further eating disorders. Following physiological approaches, various psychological approaches to the treatment of obesity have been attempted. These have included: behaviour therapy, cognitive–behavioural therapy, relaxation, group therapy and self-help methods. The lack of success in some treatment approaches has led researchers to consider new approaches, e.g. Galbraith and Wilson (1992) have tried changing the eating habits and lifestyles of adolescent obese individuals. Others have concentrated on metabolic issues, such as insulin and glucose levels, body fat distribution and obesity in diabetics (e.g. Heffner et al., 1990), or on the incidence of obesity amongst sufferers of identifiable syndromes, for example, polycystic ovary syndrome (Nestler et al., 1991). Four areas of research will now be reviewed and discussed. Specific methodologies are not presented here since these areas are particularly well documented. Instead, the reader is referred to the Further Reading section at the end of this chapter where original sources are cited. Several studies in each of the four topics are discussed, thus providing an overview of the following areas: cognitive aspects of taste perception in obesity (e.g. Drewnowski, 1981); anorectic agents and the modulation of intestinal absorption through drug therapy (e.g. Sullivan, Baruth and Cheng, 1980; Danforth and

Landsberg, 1983); adipose tissue in obesity (e.g. Björntorp, 1981; Björntorp, Cairella and Howard, 1981); mortality, morbidity and obesity (e.g. Hulley *et al.*, 1980; Keys, 1980a,b; Brunzell and Miller, 1981).

COGNITIVE ASPECTS OF TASTE PERCEPTION IN OBESITY

Cognitive and physiological factors appear to be involved in the estimation of taste preference (Drewnowski, 1981). While it is true that some taste preferences or aversions are innate (Drewnowski, 1983), most appear to be learned and even initially aversive stimuli may eventually become palatable (Rozin and Kalat, 1971). Moreover, a person's estimates of palatability or pleasantness vary both with short term metabolic status and with long term levels of fat storage (Cabanac, 1971).

Bray (1978) reported several studies that have been directed at the postulated hyper-responsiveness of obese individuals towards highly palatable stimuli. Some studies have shown that the obese consume more good-tasting foods than poor-tasting foods (Nisbett, 1972) and particularly crave sweets and desserts (Wurtman, Wurtman and Growdon, 1981). However, these studies have often used food intake as a measure of taste responsiveness and so did not address the issue of how taste responsiveness can affect food intake. Therefore, it is important to separate taste responses from actual food consumption and to distinguish between taste sensitivity and taste preference.

In a signal detection procedure, Grinker (1973) showed that obese individuals did not differ from normal weight subjects in their ability to discriminate a weak sucrose solution from distilled water. In a related experiment (Grinker, 1978), the obese and normal subjects did not differ in their ability to judge increasing intensity of sucrose solutions using magnitude estimation procedures, or in their judgements of red coloured sucrose solutions as sweeter than clear ones.

Generally, studies on taste preferences in obesity have focused on sweet taste, with inconclusive results: it would seem that obese individuals show no abnormalities in their psychophysiological taste functions. Some researchers (e.g. Rodin, Moskowitz and Bray, 1976), though, have found that obese subjects like sweet solutions of increasing concentration more than normal weight subjects do and some have found that they like them less (e.g. Novin, Wyrwicka and Bray, 1976; Grinker, 1978).

Pleasantness ratings for sweet solutions have been related to short term energy supply, level of fat storage and satiety; and such ratings for sucrose solutions by normal weight subjects have been found to decline following a glucose preload (Cabanac and Duclaux, 1970; Cabanac, 1971). This phenomenon was also evidenced in the obese by Grinker (1978) but was found to be absent in the obese by Cabanac and Duclaux (1970). There is additional evidence that a drop in pleasantness ratings following a sweet preload may be due to the 'cloying' effect (i.e. satiation) of sweetness rather than to calories. Wooley, Wooley and Dunham (1972) obtained a drop in ratings for sweet solutions following both glucose and cyclamate preloads. Drewnowski (1983) suggests that ratings would appear to be influenced not only by the metabolic status of the product but also by metabolic expectancies developed on the basis of prior learning. Malcolm, O'Neil and Hirsch (1980) and Witherly, Pangborn and Stern (1980) propose that studies of taste preference should extend beyond the four basic tastes towards more foodlike combinations of textures and flavours.

ANORECTIC AGENTS AND THE MODULATION OF INTESTINAL ABSORPTION THROUGH DRUG THERAPY

Anorectic agents

The clinical use of anorectic agents as an adjunct to dietary restriction of caloric intake has met with only limited success in the pharmacological treatment of obesity. The main disadvantages of many of the anorectic agents are a tendency towards the development of tolerance, their poorly documented ability to maintain sustained weight loss, their central nervous system side effects and, in certain cases, their potential for drug abuse (Danforth and Landsberg, 1983).

Several reviews have discussed the various aspects of appetite suppressants (e.g. Garattini and Samanin, 1978; Sullivan and Comai, 1978; Peters *et al.*, 1979; Sullivan, Baruth and Cheng, 1980). Anorectic drugs either have a central site of action or a peripheral site of action. Among those with a central site of action are two subgroups: amphetamine with its derivatives (e.g. phentermine) and fenfluramine. Much research has contributed to the current knowledge that these drugs exert their anorectic effect through interaction with or modulation of specific brain monoamine neurotransmitters, e.g. norepinephrine, dopamine and serotonin. Some studies have also shown that gamma-aminobutyric acid (GABA) may also be involved in the regulation of ingestive behaviour (e.g. Roberts, Chase and Towers, 1976; Kelly *et al.*, 1977).

The site of action of amphetamine appears to be the lateral hypothalamus and the drug exerts its anorectic effect through the mediation of brain catecholamines (Hathcock and Coon, 1978). Production of lesions in the brain stem noradrenergic area (Carey, 1976) or the ventral noradrenergic bundle (Borsini, Bendotti and Corli, 1979) resulted in selected depletion of norepinephrine in the brain and attenuated the anorectic effect of amphetamine and diethylpropion. A dopaminergic mechanism of amphetamine anorexia has also been demonstrated by several studies (e.g. Abdallah *et al.*, 1976). Dobrzanski and Doggett (1979) showed that pimozide, a drug which blocks dopamine receptors, antagonized the anorectic effect of dextroamphetamine in mice, suggesting that dextroamphetamine exerted its anorectic effects by acting as a dopamine receptor agonist. Apart from the serious ethical issues surrounding animal experimentation and debatable suggestions of the transferability of findings to humans, pimozide does not seem to have withstood similar trials in human beings and there was no significant effect on dextroamphetamine-induced anorexia (Silverstone *et al.*, 1980).

Weight loss, however, has been observed in aged patients following long term treatment with levodopa (Vardi, Oberman and Rabey, 1976), a drug commonly used for the treatment of Parkinsonism. Both levodopa and amphetamine produced anorexia in rats (Sanghvi *et al.*, 1975). The putative mechanism of action of the hypophagic effect of the two drugs appeared to be similar. Levodopa exerted its appetite suppressant effect, at least in part, through increased catecholamine synthesis specifically within dopaminergic and adrenergic neurones of the perifornical hypothalamic region (Leibowitz and Rossakis, 1979). Hemmes, Pack and Hirsch (1979; 1980) demonstrated that levodopa caused sustained body weight decline in rats in spite of a near normal food consumption. It was suggested that the anti-obesity effect of levodopa required an intact sympathetic nervous system.

Fenfluramine seems to differ from many of the other anorectic agents in that its action is believed to be mediated by a central serotonergic satiety system and it is devoid of a central stimulant effect (Duhault, Beregi and du Boistesselin, 1979). The anorectic activity of fenfluramine appears to depend upon an intact brain serotonergic system since the administration of serotonin antagonists (e.g. methergoline, cyproheptadine, cinanserin) or production of lesions in the **raphe nucleus** (an area rich in serotonin neurones) selectively depleted brain serotonin levels and inhibited the fenfluramine anorexia. The release of endogenous serotonin from central neurones and the inhibition of neuronal serotonin uptake appeared to be obligatory for the anorectic effect of fenfluramine. However, several authors have reported that chronic treatment with fenfluramine caused a significant reduction of serotonin binding sites in the cortex of rats (e.g. Samanin *et al.*, 1980) and that other compounds with a serotonin-mimetic action, such as quipazine, also reduced food consumption in rats (Clineschmidt, 1979; Samanin, Caccia and Bendotti, 1980). Pre-treatment with methergoline was found to prevent the anorectic effects of these agents. These compounds all showed a specific interaction with brain serotonin and perhaps an understanding of the differential potency of this interaction can be of importance for the development of novel anorectic agents with enhanced efficacy and safety (Danforth and Landsberg, 1983).

Modulating intestinal absorption

The small intestine is the major site of absorption of dietary nutrients. Limiting the availability of these nutrients to the body by a selective modification of the absorption of dietary lipid or carbohydrate through pharmacological intervention could create a chemical 'bypass' (Danforth and Landsberg, 1983). This type of therapy has potentially many advantages over conventional surgical bypass procedures. The degree of alteration of the absorption can be regulated by dosage and treatment can be reversed as secondary by withdrawal of the therapy. Non-absorbable orally active drugs which suppress lipid or carbohydrate absorption are particularly attractive and the side effects produced could be steatorrhoea (i.e. presence of fat in faeces) caused by lipid absorption inhibitors or carbohydrate absorption.

Several compounds have been reported to selectively reduce the absorption of dietary fat. Pluronic L-101 has been identified as a potent *in vivo* inhibitor of human pancreatic lipase (Comai and Sullivan, 1980), the enzyme which acts in the small intestine to hydrolyse and thus promote absorption of long-chain dietary triglycerides. High doses of fenfluramine also reduced intestinal lipid absorption (Comai, Triscari and Sullivan, 1978; Garattini, Caccia and Mennini, 1979; Curtis-Prior, Oblin and Tan, 1980). This decrease in fat absorption was dose-dependent and probably could also be explained through an inhibition of pancreatic lipase (Comai, Triscari and Sullivan, 1978; Borgström and Wollesen, 1981). However, the contribution of this mechanism to the fenfluramine-induced weight reduction in obese patients is probably minimal, since the major anti-obesity action of the compound at the therapeutic doses employed in obesity management is due to anorexia.

Cholestyramine, a bile salt sequestering (i.e. 'clustering') agent, produces steatorrhoea in humans at high doses, i.e. 30–36 g per day (Smith, 1976). Neomycin, an antibiotic, has also been shown to cause a marked decrease in fat absorption in obese subjects (e.g. Faloon, Paes and Woolfolk, 1966). The apparent mechanism of this effect was a precipitation of micellar lipid in the small intestine (Thompson *et al.*, 1971). However, at the dosage necessary for production of steatorrhoea, neomycin caused alterations in the intestinal mucosa, thus preventing its use on a chronic basis (Dobbins *et al.*, 1968).

Retardation or inhibition of the availability of dietary carbohydrates has also been investigated and considered as a possible facilitator of diminished lipogenesis (thus limiting the accumulation of fat in adipose tissue). Inhibitors of alpha-amylase, alpha-glucosidase (maltase) and sucrase have been identified. The use of these inhibitors in attenuating carbohydrate digestion with a subsequent decrease in the rate of glucose absorption offers an attractive approach to the treatment of obesity. An alpha-amylase inhibitor from wheat, **Bay d 7791**, and one from microbial origin, **Bay e 4609**, have both been found to decrease digestion of starch (Puls and Keup, 1973), and to attenuate the hypoglycaemic and serum insulin response to starch ingestion in healthy volunteers and diabetic patients (Frerichs, Daweke and Gries, 1973; Keup and Puls, 1975). **Acarbose**, an inhibitor of beta-amylase, sucrase and alpha-glucosidase, was derived from micro-organisms (Schmidt, Frommer and Junge, 1977) and retarded starch and sucrose digestion in rats. Furthermore, acarbose diminished body weight gain as well as blood and body lipid content in obese Zucker rats (Puls, Keup and Krause, 1977). Sucrose absorption and utilization in humans were retarded after the ingestion of acarbose (Caspary, 1978; Iselin, Ravussin and Maeder, 1978) and blood sucrose concentration was reduced effectively (Laube *et al.*, 1980). Haraczkiewicz and Vasselli (1981) have demonstrated that the compound decreased body weight gain in rats maintained on a high carbohydrate diet and Glick and Bray (1981) reported that it diminished food intake without preventing weight gain in those rats fed on a high fat diet. However, the equivalent human trials have not revealed significant results with many remaining unreported or unpublished. The biguanides, however, have received scrutiny amongst the human research literature. Phenethylbiguanide and butylbiguanide have been shown to inhibit intestinal glucose absorption in human beings (Czyzyk *et al.*, 1968; Hollobaugh, Rao and Kruger, 1970). A reduction of body weight was observed in obese diabetics treated with phenethylbiguanide or 'phenformin' (Patel and Stowers, 1964) and in obese children treated with dimethylbiguanide or 'metformin' (Lutjens and Smit, 1977). These drugs appeared to have improved glucose tolerance (Cesar *et al.*, 1980). Fifty nine percent of patients with maturity onset diabetes given long term phenformin therapy lost weight; the weight loss exceeded 10 kg in 50% of those who lost weight (Nunes-Correa *et al.*, 1980). Phenformin controlled excessive body weight gain probably through a normalization of hyperinsulinaemia, thereby decreasing the lipogenic or antilipolytic effects of insulin and thus leading to a reduction of body lipid deposits (Danowski, 1967).

ADIPOSE TISSUE IN OBESITY

Adipose tissue mass in an ordinary person is in the order of 10–20 kg (Björntorp, 1981). It is able to regulate its mass by a factor of about 1000. An adipose tissue consists of cells with the approximate size and density of lymphocytes, with approximately 3×10^{10} adipocytes in a tissue of the size mentioned. These cells empty would have much the same mass as a kidney; or, with all cells for supply and support of adipocytes, perhaps the mass of the liver (Björntorp, 1983). The empty adipose tissue would be stretched out as a thin sheath in the subcutaneous tissue and among the visceral organs. Filling up the adipocytes with triglycerides to their capacity would mean a resulting adipose tissue mass which is about 100-fold larger. Increasing the number of fat cells to further enhance triglyceride storage capacity might produce an enlargement factor in the order of 1000-fold.

Researchers in the 1950s started to be actively interested in these dramatic characteristics of the fat cell in relation to obesity (e.g. Reh, 1953; Bjurulf, 1959). Both these early studies indicate that obesity in humans is indeed the result of an increase in body fat mass produced both by an enlargement of fat cells and by an increased number of these cells. In the late 1970s, accurate, reproducible measurements of adipocytes were made possible (e.g. Sjöström, Björntorp and Vrana, 1971; Hirsch and Gallian, 1978) with non-traumatic sampling of adipose tissue (Hirsch and Goldrick, 1964). Since internal fat cells are not easily measured, small adipocytes or unfilled cells might be missed in a count of body fat cells. The combination of body fat cell hypertrophy and fat cell hyperplasia to adipose tissue enlargement has thus been questioned on a number of occasions (e.g. Brook, Lloyd and Wolf, 1972; Salans, Cushman and Weismann, 1973; Jung *et al.*, 1978).

Fat cell number is calculated by dividing the total body fat by the average fat cell size: internal fat is included in the total body fat measurements, but the *size* of the internal fat cells is not included in the calculation of an average fat cell size. If the internal fat cells have approximately the same size as those measured in the subcutaneous adipose tissues, this error is negligible, even in severely obese individuals (Hirsch and Knittle, 1970). With regard to the situation in non-obese individuals, again internal fat is included in total fat measurements but adipocyte size is not included. The internal fat cells are, indeed, much smaller than the subcutaneous fat cells (Goldrick and McLoughlin, 1970; Jung *et al.*, 1978). Therefore, it is argued that the number of fat cells calculated from the subcutaneous fat cell size results in an underestimation. As Björntorp, Cairella and Howard (1981) suggest, the degree of this error is, to a large extent, dependent on the mass of internal fat (i.e. the contribution of internal fat cells to the total fat cell number). Internal fat is difficult to quantify precisely in living humans (Björntorp, 1983); if the majority of body fat were internal the consequence would be that the fat cell number would be the same in the non-obese individual as in the severely obese individual, which would clearly bias results.

Understandably, the postulated error discussed has led to some controversy and delays in the attempts to clarify obesity in terms of adipose cellularity in the moderately obese. Salans et al. (1973) have felt that there was no question about the existence of hyperplastic obesity when examining extremely obese persons; however, these types of people are not frequently seen in the general population but do constitute a severe problem in obesity clinics since their prognosis for treatment is often very poor.

Measuring adipocytes in order to assess obesity status has undergone significant reviews. It was thought that adipose tissue grew by fat cell multiplication only during an initial period before adulthood. This was based on observations in the laboratory animal where even in the most extreme overfeeding situations only fat cell size seemed to increase with obesity produced at the adult age (Hirsch and Han, 1969). Evidence in humans for a critical period was lacking, but from examination of the animal data it was tentatively assumed that an analogous situation existed with human adipose tissue (Björntorp, 1983). Lemonnier (1972) then found that new adipocytes were formed in fat-fed adult rats. Faust et al. (1978) reported that this was the case also in other overfeeding situations and occurred in several depots and in different rat strains. Evidence that revised the concept of a critical period for new adipocyte formation was also provided by other types of experiments. Such studies examined the precursor cell conversion to adipocytes (e.g. Van et al. 1976) and found that these cells were able to multiply freely in tissue culture systems.

Advances in technology have made it possible to examine more closely the chain of events leading to the production of mature fat cells. With fat overfeeding, the available fat cells fill up to a certain critical size but long before this occurs, non-determined adipocyte precursor cells as well as cells for supply and support of adipocytes start to multiply (Klyde and Hirsch, 1979; Björntorp, 1981). These adipocyte precursor cells are, however, not committed to adipocytes until they are needed, i.e. when available adipocytes are full. At this stage, undetermined precursors change irreversibly to determined precursor cells and then to adipocytes, which fill up with triglyceride and are detected among the other adipocytes (Faust *et al.*, 1978; Björntorp, 1981). Then, the picture is of a tissue which has an easily triggered, generalized ability to form new cells including new fat cell precursors, a flexible response to the potential of overfilling and not, as previously believed, a static picture of adipocyte filling only.

It would seem likely that there is a mechanism or activating signal present in the human blood circulation. Indeed, Green (1979) has shown the presence of such **adipogenic** factor or factors in the serum or plasma of certain species. However, Björntorp (1983) speculates that the local triggering of determination of adipocyte precursors to mature adipocytes most probably occurs via regional adipose tissue signals. Further research into this complex area of adipocyte cell division is underway.

MORTALITY, MORBIDITY AND OBESITY

In 1959, the Build and Blood Pressure Study (Society of Actuaries, 1960) suggested that the risk of increased weight for height increased linearly over the range of relative body weight for both men and women and tables were developed at this time to calculate ideal body weight for height from these data. In later years, this study has been criticized for being unrepresentative of the general population in the United States where the study was conducted, since individuals in the study weighed less than the average American. Conflicting evidence relating obesity with mortality has been reported by Bray (1976c) and Larsson, Björntorp and Tibblin (1981), who found (a) no apparent increased risk for mortality, and (b) a universal increase in mortality, with excess weight, respectively.

Andres (1980) provided a possible explanation for the apparent discrepancies of a number of studies relating body weight with mortality. By re-analysis of previous data, he suggested that there was excess mortality at both low body weights for height and high body weights for height. Indeed, Bray, Davidson and Drenick (1972) had demonstrated such a U-shaped curve for mortality, especially for men, from the data from the Build and Blood Pressure Study. Lew and Garfinkel (1979) demonstrated a similar U-shaped curve for mortality in a study of 750 000 men and women screened by questionnaire by American Cancer Society volunteers who were followed for 13 years. When Keys (1980b) re-analysed the data from the Chicago Peoples' Gas Company, the United States railroad men, and males in Northern and Southern Europe (Keys, 1980a), he found similar U-shaped curves for mortality in each group. This excess mortality for low weight and high weight men was present even though the data were corrected for the independent effects of blood pressure. This analysis seems to explain some of the disparate results that previously were known to exist between these groups (Keys, 1980b).

Analysis of the mortality data from the Framingham study also demonstrates increased mortality at both low and high relative body weights (Sorlie, Gordon and Kannel, 1980). It would appear that individuals who are below average body weight and those above average body weight are at increased risk for mortality. However, it is important to note that the curves drawn from data in this study represent small numbers of individuals, i.e. 5–10% of individuals at each end of the curve. The increased incidence of death at low body weight (see Chapter 1 for a discussion of low body weight and health implications in anorexia nervosa) does not seem to be explained by increased smoking in this group of individuals (e.g. Lew and Garfinkel, 1979; Sorlie, Gordon and Kannel, 1980; see also Garrison *et al.*, 1978, on cigarette smoking and cholesterol levels) or by the presence of pre-existing cancer or other diseases (Lew and Garfinkel, 1979). Thus, the 'ideal' or 'desirable' weights calculated from the Metropolitan Life Insurance Tables (1959) seem to be neither ideal nor desirable for adults of 30 to 59 years of age, as previously suggested.

An increase in cardiovascular morbidity and mortality in obese individuals has been demonstrated in many studies (e.g. Castelli *et al.*, 1977; Brunzell and Miller, 1981). Rimm *et al.* (1972) and Marks (1960) showed an increase in the incidence and in death, respectively, following gall bladder disease in obese men and women; and Larsson, Björntorp and Tibblin (1981) reported that patients with gall stones were more obese than those without them. Lew and Garfinkel (1979) have also shown an increased mortality due to digestive diseases in obese individuals in a prospective study of 750 000 individuals who were followed for 13 years in the American Cancer Society study.

Precursors of diseases that may lead to death, such as atherosclerosis and hypertensive vascular disease, have been examined in several follow-up studies of obese patients (Abraham, Collins and Nordsiech, 1960; Paffenbarger and Wing, 1969) and the finding linking obesity with coronary heart disease or myocardial infarction has been reported by Pell and Alonzo (1963) and Chapman *et al.* (1971). While body weight may relate to the risk for premature cardiovascular disease and other disorders, it has been demonstrated that body weight is also associated in various ways with most of the known risk factors for atherosclerosis such as blood pressure, cigarette smoking, high density lipoprotein (HDL) cholesterol (Castelli *et al.*, 1977), total plasma cholesterol, plasma glucose levels and total plasma triglycerides (Hulley *et al.*, 1980). Elevated systolic and diastolic blood pressure would appear to be associated with increased risk for coronary heart disease at all ages and is more prevalent in the obese.

Cigarette smoking is associated with decreased HDL cholesterol levels (Garrison *et al.*, 1978) and the effect of cigarette smoking on the risk of coronary artery disease seems to be entirely reversible by cessation of smoking (Pooling Project Research Group, 1978). Decreased HDL cholesterol levels are associated with increased risk of coronary artery disease in older (Castelli *et al.*, 1977) and younger individuals (Miller *et al.*, 1977). HDL cholesterol levels are decreased in obesity (Garrison *et al.*, 1978), in those individuals with elevated glucose levels (Lopez-Virella, Stone and Colwell, 1977) and in those with elevated levels of triglyceride (Schaeffer *et al.*, 1978). Cigarette smokers, however, weigh less than non-smokers (Comstock and Stone, 1972). While smoking, increased blood pressure and increased total plasma cholesterol can be shown to be independent risk factors for coronary artery disease (Pooling Project Research Group, 1978), the complex interaction of these factors with others, such as excessive overweight, may be potentially hazardous to any individual, but also makes investigations particularly difficult in teasing out their relative importance in contributing to a person's health (or ill health).

FURTHER READING

Eating habits and lifestyles

Galbraith, L. and Wilson, A. (1992) Adolescent obesity – a new treatment programme in Ninewells Hospital, Dundee. *BPS Scottish Branch Newsletter*, **14**, 10–12.

Metabolic issues in obese diabetics

Heffner, S.M., Stern, M.P., Mitchell, B.D., Hazuda, H.P. and Patterson, J.K. (1990) Incidence of type II diabetes in Mexican Americans predicted by fasting insulin and glucose levels, obesity and body-fat distribution. *Diabetes*, **39**(3), 283–8.

Polycystic ovary syndrome

Nestler, J.E., Powers, L.P., Matt, D.W. *et al.* (1991) A direct effect of hyperinsulinemia on serum sex hormone-binding globulin levels in obese women with the polycystic ovary syndrome. *Journal of Clinical Endocrinology and Metabolism*, **71**(1), 83–9.

Cognitive aspects of taste perception in obesity

Drewnowski, A. (1981) *Cognitive Aspects of Taste Perception in Obesity*. Paper presented at Eastern Psychological Association Meeting, New York.

Anorectic agents and the modulation of intestinal absorption through drug therapy

Danforth, E. Jr. and Landsberg, L. (1983) Energy expenditure and its regulation, in *Obesity*, (ed M.R.C. Greenwood), Churchill Livingstone, New York, pp. 103–21.

Sullivan, A.C., Baruth, H.W. and Cheng, L. (1980) Recent advances in the design and development of antiobesity agents. *Annual Reports in Medicine and Chemistry*, **15**, 172–81.

Adipose tissue in obesity

Björntorp, P. (1981) Adipocyte precursor cells, in *Recent Advances in Obesity Research*, (eds P. Björntorp, M. Cairella and A.N. Howard), John Libbey, London, p. 58.

Björntorp, P., Cairella, M. and Howard, A.N. (1981) *Recent Advances in Obesity Research*, John Libbey, London.

Mortality, morbidity and obesity

Brunzell, J.D. and Miller, N.E. (1981) Atherosclerosis in inherited and acquired disorders of plasma lipoprotein metabolism, in *Lipoproteins, Atherosclerosis and Coronary Heart Disease*, (eds N.E. Miller and B. Lewis), Elsevier, Amsterdam, pp. 73–88.

Hulley, S.B., Rosenman, R.H., Bawol, R.D. and Brand, R.J. (1980) Epidemiology as a guide to clinical decisions. The association between triglyceride and coronary heart disease. *New England Journal of Medicine*, **302**, 1383–9.

Keys, A. (1980b) Overweight, obesity, coronary heart disease and mortality. *Nutrition Review*, **38**, 297–307.

10

Eating and feeding disorders in people with a learning disability

INTRODUCTION

There has been much debate over the use of the term 'learning disability' as, indeed, there has been over the term 'mental handicap'. Since there is majority support in the literature, and for the purposes of this book, the former label will be adopted. Similarly, the terms 'eating' and 'feeding' have sometimes been used interchangeably, though in this case, incorrectly. In fact, the former refers to the digestion and absorption of food whilst the latter is the ingestion (or putting in the mouth) of food.

This chapter is not intended to provide a comprehensive guide to learning disabilities nor is it intended as a comprehensive work on 'eating and feeding disorders in people with learning disabilities' since these areas would probably justify an entire book of their own. Instead, it hopefully provides the reader with a 'taste' (!) of eating and feeding disorders in this specialized setting and describes some of the problems health professionals face in managing and treating such problems. Finally, the term 'client' is sometimes used to refer to 'patient'. This is intentional and reflects the use of the more common term in both institutional and community settings that provide services for people with learning disabilities.

DEFINITION OF LEARNING DISABILITY

One of the most frequently observed forms of learning disability is Down's syndrome or mongolism. The former term is used more often clinically and was first described by Langdon Down as a separate entity in 1866 (Down, 1866) and independently in the same year by Seguin (Seguin, 1866). Seguin referred to the disorder as 'furfuraceous cretinism', emphasizing an assumed relationship to cretinism, while Down, struck by some aspects of the physiognomy of the patients which were superficially similar to those of people in outer Mongolia, called it Mongolian idiocy. Thankfully, today people with such disorders are more commonly referred to by their first names, thus recognizing the fact that there is a person behind such stigmatized labels.

'Learning disability' or 'mental handicap' is a very broad term and has been used to describe people with an intelligence quotient (IQ) below 70. Both terms commonly describe people who, in fact, may have a range of difficulties which might include approaches to problem-solving, coordination difficult-ies, problems with speech or comprehension, cognitive delay, or slowness or inability to perform daily routines, such as hygiene or feeding (Thompson, 1993b). The range or number of disabilities an individual may have can be very large or equally, very small. Increasingly, therefore, it is useful to state a person's *abilities* rather than emphasizing their negative *dis-abilities*. With the promotion of community living, definitions of learning disability have come to include the extent of a person's ability to live alone or his or her 'independence'. Therefore, such a definition has been assumed for the discussions in this chapter and is stated as follows:

> A person with a learning disability is someone who is, to a varying degree, dependent on others for their living needs because of a cognitive impairment resulting from hereditary abnormalities or directly following (or during) birth. They may (or may not) also have associated physical/sensory/behavioural/medical disabilities.

Other researchers and clinicians working in this field may also feel that people with acquired brain damage (e.g. Sarason and Doris, 1969); sufferers of dyslexia and some types of dementia or other syndromes, e.g. autism (Sarason and Gladwin, 1958); alkaptonuria (Garrod, 1902; Knox, 1958); phenylketonuria – PKU (Knox, 1960) should also be included in this category. Clearly, this is a subject for debate. One category of disabilities in particular, eating disorders, is commonly observed with a learning disability and will be discussed in this chapter. The reader is referred to the Further Reading section at the end of the chapter for sources of reference on other areas of learning disability.

TYPES OF EATING AND FEEDING DISORDERS

Almost any kind of behaviour can occur in association with feeding: non-compliance, aggressive behaviour, self-injurious behaviour and stereotyped behaviour (Presland, 1989). A problem related to eating is stealing food. This has been reported most commonly at mealtimes where it frequently takes the form of grabbing handfuls of food that is intended for others (Smith *et al.*, 1983), especially in institutionalized settings. A related problem, scavenging or 'pica', is also evidenced in these environments and is commonly defined as eating non-nutritive substances such as string, sweet wrappers, needles, items from refuse containers, pills, paper, soil, cigarette ends, stones, etc. Some authors include in the definition of pica the eating of food obtained from the wrong places, e.g. by picking it up from the floor. There are also some people with learning disabilities who consume their faeces, a behaviour termed **coprophagy**.

Other types of disorders of feeding include vomiting (Azrin, Jammer and Besalel, 1986) and rumination (Rast *et al.*, 1985) which tend to occur after eating. The distinction between these terms is not consistent in the literature. If the term *vomiting* is used it implies that the regurgitated matter is immediately ejected from the mouth. *Rumination* usually implies that it is retained in the mouth for a while, perhaps chewed and then either re-swallowed, allowed to run out of the mouth or ejected.

Whilst many of these disorders are problems that face clients and carers in institutions, they are not always the result of a poor care setting, i.e. inadequate attention or care from staff; poor facilities for the clients; an unvaried, uninteresting diet; a dull environment in which to consume meals, etc. Problem behaviours can originate from care during childhood or may simply be because of an ignorance of personal hygiene and self-care, etc. It is sometimes because of these reasons that people (whether or not possessing a learning disability) decide to refuse to eat altogether. A person with a learning disability may put up a hand to fend off food, turn their head away, cry or scream. It is understandable how some people begin to fast and lose weight because of disharmony in the care setting or because of some other feelings that they may have and which they may not be able to express to others. Although anorexia nervosa and bulimia are not well documented in people with learning disabilities, there is evidence to suggest that behavioural problems do occur in association with eating and diets (e.g. Oliver, 1986; Cole, 1990) and perhaps for similar reasons as for the general population. Obesity, on the other hand, seems to appear often in the research literature (e.g. Fox *et al.*, 1985) and has been commonly associated with people suffering from Down's syndrome or Prader–Willi syndrome (Page *et al.*, 1983a,b).

Other problems related to food seen in people with learning disabilities include: eating too fast; eating without utensils; spilling food; eating directly off the plate; throwing food; and over-eating. Though rarely serious, these problems or disorders can sometimes pose difficulties which disrupt or prevent a person learning even basic self-care skills that would increase the possibilities of their independent living.

EPIDEMIOLOGY OF EATING AND FEEDING DISORDERS

There are some medical conditions, such as the Prader–Willi syndrome, which have recognized genetic origins, i.e. chromosomal abnormalities. People with this syndrome often have a mild learning disability, eat to excess and are usually overweight (Presland, 1989). Sufferers also often forage for food (and even steal food) or eat things of no nutritive value.

Pica, on the other hand, has sometimes been claimed to be the result of iron deficiency. However, grounds for this claim are dubious and complicated; pica can also cause iron deficiency, which makes cause and effect difficult to discern. Likewise, authors have used the terms **rumination** and **regurgitation** interchangeably; both in fact can have medical causes but causes of the former are more likely to be behavioural. The latter is a gastro-oesaphageal reflux in which the stomach contents are ejected into the oesophagus, because of abnormalities of the muscles joining these entities. However, stomach and intestinal infections can also have similar effects.

Refusing food and overselectivity of food can be the cause of various abnormalities of muscular function. For example, one study claimed that of 52 cases of delay in taking solid food, nearly 80% were the result of neuromuscular disorders (Presland, 1989), such as cerebral palsy. Often these difficulties may be regarded as 'difficult behaviours' rather than a medical condition; indeed, some people display tantrums when pressed about food refusal even when the food may have been tolerated in the past. In particular, anorexia nervosa is thought to have a variety of origins (see Chapter 1 for a full discussion of the epidemiology of anorexia nervosa) which may be different amongst people with learning disabilities because of their socioeconomic background and intellectual development. With the growing evidence in support of an organic origin for anorexia nervosa (Holden, 1990; Thompson, 1991b,c; 1992a; 1993a; and also see Chapter 3 for a discussion on the research literature), there may be other reasons for the establishment and maintenance of this disorder in sufferers. Similarly, bulimia may too have causes that were not previously thought to be organic in origin (see Chapter 4 for a discussion of the epidemiology and theories of bulimia).

In the population of people with learning disabilities, there can be numerous reasons for food-related disorders that are directly linked with their medication. For example, in the control of epilepsy, phenytoin is known to reduce the sensations of taste in some people and has also been known to cause gastric upset and gum disorders (Thompson, North and Pentland, 1992). Other drugs used in the control or management of behavioural disorders may have side effects which influence food intake, such as a dry mouth, headache or nausea. Some drugs can even lead to vomiting.

Other reasons for food-related disorders in people with learning disabilities also concern the access to reinforcers. This might apply particularly to people with severe learning disabilities where food acts as an important positive reinforcer, so much so that it can lead to over-indulgence in food intake and subsequent obesity. There is also some evidence to suggest that sensations derived from having food in the mouth and chewing it are positively reinforcing; though this is clearly the opposite case in sufferers of anorexia nervosa or bulimia.

People living in long-stay institutions often have a variety of behavioural disorders and pica is one that is commonly found in this population. Presland (1989) reported the occurrence of pica in institutions from two studies: 8% and 26% respectively.

Rumination was found to occur in 5.3–9.6% of such populations and vomiting in up to 25% of institutions surveyed. Over-eating seems to be less evident in populations with a severe versus mild learning disability but there is little reliable evidence in the research literature. It is clear, however, that some feeding problems are so severe that they threaten life; rumination, for instance, can lead to dehydration and malnutrition and refusal to eat and disorders such as anorexia nervosa and obesity have been evidenced as contributors to mortality rates in the population.

HOW TO ASSESS

The first step in any intervention technique should be an assessment of the problem. Whether in an institutional setting or in the community, care staff and, where appropriate, the client and family should be consulted in order to acquire an accurate picture of the problem. Observational techniques are particularly useful to assess a person's difficulty during feeding; video cameras have come into their own in this area, but it should be borne in mind that the client's or an advocate's consent should be sought. Also, some people react in a different way when they are being filmed!

ABC chart

The 'ABC' or antecedents, behaviour and consequences chart is a useful way to record and assess behaviour. In the feeding situation, clients may be usefully observed and their behaviour before, during and after feeding recorded for later analysis. Sometimes it is the behaviour or actions of others that precedes an event that is important to know in order to rectify or modify an abnormal behaviour or to assist with some difficulty which the client may be experiencing. With the ABC chart, the actions or events before feeding are recorded, then the client's behaviour during feeding, followed by the consequences of the client's behaviour. An example of this might be:

> Gary dislikes eating in the dining room with others because the noise of other people talking disturbs his concentration. He responds by verbalizing annoyance at the dining table

and throws his food onto the floor. The staff, not under-standing his behaviour, do not replenish any food supplies he has ejected and subsequently he eats a very small meal. After the meal, he is observed by staff to forage for food from the kitchen or from anyone who is having a snack, probably because he is still hungry.

This is a simplified example but demonstrates a scenario which has the benefit of hindsight: Gary dislikes excessive noise while feeding. By using the ABC chart or other methods of observation, staff may be able to observe any patterns in his behaviour. The next step might be to observe Gary in a dif-ferent environment to see if it is truly noise, or only noise, that predicts his consequent food refusal.

Sampling methods and diet diaries

Other methods of assessing clients' behaviour include time sampling. This is when the behaviour being observed is re-corded over a period of time; interval sampling is when this behaviour is recorded at set intervals, e.g. at mealtimes only, or at a set time, e.g. every tenth minute for one minute dur-ation, etc. There are variations on these observational tech-niques such as time lag sampling and interval lag sampling when specific behaviour may be observed or when there is a wish to exclude other behaviour from the recording. These tech-niques can be used for a variety of behaviours but sometimes it is useful to record behaviour which is not being observed. In this case, a diet diary or weekly record of diet-related behaviour may be kept. Depending on the intellectual level of the client, it is important to ensure that instructions for making these recordings are kept as simple as possible. Asking a member of the care staff to assist the client in completing the record is sometimes a useful option.

There are specific difficulties with some types of eating dis-orders. For example, bulimics usually display highly secretive behaviour and it is difficult, therefore, to encourage them to record this behaviour. Likewise, for some clients, it is difficult to replace food with another positive reinforcer which has the same success of promoting a given behaviour. Food, indeed, is very reinforcing to some people, although in some disorders like anorexia nervosa, the converse is true when feeling empty or purging (as in bulimia) is very reinforcing for the behaviour.

Physical recording measures

Sometimes it is useful to make direct physical measures in order to assess a client's behaviour. Weighing people is perhaps the most obvious method, though it may be useful not to reveal to the client his or her weight especially if the client is intending to lose weight at any cost! Measuring the caloric value of food, weighing food itself or counting the number of items of food in a diet may be a useful standard for assessing change in eating and feeding behaviours. Handfuls of food is a rough measure but may be a useful guide in assessing a client's tendency to grab and steal food from another's plate.

In summary, there are many assessment tools available to the clinician for assessing eating and feeding behaviour in people with learning disabilities. The reader is referred to the assessment section of Chapters 2, 5 and 7 where a discussion is made of the procedures involved in assessing anorexia nervosa, bulimia and obesity, respectively. Although similar, the procedures involved in assessing these disorders in people with learning disabilities may have to be adapted in order to accommodate the differences in intellectual functioning and life experiences. Clear, simple instructions, though, are always preferable to long, complicated or over-expansive requests for any client group.

HOW TO TREAT

Premack Principle

Following the use of ABC charts to assess the client's feeding behaviour, a decision can be made over which problem behaviours should be removed, modified or used in different ways. One method of identifying such behaviours to be reinforced or selected is the Premack Principle. This states that 'any behaviour is reinforced by subsequent participation in any other behaviour which is of more frequent natural occurrence' (Premack, 1959). Using this principle, it is necessary first to choose the behaviour whose occurrence is to be increased and

then to select any behaviour from further up the list of behaviours recorded to use as a reinforcing consequence. The
principle could be extended to assert that any behaviour lower
down the list (in order of frequency – highest frequency at the
top of the list) could be enforced as a reducing consequence for
a behaviour whose occurrence is to be decreased (Premack,
1971).

However, some of the research conducted does not support
the concept (e.g. Hulse *et al.*, 1981) and little is known about
how it could apply to people with severe learning disabilities.
One study has even reported that people engage in frequent
behaviours as a reducing consequence and do not decrease the
frequency of occurrence of more frequent behaviours (Krivacek
and Powell, 1978). It would seem that this principle is likely to
apply directly only to reinforcers which constitute an activity in
which someone participates; and it is difficult, moreover, to
determine the 'natural' rate of a behaviour.

Behaviour modification

Modifying a person's behaviour can take a variety of forms. In
people with learning disabilities, this encompasses a variety of
methods, e.g. shaping behaviour; extinguishing undesirable behaviour; prompting behaviour; use of time-out from activities;
deprivation; overcorrection; chaining; positive and negative reinforcing (Thompson, 1991a). In altering a person's feeding
behaviour, several of these methods may be used at the intervention stage of treatment. For example, in the Thompson and
Gittins (1989a,b) studies, prompting was used to increase the
independence in feeding of a woman with a profound learning
disability. This took the form of verbal praise or physical assistance to raise or lower a utensil used in feeding. Prompting
behaviour in this way increased the occurrence of the client
performing these tasks herself. The success of this procedure
was partly attributable to the dedicated care staff and also to
reinforcing her behaviours *in situ*, since there is sometimes the
difficulty of clients generalizing specific skills learned outside
the task situation or environment.

Chaining a sequence of behaviours is a technique also used
to modify behaviour. This is done when a series of behaviours
is to be linked together in sequence. Often the end result or

final behaviour is taught first so that the client can see the final goal to be attained. The earlier behaviours in the sequence are then taught so that the client builds up a picture of the behaviours that must be performed before the goal is reached. This method is commonly referred to as 'backward chaining'.

Other techniques may also be incorporated in backward chaining. For instance, 'shaping' a response can sometimes help the client to learn an approximate response or behaviour to a situation. This response can then be modified or shaped until it is the desirable response. An example of this may be the altering of a client's grip on a spoon as s/he uses it to feed. Reinforcing the behaviour at this stage can be an important step to promoting further occurrences of the desired behaviour and the reader is referred to the Thompson and Gittins (1989a) study where a discussion is made of the selection of preferential reinforcers for a client to increase her independence in feeding.

Use of reinforcers

A positive reinforcement is where an action or behaviour increases the occurrence of another behaviour. For example, a person may be given verbal praise in order to increase the probability of the client performing an action once again. If, however, the verbal praise is not understood, is given in the wrong context or for some other reason is inappropriate, then it may not produce the desired behavioural consequence. A negative reinforcer, on the other hand, is one that removes an undesired behaviour; and extinction is the gradual reduction of a (possibly undesired) behaviour. Aversive stimuli or the use of punishment is sometimes confused with negative reinforcement and sometimes has similar effects but for different reasons. To illustrate the use of these reinforcers, a food-related example will be given:

> Elisabeth is making a continuous gurgling noise with a cup of water which is causing extreme annoyance to her father. If he slapped her with his hand (an aversive stimulus, i.e. punishment), she might start crying which would stop the gurgling noise but replace it with another, perhaps equally annoying noise. The slap would then have acted in an aversive way, being paired with the occurrence of the gurgling noise (or with Elisabeth crying). If, on the other hand, he

took away the cup of water, this action would act as a negative reinforcer to Elisabeth; if he praised her for gurgling which encouraged her to gurgle more, then the praise would have acted as a positive reinforcer since it increased the occurrence (or probability) of the gurgling. Alternatively, he might have offered her some chocolate, which she likes, and the gurgling noise may have given way to her consuming the chocolate!

There are numerous examples but this one is intended to illustrate how reinforcers are viewed differently accordingly to the perspective of the client or carer. Several researchers have examined the effects of reinforcers in treating eating and feeding disorders in people with learning disabilities: e.g. Michael, 1975; Green, 1977; Pace *et al.*, 1985; Wacker *et al.*, 1985; Green *et al.*, 1988; Yarnall and Dodgion-Ensor, 1980; Thompson and Gittins, 1989a,b; Johnston *et al.*, 1991. Reinforcing consequences for appropriate behaviours can be used in two main ways: to reinforce abstaining (that is, engaging in any behaviour *other* than one that is a problem); and to reinforce specific behaviours incompatible with, or with the same purpose as, the problem behaviour. Presland (1989) gives several examples including how differential reinforcement of behaviour (DRO) is used to decrease the incidence of food stealing in a woman with a severe learning disability by giving her tokens (exchangeable for various items of more concrete value) for periods of abstaining; and an application of the same procedure for rumination in a young man with a profound learning disability, who was reinforced with food for periods of not ruminating.

Other treatment methods

An antecedent device which has been used specifically for reinforcing to eat certain kinds of food is to camouflage those foods with something more appealing (Presland, 1989). Other methods have used exclusion diets (Oliver, 1986) to combat obesity; a 'mini-meal' (Azrin and Armstrong, 1973) to teach eating skills to people with learning disabilities; pharmaco-therapy (Aman and Singh, 1983; Aman, 1985); and a 'gentle teaching' (McGee *et al.*, 1987; Caldwell, 1991) approach recognizing and emphasizing a person's achievements and skills instead of their disabilities. Medication procedures have sometimes been used for food-related problems that do not have known medical causes. Food refusal, for instance, has been treated by forced feeding, intravenous feeding and tubes inserted directly into the stomach or intestine. These methods do not tend to promote effective eating habits and the insertion of tubes (as discussed in Chapter 2 concerning an optional inpatient treatment intervention for anorexia nervosa) brings health risks of its own. Similarly, medication has been used in the context of vomiting, but again, there is no clear evidence that it is helpful for people in whom no medical cause of vomiting has been found.

OUTCOME OF TREATMENT

It is difficult to discuss the outcome of treatment unless specific circumstances are described. The outcome of interventions is dependent upon the individual; this is especially the case with people with learning disabilities since there can be a very great variation in the individual's intellectual abilities and background. Generally, the same conditions for outcome apply as with the general population, but with some notable differences: for any treatment with a hope of success, compliance must be sought from the individual patient. This usually implies some level of understanding of the procedure involved, though this is not necessarily the case. For people with learning disabilities, comprehending intervention techniques may be difficult and so simplification or explanations at a level appropriate to the individual should be given. In essence, the major differences in treating people with learning disabilities and those who do not have such disabilities are that the individual may take longer to accept or understand the information being imparted. Also, the former category of patient may be so severely affected that only behavioural techniques are effective with little explanation being possible.

There has so far been no discussion on the use of cognitive–behavioural techniques or cognitive therapy for the treatment of eating disorders in people with learning disabilities. This is mainly because of the lack of scientific research on the subject and not because it is particularly excluded. Again, it depends on the intellectual functioning of the individual: if the client is able to accept the concepts used in cognitive therapy then it is potentially effective in any client group. However, it would seem that behavioural methods tend to be preferred in people with learning disabilities because these people generally do not have the level of functioning commonly believed to be necessary for success with this method of therapy. That is not to say, however, that there will not be future evidence showing its usefulness as a therapeutic tool for this client group as some researchers would agree that the level of functioning required is little more than that required in other therapies successfully used with this client group, such as some progressive muscle relaxation methods that involve the use of imagination. The question remains whether disorders like anorexia nervosa and bulimia, generally thought to occur in people with a higher than average intelligence quotient, are present in people with learning disabilities because of an organic abnormality. The prevalence of eating disorders in this client group is, indeed, stimulation for further research.

RESEARCH

This chapter will again deviate slightly in layout from the rest of the book (i.e. Chapters 1–9) by including a selection of contemporary areas of research. It is recognized that there is a lot of useful and interesting work documented on the general area of people with learning disabilities; in recognition of this fact, a selective list of references has been included under the research section of Further Reading. However, since it is not possible to present all of these works here, four areas of research are now presented and discussed. The first is a description of the Thompson and Gittins (1989b) study, which describes a feeding programme for a person with a profound learning disability. The second study discusses some lessons learned from teaching people with learning disabilities how to manage their own 'special' diets (Cole, 1990). In the third study, by Hinds and Oliver (1985), a treatment approach to chronic vomiting in this client group is discussed. The fourth study (Thompson, Smith and Muir, 1992) describes an investigation into apparent low weight gain in clients with learning disabilities, in spite of dietary intervention.

INCREASING INDEPENDENCE IN FEEDING

The search for appropriate reinforcers for prompting behaviours in people with learning disabilities is well known (Favell and Cannon, 1976; Johnson, Firth and Davey, 1978; Pace *et al.*, 1985; Wacker *et al.*, 1985; Green *et al.*, 1988). However, the use of a Pethna to provide systematic auditory and visual reinforcement during feeding is less well documented (Thompson and Gittins, 1989b). Indeed, there is limited reference concerning feeding clients with severe learning disabilities (e.g. Ohwaki and Zingarelli, 1988) and the use and effectiveness of such devices as the Pethna (Woods and Parry, 1981; Sturmey, Woods and Crisp, 1984).

The Thompson and Gittins (1989b) study focused on the use of a Pethna to provide two types of reinforcement, namely auditory (music) and visual (flashing lights), to improve the feeding skills of a 22 year old woman with a profound learning disability. The Pethna, in conjunction with fairground music, was found to be reinforcing to the woman. This had been confirmed from two sources: (i) the parents had seen their daughter's enjoyment (smiling, vocalizing and moving arms in the air, etc.) in response to hearing and seeing a fairground organ, and (ii) from using the flashing lights of the Pethna while playing popular music to the client in the quiet 'dark' room in the Special Care Unit of the day centre. For these reasons a combination of fairground music and flashing lights, as provided by the Pethna, was used to reinforce and increase the client's feeding skills. A detailed task analysis of those skills required during feeding was also completed in order to decide which parts of the feeding sequence could most effectively be reinforced and consent for the woman's participation in the study was obtained from the parents who acted as her advocates.

A brief description of the equipment will be detailed here but the reader is referred to Woods and Parry (1981) for a fuller description of the Pethna. It incorporates two interchangeable components which the designers have called the 'in-box' and the 'out-box'. An 'in-box' consists of a device that has to be operated in some way by the disabled person and an 'out-box' provides a reward of some kind. Electronic components are housed in the 'out-box' and are powered by replaceable (or rechargeable) batteries. The interchangeable 'in-boxes' and 'out-boxes' are fastened together and connected by plug and socket systems.

'Out-boxes' can deliver one form of stimulation or combinations of different forms. Operating an 'in-box' switches on the stimulation from an 'out-box' for several seconds. A timer switch inside the 'out-box' enables the length of a bout of stimulation to be selected (over a range from 2 to 30 seconds).

A cassette player is housed in the 'out-box' so that any auditory stimulus can be taped and inserted into the Pethna. Easily accessible controls inside the Pethna enable the volume and the duration of the cassette play to be adjusted.

In this study, a task analysis was completed for the woman's feeding episode and a chart constructed for manual recording of events during the baseline, intervention and assessment phases of the study. Each column of the task analysis chart carried a heading appropriate to the degree of dependence of the observed behaviour, e.g. 'HELPER' indicated that the observed behaviour (which may have been 'scoops up food with spoon') was performed solely by the helper who was assisting the woman during feeding. A 'PHYSICAL PROMPT' meant that it was considered necessary by the helper to issue some physical prompting to the client (i.e. nudging elbow; moving feeding arm towards spoon; gripping client's fingers around spoon handle, etc.); 'INDEPENDENT' meant that the client performed the task without any physical prompt from the helper.

A hypothesis proposed that the woman would become independent (i.e. would perform without physical prompting by the helper) following training with the Pethna in the following tasks: moving her left hand towards the spoon; gripping handle of spoon; picking up spoon; lifting spoon away from dish; moving spoon towards mouth to touch lips.

A baseline period of the initial seven minutes of 11 feeding situations were videotaped and manually recorded using the task analysis chart. It was considered sufficient to record for the initial seven minutes of each feeding situation since the woman displayed most independence during this time with the average duration of these meals being 15 minutes. This provided a picture of the woman's initial extent of independence during feeding. The woman was seen at the same time for her mid-day meal throughout the study. An instructor and a general assistant, one male and one female, who regularly helped the woman to feed were collaborators in this study and continued to assist the client during the feeding sessions without their routine or method being altered by the intervention.

The woman was seen in the usual dining area seated in a wheelchair in front of a table shared by three other clients. The two researchers were situated behind a counter out of sight of the woman about ten metres distance from the woman. Hidden video equipment was located in this area with a video camera focused on the woman. The intervention period (14 feeding sessions) was conducted in the Special Care Unit of the day centre with the woman situated again at a table but in this case not shared with other clients. The Pethna was placed directly in front of the woman on the table with the dish placed between the client and the Pethna. The researchers were seated either side of the Pethna, being as unobtrusive as possible: one to record events (on task analysis charts) and the other to operate the 'out-box' of the Pethna in order to provide reinforcement for the woman's feeding behaviour.

For the final assessment, four feeding situations were video-taped on returning the woman to the usual dining area and these were analysed using the task analysis chart by another colleague who was naïve to the study.

The Wilcoxon Signed Ranks Test was used to test the significance between the woman's independence in feeding at the baseline with the woman's independence on assessment. There was no significant difference (at the 5% level, two-tailed) using this test. However, using the median and grand total medians over all sessions for the five identified behaviours, an 8.3% improvement was found in the independence of the client from baseline to assessment (Figure 10.1). Learning curves drawn from data collected during nine of the 14 intervention sessions also evidenced improvement in independence, particularly in the client's frequency in three out of five of the behaviours: (a) grips spoon with left hand, (b) picks up spoon, and (c) lifts spoon from dish. Hence, there was a 60% improvement in the client's independence from baseline to assessment in three of these behaviours.

Although anecdotal evidence is not scientifically sound, it can often provide a useful insight into situations. Such was the

	Median rating over 11 baseline sessions	Median rating over 4 assessment sessions
	15	19.5
Median of grand total over all sessions	36	39
Rating of selected behaviours as a percentage of the total	41.7%	50.0%

Figure 10.1 Independence of client during feeding sessions for five selected behaviours assessed by task analysis (Thompson and Gittins, 1989b).

case when the client apparently showed less interest in the Pethna reinforcement in week 15 of the research. It is possible that such reinforcers may lose their potency and that a change in reinforcer could have been more effective in increasing the woman's independence during feeding. For this reason, a further period of study considered other potentially reinforcing agents.

TEACHING PEOPLE TO MANAGE SPECIAL DIETS

Anyone can develop health problems which result in the need to follow a particular type of diet in order to stay well. If this happens, having the opportunity to learn how to manage their health through their diet can mean the difference between a lifestyle that is relatively independent from the medical profession and one that is not. People who have learning disabilities may require increased assistance to learn dietary control of their health and there may be risks involved (Cole, 1990).

For people with learning disabilities who need a 'special' diet because of health problems there are factors which complicate the process of teaching dietary self-management. Controlling health through diet is often complicated and difficult to understand (see Oliver, 1986, on exclusion diets for people with learning disabilities). For example, with diabetes 'fine-tuning' is often required to adjust sugar levels in the body. For most people, awareness and vigilance over food and drink intake become almost second nature over time. This, however, is a learned response which people who have learning disabilities may need extra help to develop. As Cole (1990) suggests, this help must be offered in the most appropriate way in order that learning can occur. Some workers in the field hold the view that all people, in fact, are capable of personal growth, given the right conditions (Mental Handicap in Wales Applied Research Unit, 1985). Without the 'right conditions', people who have learning disabilities will be denied the opportunity and will, therefore, remain dependent upon others (see also Wolfensberger, 1972, on the principle of normalization and people with learning disabilities).

Cole (1990) drew on information from the case of a young girl who suffered from diabetes mellitus. She identified the following problems which required help:

1. **Choice of foods**: the right to choose what we eat is one valued by most people in Western society and this is reflected in the concept of 'exchange' in diets for people with diabetes. For people who have learning disabilities, however, making choices can be problematic. Many have been in a dependent role for a long time, either within the family or in an institution, where their opportunities to make choices have been limited. Therefore, the concept may be new to them and the practice of making choices may need to be learned.
2. **Information about diets**: most people with learning disabilities, by virtue of the difficulties they experience with learning, have been unable to develop competent reading and writing skills. Thus, fundamental problems are posed by diet sheets which rely on the written word to communicate their content. Such sheets are only of use when they are in the presence of another person who can read. This situation, therefore, places a person with learning disabilities in a dependent role.
3. **Recalling and retrieving dietary information**: although most people who have a 'special' diet have diet sheets and information to hand, these are needed progressively less as they become familiar with what is required in order to maintain health. This is a function of memory and a process of learning. People who have learning disabilities are likely to take significantly longer to achieve this skill and ready

access to understandable information (or information obtained from another person) becomes essential.

4. **Terminology**: dietary control of medical conditions may require an understanding of more than just food. For example, 'energy', 'carbohydrates' or even 'grams' are words that may be very unfamiliar to a person with learning disabilities; likewise, their intrinsic meanings may be equally unfamiliar.

5. **Financial concerns**: people living independently in the community may have very limited financial resources (Cole, 1990), although it is debatable whether or not healthy eating is more or less expensive than eating 'convenience' foods.

6. **Information for people in the support network**: it is essential that a coordinated and accurate picture of a person's dietary situation be presented in order to avoid 'misinformation (!)' being imparted to the client.

7. **Information for living companions**: especially in community living, the need for others to be aware of a person's special dietary needs becomes important. Complications can occur when turns are taken in cooking rotas or in the purchasing of special foods.

Cole (1990) illustrated short-term and long-term goals for her client in which a series of steps indicated the goals, actions and aids used to facilitate these steps. For example, the short-term goal set in one of the steps was for people in the support network to understand what her client liked to eat (and what she did not like to eat) and the amount of her food budget. The action taken was to talk with her client about her likes and dislikes, where she liked to shop and what she liked to purchase, etc. It was important to remember and observe her client's rights and confidentiality and to involve her in any decisions made concerning purchases and diet planning. Other steps involved teaching her client cooking skills and learning how to recognize the 'danger' signs of diabetes, etc.

Cole (1990) comments that for those with particular dietary needs, restraint and control over their diet may seem contradictory to their lifestyle. Teaching people how to manage their own diets in their new settings produces thought-provoking dilemmas:

Jane knows that chocolate is not a wise thing to eat, but she likes chocolate. Diabetic chocolate is expensive, and doesn't taste so good, so she secretly eats ordinary chocolate . . . (Cole, 1990)

Here she is making a choice, but is it an informed choice? Does Jane really understand the consequences of her choices or what 'coma' really means? In such a situation, it is all too easy to conclude that the client cannot cope independently and therefore start to deny her some of that independence.

People with learning disabilities experience problems in recognizing, retaining and retrieving information. As Drumm and Schade (1986) have written: 'Some of the prerequisite skills called upon for adherence to diabetes programmes, and taken for granted by the health care professional, are the ability to integrate information into meaningful concepts, to sequence, to remember and retrieve information, to problem-solve and reason beyond immediate conditions'. These cannot be taken for granted when trying to teach people with learning disabilities the skills of dietary self-management.

Rather than outlining the successes in teaching her client dietary self-management, Cole (1990) outlines three important requirements for teaching people to manage their own 'special' diets:

1. Education programmes must be designed to develop learning at a pace suitable for the client (i.e. comprehension, choice, financial circumstances, etc.). A goal planning approach should involve an analysis of the knowledge and tasks to be learned in order to achieve the overall goal of dietary self-management.
2. Verbal and written information should be given in language and form that is understandable and relevant to each individual's experience of life (i.e. braille may be appropriate for partially sighted clients; written information might be a useful reminder for care staff to read out to the client if the client cannot read, etc.). Signs such as those found in pictorial cookery books for adults may also be helpful (Day and Hollins, 1985). Reminder cards showing appropriate foods which may be easily carried by the person to the shops may help in the recall of information.

3. Everyone in the support network needs to be educated in the dietary needs of everyone requiring a 'special' diet.

A TREATMENT APPROACH TO CHRONIC VOMITING

Rumination, regurgitation and vomiting are all terms used to describe processes in which food is 'manoeuvred' by the individual. **Vomiting** usually implies that regurgitated matter is immediately ejected from the mouth; **rumination** usually implies that it is retained in the mouth for a while and then either re-swallowed, allowed to run out of the mouth or ejected. **Regurgitation** is the process whereby previously swallowed matter is returned to the mouth. These are all processes that can be seen in some disorders of feeding (and eating) in people with learning disabilities.

Behavioural management of food regurgitation in children who have learning disabilities has received little systematic attention. Temporary suppression of self-induced vomiting has been demonstrated by Becker, Turner and Sajwaj (1978) and Hogg (1982) who used lemon juice as an aversive stimulus. Other methods have included collaborative approaches involving parents, clinical psychologists and community nurses in agreeing to verbal contracts for behavioural treatment programmes (Hewitt and Burden, 1984).

Chronic vomiting has been defined as the 'bringing up of food without nausea, retching or disgust. The food is then ejected from the mouth . . . or re-swallowed' (Kanner, 1972). It is a severe problem in 5.3% of people with learning disabilities living in institutions (Ball *et al.*, 1974). In addition to medical side effects such as dehydration and weight loss, the practice is repulsive to observers and reduces social contact.

There is usually no organic cause for the vomiting (Hinds and Oliver, 1985). Behavioural studies have shown that its frequency may be varied by altering its social or stimulatory effects (Wolf *et al.*, 1966; Smeets, 1970). In some people, it has been shown that vomiting increases if it results in them being given attention or tangible rewards (i.e. positive reinforcement). In others, it increases if it results in them avoiding an undesirable event (i.e. negative reinforcement). For some people, vomiting is self-stimulatory (the stimulation being a positive reinforcement). Hinds and Oliver (1985) conclude that the persistence and frequency of vomiting, therefore, is influenced by its effectiveness as a means of gaining reinforcer(s).

It is important to establish the function of each person's vomiting behaviour as different functions suggest different treatments (Hinds and Oliver, 1985). If vomiting is maintained by social attention alone (positive reinforcement) then removal of attention resulting from vomiting should reduce the frequency of behaviour (extinction). However, if vomiting is maintained by the removal of demands or tasks (negative reinforcement), removing attention resulting from vomiting would be inappropriate as it would lead to an increase in the behaviour as the demand or task would also be removed (Wolf *et al.*, 1966). Extinction in this case would mean continuation of the task, as the reinforcer (task removal) is not given (Hinds and Oliver, 1985). If vomiting is maintained by the stimulation it provides, this should be reduced if possible, perhaps by feeding with bland and/or textureless foods. It can be seen from these examples that there is no single method of treatment. The treatment chosen for each person will need to be determined according to the function of that person's vomiting behaviour.

Once a function of vomiting has been determined, treatment selection is a logical process (Hinds and Oliver, 1985). Vomiting which is maintained by attention can be modified by giving no attention following vomiting (Smeets, 1970). Vomiting maintained by the removal of demands can be modified by the continued presentation of the demands (Wolf *et al.*, 1966). Vomiting maintained by stimulation can be treated by reducing the resultant stimulation or providing alternative forms of stimulation. For example, other forms of stimulation providing a sensation similar to that of vomitus held in the mouth, such as mouth play and finger feeding, may reduce the frequency of vomiting. Satiation and small feeds given at short, regular intervals have also been used to good effect (Libby and Phillips, 1979).

Where vomiting has elicited a reduction in demands or increased attention, it is crucial to replace it with another, more appropriate behaviour if it is not to recur. The persistence of a person's vomiting testifies to success in achieving its purpose. Reinforcement of alternative behaviours is therefore essential (Hinds and Oliver, 1985). Ideally these behaviours should be incompatible with vomiting and should also satisfy the function (attention, stimulation or reduced demands) that vomiting previously served.

Hinds and Oliver (1985) comment that in severe cases (though not defined by them) punitive methods may be necessary, such as overcorrection, time out, aversive tastes and smells and electric shocks, but these should only be used after the logical treatments have failed. However, the use of these methods is debatable on ethical grounds and Hinds and Oliver (1985) do not state the relative successes of these suggested interventions (Rapoff, Altman and Christophersen (1980) have discussed a method of determining the least restrictive procedure). It would seem that aversive tastes have become more common in treatment, presumably because they are quick and efficient, but they may not be necessary if a careful functional analysis is conducted before trying logical, adaptable treatment procedures. Davis and Curo (1980), in a review of treatment procedures, mentioned very few treatments that included a functional analysis of the behaviour preceding treatment and treatments using aversive techniques seemed to appear more commonly than necessary or appropriate.

Hinds and Oliver (1985) reported that sometimes there was no appreciable decline in vomiting in spite of clinical intervention. They provided several reasons for such apparent treatment 'failures': the functional analysis of the behaviour may have been incorrect or insensitive, or some functions of the behaviour may have been unrecognized so that the treatment strategy may not always have been appropriate. For example, if exclusionary time out (the procedure which effectively reduces demands whilst it is being carried out) is indiscriminately applied to vomiting previously negatively reinforced by demand reduction, it may increase the frequency of vomiting by acting as a positive reinforcer. If aversive tastes and smells are to be used it must be ensured that they are disliked by the person concerned as not all are aversive to everyone. Hinds and Oliver (1985) conclude that in devising extinction programmes, the long reinforcement history of the behaviour and its power to naturally elicit attention, demand reduction or stimulation must be remembered.

DIETARY INTERVENTION AND LOW WEIGHT GAIN

There have been numerous articles on planning diets for obese people and advice written on how we should select foods and prepare them for consumption. There has been less written on how people with learning disabilities cope with these choices (Cole, 1990) despite the philosophy of normalization (Wolfensberger, 1972) and past policies of care (DHSS, 1981) which have seen many people with learning disabilities achieve increased independence through moves to ordinary housing.

In the past, researchers have tended to focus on problems with managing clients' behaviour in 'long-stay' or residential institutions; these have typically included strategies for coping with food regurgitation (Hewitt and Burden, 1984), chronic vomiting (Hinds and Oliver, 1985) or the effects of caloric level (Johnston *et al.*, 1991) and food consistency on ruminative behaviour (Johnston *et al.*, 1990; Greene *et al.*, 1991). There has been little reported on exclusion diets for people with learning disabilities (Oliver, 1986) or the prevalence of eating disorders in this population. Part of the reason may be because of the wide range of disabilities that are included in the definition of 'learning disability'. Also, there is sometimes a confusing picture presented when other psychiatric illnesses are present. There is no doubt that this area of research is justifiable if only to enable the provision of appropriate care and treatment for these people. Clearly there is a need for further clinical investigation especially since it seems that our Western culture is already beginning another wave of fashionable diets and healthy living.

In the Thompson, Smith and Muir (1992) study, a number of referrals had been received by the Department of Nutrition and Dietetics requiring dietary intervention for clients with a range of learning disabilities on wards in Lynebank Hospital, Dunfermline, Scotland. The senior dietitian was involved with advising nursing staff and in compiling diet plans for these clients. Apart from overcoming some of the difficulties of standard hospital procedures (such as diet substitutes* being issued on the ward by nursing staff rather than by a designated diet kitchen), these clients had gained very little weight, despite dietary intervention.

---

* The term 'diet substitute' has been used to mean a 'nutritional supplement' that is given in place of foodstuffs where the client is unable to consume certain foods, for example, because of a difficulty in chewing or swallowing. Supplements such as 'vitamin supplements' are those given in addition to the diet in order to provide the client with the total dietary requirement.

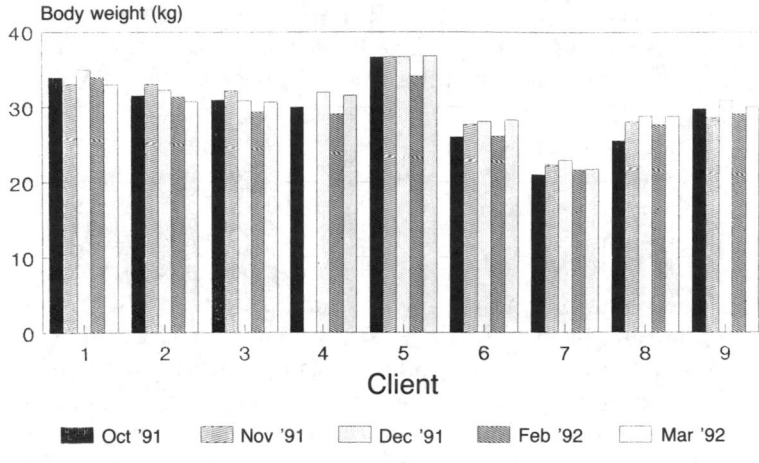

Missing data: Nov '91 (C4); Jan '92

Figure 10.2 Weight change in clients over a 6-month period.

Investigation into apparent small weight gain following dietary intervention

Screening Questionnaire
(Information to be collected from nurses' notes, medical notes and nursing staff).

Client's name: _____   Nursing staff _____

Grade _____

1. To what extent is the client dependent on nursing staff for feeding?

_____

2. What medication does the client receive? Does any of this affect appetite or cause the patient to vomit, or have bowel disturbance in any way?

_____

3. What are the times of the client's meals? (Is the client the first person to be fed, etc.?)

_____

4. When does the client receive snacks? (times)

_____

5. Details of past personal/medical history relevant to eating/feeding? (History of disorders?)

_____

Figure 10.3 Screening questionnaire.

6. Any observations/comments that the nursing staff have made concerning the client's behaviour before, after or during mealtimes?

_____

7. What is the client's ability to respond/comprehend to requests made by nursing staff?

_____

8. Any language/special disabilities?

_____

9. Does the client have any physical disabilities or disfigurements that make *independent* feeding difficult?

_____

10. Any previous involvement of the client with speech therapy or physiotherapy? (Specify with dates)

_____

11. Staff–client ratio on ward during mealtimes

_____

12. Client's daytime activities (am/pm)?

Mon	Tue	Wed	Thu	Fri	Sat	Sun

13. Client's diagnosis (borderline learning disability; mild; moderate; severe; profound; unspecified)?

_____

14. Specific syndrome (Down's; autism; prenatal; perinatal; postnatal; not known)?

_____

15. Length of hospitalization?

_____

Figure 10.3 *Continued*

A collaborative project was set up with the Department of Nutrition and Dietetics and the Department of Clinical Psychology to investigate diet- and weight-related issues with these clients. In addition, an examination was made of staff–client ratios and clients' behaviour before, during and after mealtimes on the hospital ward.

Ten clients (aged 26–59 years; average 35 years; mode 32 years) from the Special Needs ward were selected from referrals to the hospital dietitian. All of these clients had been reported by nursing staff as having low body weight and little or no weight gain over a six month period (Figure 10.2). The first step was to collect as much information as possible about these clients from nursing and medical notes and also directly from the care staff on the ward. This was achieved in a systematic way by designing a simple 'screening' questionnaire which would hopefully reveal relevant or important information about each client (Figure 10.3). The questionnaire was completed by a clinical psychologist and a nurse, the latter being a person who was presently working with and who had knowledge of the particular client in question. Reference to medical and nursing notes was made during the completion of this questionnaire so that information concerning past personal or medical history could be accurately recorded.

Investigation into apparent small weight gain following dietary intervention

Today's date:

Times of observations:

Name of client:

Name of meal:

Name of observer:

What does it comprise:

Drinks:

Location of observation:

Staff-to-client ratio at this mealtime:

Figure 10.4 Checklist of behaviours observed at mealtimes.

Checklist	Description/comments
1. Behaviour during 5 minutes prior to feeding session?	
2. Amount of time client is left on own?	
3. Does client attempt to feed self whilst left on own (or when being helped)? Specify	*Whilst being helped*: *Left alone (Is food available?)*:
4. Quantity (¼ segments/ ¼ cupfuls) of food *and* drink remaining at end of feeding session?	*Food*: *Drink*:
5. Quantity (¼ segments/ ¼ cupfuls) of food *and* drink discarded (eg on floor; removed by staff; left on table) at end of feeding session?	*Food*: *Drink*:
6. Duration of client's feeding session?	
7. Behaviour during 5 minutes after feeding session? (eg self-induced vomiting; visits toilet)	
8. Any other behaviour observed before, during or after feeding session?	
Comments:	

Figure 10.4 *Continued*

The results of these questionnaires revealed that of the ten clients selected, three clients had severe learning disabilities and could not respond to requests by the nursing staff. The remaining seven clients had very little ability to respond to requests from nursing staff. In addition, all ten clients had no verbal communication skills. Although the results of the questionnaires were only used as a 'rough' guide to the abilities of these clients, they were useful in deciding which sorts of measures might be used best for investigating the problems faced. For example, since all of these clients had no spoken language, psychological tests that required a recognizable verbal response were not helpful. Likewise, it would have been difficult to know whether or not a client's response was by chance or was the appropriate response, if his or her comprehension of the task was in doubt. For these reasons, it was decided that direct observations of the clients would probably be the only reliable measures of their abilities.

A checklist was devised (Figures 10.4 and 10.5) to help with these observations which were made at mealtimes on a number of occasions. In addition, a task analysis was produced from initial observations of clients on the ward of a typical sequence of feeding behaviour (Figure 10.6). This allowed the observer to assess the degree of independence/dependence the client exhibited at mealtimes. Note was taken of the fact that some clients had never been given the opportunity to learn an appropriate sequence of feeding behaviour and therefore, these observations were not necessarily an accurate reflection of their abilities, but rather of their current behaviour in these feeding situations. Consideration was also given to clients who had a history of a longstanding problem with maintaining their correct body weight or who had other related medical conditions affecting weight gain – see Figures 10.7 and 10.8.

Each client was observed by two psychologists, discreetly seated in parts of the ward out of sight of the client during mealtimes. Eighteen lunchtime meals were observed (two for each client) over a 4-week period by each observer – sometimes simultaneously so that inter-observer reliability could be assessed (Figure 10.9). During a further 4-week period, nine breakfasts, nine dinners and nine snacks were observed for each client. Data from mid-afternoon snacks and following meals (e.g. evidence of self-induced vomiting; visits to the

Client's name: [   ]   Today's date: [   ]

Type of meal
(i.e. breakfast, lunch,   [   ]   Time of meal: [   ]
dinner, snack):   am/pm

What does the meal comprise? | Food: |
(include any *diet supplements*) | Drink: |
                                  | Diet supplements: |

Please indicate, as accurately as possible, the following information for this client by *shading areas* on the diagrams of *food bowls* and *drinking cups* below:

1. How much food remains
   (i.e. uneaten) at end of meal?

2. How much food was discarded
   (i.e. on floor; regurgitated; etc.)?

3. How much drink remains
   (i.e. not drunk) at end of meal?

4. How much drink was discarded
   (i.e. on floor; spilt; regurgitated; etc.)?

5. Did the client visit the toilet (or become incontinent), vomit, regurgitate or eject any food or drink *after* the meal? Please give details:

Figure 10.5 Assessment of client's food/drink intake.

toilet; amount of food discarded; etc.) were recorded by nursing staff. In addition, the dietitian weighted all of the clients at monthly intervals over the study period in order to monitor weight gain or loss. Clients' heights and skinfold thicknesses at standardized sites were also recorded each month using skinfold calipers and clients' dietary intake was accurately weighed by the dietitian. Unfortunately, one of these clients had sustained a tibial fracture and due to difficulties on the ward for weighing her, information concerning body weight

Check on sequence of behaviour	Requires verbal prompt? yes/no	(Specify if *yes*)	Requires physical prompt? yes/no
1. Reaches out hand towards spoon on table			
2. Grips handle of spoon			
3. Raises spoon above table			
4. Moves spoon to dish			
5. Scoops up food in dish with spoon			
6. Moves spoon towards mouth			
7. Opens mouth			
8. Moves spoon into mouth			
9. Closes mouth over spoon			
10. Withdraws spoon from mouth			
11. Moves spoon towards dish			
12. Go to *5* or *13*			
13. Places spoon in dish			
14. Releases grip around handle of spoon			
15. Withdraws hand from spoon			

Figure 10.6 Task analysis of feeding behaviour.

(Specify if *yes*)	Action achieved successfully? yes/no	(Specify if *no*)	Food on spoon? yes/no	(Specify)

Client	Diet supplement/medication	Qty/dosage
C1	Carbamazepine tabs	500 mg
	Gaviscon liq.	10 ml
C2	Algicon liq.	10 ml
	Multivitamin caps	–
	Pirenzepine tabs	50 mg
	Thioridazine syrup	25 ml
C3	Haloperidol tabs	3 mg
	Procyclidine tabs	7.5 mg
C4	Acetazolamide	250 mg
	Carbamazepine	800 mg
	Fersamal syrup	140 ml
	Ketovite liq.	5 ml
	Ketovite tabs	–
	Lactulose	15 ml
	Vigabatrin tabs	2 g
C5	Carbamazepine liq.	4 ml
	Carbamazepine liq.	6 ml
C6	Carbamazepine tabs	400 mg
	Diazepam tabs	10 mg
	Gaviscon liq.	10 ml
	Pirenzepine tabs.	50 mg
C7	None	–
C8	Gaviscon liq.	10 ml
	Haloperidol tabs	3 mg
	Multivitamin tabs	–
	Pirenzepine tabs	50 mg
	Procyclidine tabs	5 mg
	Ranitidine tabs	150 mg
C9	Dicyclomine	10 mg
	Fybogel liq.	5 ml
	Lactulose	10 ml

KEY: b.d. = twice/day; t.d. = thrice/day; q.d. = four times/day; nocte = night-time; P.R.N. = as required; liq. = liquid; tabs = tablets.

Figure 10.7 Diet supplements and medication administered to clients.

Administration	Reason/description
b.d.	Anticonvulsant
After meals t.d.	Reflux oesophagitis
After meals q.d.	Reflux oesophagitis
Once/daily	Vitamins
Before meals b.d.	Gastric, duodenal ulceration
t.d.	Neuroleptic (tranquillizer)
t.d.	Choreographic movements
t.d.	Parkinsonian symptoms
b.d.	Reduce intra-occular pressure
b.d.	Anticonvulsant
b.d.	Iron
Once/daily	Vitamins
t.d.	Vitamins
P.R.N.	Constipation
b.d.	Anticonvulsant
a.m.	Anticonvulsant
Nocte	Anticonvulsant
Once/daily	Anticonvulsant
P.R.N.	Neuroleptic (tranquillizer)
After meals t.d.	Reflux oesophagitis
Before meals b.d.	Gastric, duodenal ulceration
—	—
After meals t.d.	Reflux oesophagitis
t.d.	Choreographic movements
b.d.	Vitamins
Before meals b.d	Reflux oesophagitis
b.d.	Parkinsonian symptoms
b.d.	Peptic ulcer
P.R.N.	Gastrointestinal distress
b.d.	Constipation
b.d.	Constipation

Client	(Q.5) History relevant to eating/feeding – from nursing/medical notes
C1	Feeding 'problems' during childhood.
C2, C3, C4, C5, C9	No eating/feeding disorders/difficulties noted.
C6	Gastrointestinal disturbance; 'habitual vomiter'; past history of chronic ricketts.
C7	Swallows air by keeping mouth wide open during feeding; history of very low body weight; distended gut; difficulties in chewing due to teeth extracted because of severe dental caries during early adulthood.
C8	Gastro-oesophageal reflux during feeding.

Figure 10.8 Clients' relevant past medical histories.

was not recorded at regular intervals. Therefore, data from the remaining nine clients were considered.

There were six set times of meals throughout the day: breakfast (08:00 am); mid-morning snack (10:00 am); lunch (12:00 pm); mid-afternoon snack (02:00 pm); dinner (05:00 pm); evening snack (07:00 pm). Snack time was used by nursing staff for the issue of 'puddings' and diet substitutes not previously issued at other mealtimes. The order in which clients were fed varied but generally the same nursing assistant or volunteer fed the same clients, except when the staff–client ratio was particularly low on the ward. However, qualified nursing staff were apparently randomly allocated to feed individual clients.

Results of using the task analysis of feeding behaviour showed that all nine clients observed were totally dependent on staff for feeding. The reliability of observers' observations was judged by three independent raters who were naïve to the study. Findings showed an overall 52.9% agreement in observers' descriptions of clients' behaviour (Figure 10.10). However, observers' agreement in ward observations of clients' food and drink intake was much higher (87.5%), making an overall agreement in 70.2% of observations. Data from mealtime observations of clients (main meals and mid-afternoon snack) can be seen in Figure 10.11. In general terms, the duration of meals was often less than ten minutes; clients seldom

Listed below are some descriptions of clients' behaviour during mealtimes. There are two sets of descriptions, one from each observer. Using your judgement, on a scale (1 to 4) please indicate how you judge the two sets of descriptions.

For example, if you judge them to be *exactly the same as each other*, then they should both give you the same picture of the behaviour that is observed. On the other hand, if each of them provides you with completely different pictures of the behaviour being observed, then you should judge them to be *completely different from each other*.

Alternatively, you may judge them to be *nearly the same as each other*, *rather different to each other*, or *'don't know'*.

Here is the scale to be used:

0 = don't know
1 = *exactly* the same as each other
2 = *nearly* the same as each other
3 = *rather* different to each other
4 = *completely* different to each other

Client: E2

Item No.	Description 1	Description 2	Your judgement (0, 1, 2, 3, 4)
1	Waiting in dining area – stereotyped circling around. Tongue out. Hanging onto staff. Sitting.	Moves around in circles continually around waiting/serving hatch area.	
2	Sitting in chair – tongue out. Hair being pulled but does not retaliate or move away.	Sits on own in chair – sticks tongue out, rocks. Hair pulled but does nothing in response.	
3	Later on was again hanging onto staff at hatch area as if looking for more food or perhaps a drink. Not independent feeder. Tongue remains out while eating – sucks air?	Sticks out tongue frequently. Sucking in air apparently.	

Figure 10.9 Questionnaire for rating inter-observer reliability.

attempted to 'finger feed' themselves if they were left on their own with food and the 'offending' mealtimes when some clients did not consume all of the food were at lunch and dinner. Snacks were considered to be the most successful in terms of

No. of observations rated	Rater 1 (%)	Rater 2 (%)	Rater 3 (%)	Mean (%)
In agreement (pt. 1 or 2)	4 (57)	5 (71)	2 (29)	3.7 (52.9)
In disagreement (pt. 3 or 4)	3 (43)	2 (29)	5 (71)	3.3 (47.1)
Too difficult to rate (pt. 0)	0 (0)	0 (0)	0 (0)	0.0 (0.0)
Total observed simultaneously by the two observers	7 (100)	7 (100)	7 (100)	7 (100)

Figure 10.10 Inter-observer reliability ratings.

intakes of diet substitutes (that were offered to the clients) and breakfasts were the most successful for foods; all meals had poor records for clients' intakes of drinks. Generally, clients were thought to receive little fluid throughout the day.

From clients' anthropometric measurements (i.e. Body Mass Index (BMI; see Garrow, 1988) and skinfold thicknesses) which can be seen in Figures 10.12–10.14, four out of nine clients had slight decreases in their BMIs over the study period. These were all below 'normal', i.e. 20 (although this figure may be much lower considering clients' low muscle mass). Slight decreases in skinfold thicknesses were also found.

A number of dependent variables were thought to influence clients' food and drink intake: liquidized versus non-liquidized food; texture, consistency and taste of food; speed with which the client was fed; whether or not the diet substitute was palatable; clients' dietary preferences; medical and psychological factors, such as oesophagitis, gastro-oesophageal reflux (Richter, 1992), swings in mood, etc. Medication was also considered to affect clients' appetites in some cases. Whilst it was very evident that there was a high standard of medical care for these clients, there was still a need to address such issues as the appearance and palatability of foods and diet substitutes. Sometimes a useful measure is whether or not the feeder is also willing to eat what is being offered to the client! The following recommendations were made for each client:

1. Re-assess client's requirements for feeding (e.g. speed of feeding; consideration of dysphagia or gastro-oesophageal reflux, referral to speech therapy, etc.).
2. Design a programme to determine, as far as possible, client's

Client		Mean duration of meal (mins)	Behaviour (Active/Passive) 5 mins		Mean time left on own (mins)	Attempt to feed on own or whilst being helped	Amount of food (0.25 segments) remaining	Amount of food (0.25 segments) discarded	Amount of drink (0.25 cupfuls) remaining	Amount of drink (0.25 cupfuls) discarded
			Before	After						
C1	Breakfast	6	Active	Active	0	No	0.00	0.00	0.00	0.00
	Lunch	5	Passive	Passive	0	No	0.00	0.00	0.25	<0.25
	Dinner	12	Active	Passive	0	No	0.00	<0.25	0.25	<0.50
C2	Breakfast	7	Active	Active	0	No	0.00	0.00	0.00	0.00
	Lunch	5	Active	Active	0	No	0.00	0.00	0.00	0.00
	Dinner	7	Active	Active	0	No	0.00	0.00	0.00	<0.25
C3	Breakfast	4	Passive	Active	0	No	0.00	0.00	0.00	0.00
	Lunch	7	Passive	Passive	0	No	>0.75	<0.25	>0.75	<0.25
	Dinner	10	Passive	Passive	0	Yes (helped) food	0.00	<0.25	0.00	0.00
C4	Breakfast	4	Active	Active	0	No	0.00	0.00	<0.25	<0.25
	Lunch	7	Passive	Passive	2	No	>0.75	<0.25	0.50	<0.25
	Dinner	17	Passive	Active	10	Yes (helped+own) food	>0.75	0.00	0.00	0.00
C5	Breakfast	8	Passive	Active	0	No	0.00	0.00	0.00	0.00
	Lunch	8	Passive	Passive	1	No	0.00	0.00	0.00	0.00
	Dinner	10	Passive	Passive	0	No	0.00	<0.25	0.00	<0.25
C6	Breakfast	5	Active	Active	1	No	0.00	0.00	<0.25	<0.25
	Lunch	7	Passive	Passive	0	No	0.00	0.00	<0.25	<0.25
	Dinner	5	Active	Active	0	Yes (own) drink	0.00	<0.25	0.00	<0.25
C7	Breakfast	6	Active	Active	0	No	0.00	0.00	<0.25	<0.25
	Lunch	12	Active	Active	1	No	>0.75	<0.25	<0.25	0.25
	Dinner	10	Passive	Passive	0	No	0.00	<0.25	0.00	0.00
C8	Breakfast	6	Active	Active	0	No	0.00	0.00	0.00	0.00
	Lunch	12	Passive	Active	2	No	0.00	<0.25	0.00	<0.25
	Dinner	10	Passive	Passive	0	No	0.00	<0.25	0.50	0.00
C9	Breakfast	12	Passive	Passive	0	No	0.00	0.00	<0.25	<0.25
	Lunch	14	Passive	Passive	1	No	<0.25	0.00	<0.25	<0.25
	Dinner	6	Passive	Passive	0	No	0.25	0.00	0.00	0.00

Figure 10.11 Results of mealtime observations of clients (mean values).

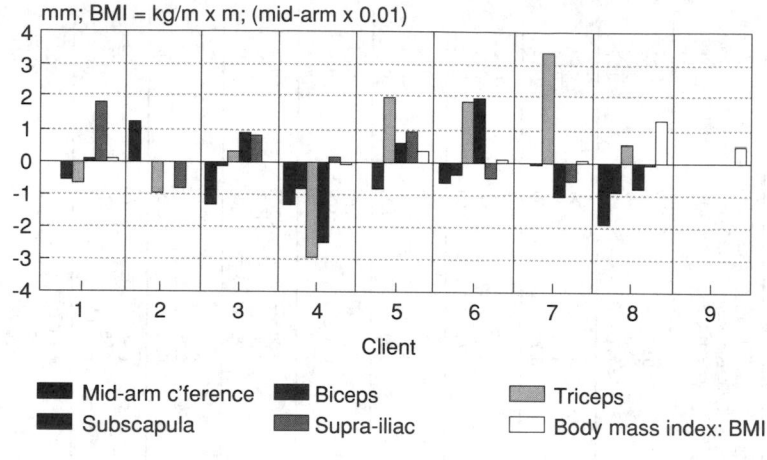

Figure 10.12 Clients' anthropometric measurements April 1992 to May 1992.

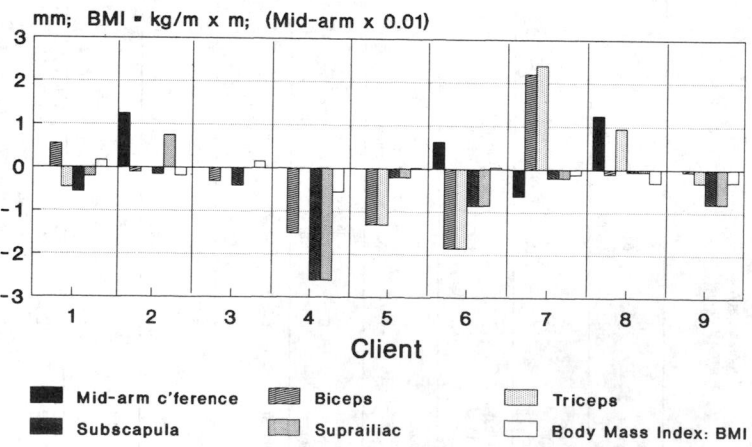

Figure 10.13 Clients' anthropometric measurements May 1992 to June 1992.

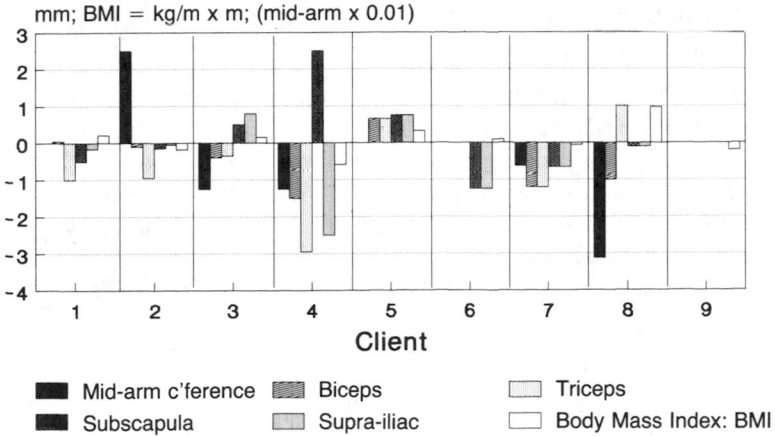

Figure 10.14 Clients' anthropometric measurements April 1992 to June 1992.

dietary preferences. (Care plans are already underway for all clients where types of specialized utensils, clients' posture and techniques for feeding are being addressed to ensure that there is a consistent approach to feeding each client.)

3. Monitor impact of issuing 'puddings' and diet substitutes at main mealtimes (i.e. breakfast, lunch, dinner) and issuing only biscuit(s) and tea (or other preferred drink) at mid-afternoon snack time.

4. Monitor adherence and accuracy of actual diets issued by catering and nursing staff (compared with the dietitian's recommendations of diets and substitutes).

5. Cease issue of diet substitutes for a period of time (e.g. one month) to see if this affects clients' weights, BMIs or food and drink intake. It is possible that the diet substitutes had become replacements for food rather than supplements in the clients' daily diets.

6. Examine clients' daytime activities in more detail with particular reference to energy expenditure, etc.

7. Continue to monitor clients' weight and skinfold thicknesses at monthly intervals.

The implementation of these recommendations would take several months to complete and would involve collaboration of the clinical psychologist, dietitian and nursing staff in a team approach to the issues raised. Following this programme, the authors envisaged a follow-up study to evaluate any gains from this research.

FURTHER READING

General

Best, A.B. (1987) *Steps to Independence: Practical Guidance on Teaching People with Mental and Sensory Handicaps*, BIMH Publications, Kidderminster.

Clarke, D. (1986) *Mentally Handicapped People: Living and Learning*, 2nd edn. Baillière Tindall, Eastbourne.

Giffin, J.C., Williams, D.F., Starke, M.P., Altmeyer, B.K. and Mason, M. (1986) Self-injurious behavior: A state-wide prevalence survey of the extent and circumstances. *Applied Research in Mental Retardation*, **7**(1), 105–16.

Gunn, M. (1986) Human rights and people with a mental handicap. *Mental Handicap*, **14**(3), 116–20.

Gunn, M. and Rosser, J. (1987) *Sex and the Law: A Brief Guide for Staff Working in the Mental Handicap Field (England and Wales only)*. Family Planning Association, London.

Harris, J. (1983) Citizen advocacy. *Mental Handicap*, **11**(4), 145–6.

Hogg, J. and Mittler, P. (1987) *Staff Training in Mental Handicap*. Croom Helm, London.

Jones, T.W. (1982) Treatment of behavior-related eating problems in retarded students: a review of the literature, in *Life-Threatening Behavior: Analysis and Intervention*, (eds J.H. Hollis and C.E. Meyers), AAMD, Washington DC, pp. 3–26.

Mental Health Act Commission (1985) *Mental Health Act 1983: Section 118: Draft Code of Practice*. Department of Health and Social Security, London.

Wolfensberger, W. (1972) *The Principle of Normalisation in Human Services*. National Institute on Mental Retardation, Toronto.

Obesity

Fox, R.A., Hartney, C.W., Rotatori, A.F. and Kurpiers, E.M. (1985) Incidence of obesity among retarded children. *Education and Training of the Mentally Retarded*, **20**(3), 175–81.

Fox, R.A., Switzky, H., Rotatori, A.F. and Vitkus, P. (1982) Successful weight loss techniques with mentally retarded children and youth. *Exceptional Children*, **49**(3), 238–44.

Page, T.J., Stanley, A.E., Richman, G.S., Deal, R.M. and Iwata, B.A. (1983) Reduction of food theft and maintenance of weight loss in a Prader Willi adult. *Journal of Behavior Therapy and Experimental Psychiatry*, **14**(3), 261–8.

Rotatori, A.F., Switzky, H.N. and Fox, R.A. (1983) Obesity in mentally retarded, psychiatric and non-handicapped individuals: A learning and biological disability, in *Advances in Learning and Behavioral Disabilities, Volume 2*, (eds K.D. Gadow and I. Bialer), JAI Press, Greenwich, Connecticut, pp. 135–78.

Whelan, E. and Speak, B.R. (1980) *Scale for Assessing Coping Skills*. Copewell Publications. Manchester.

Specific syndromes

Coupe, J., Barton, L., Barber, M., Collins, L., Levy, D. and Murphy, D. (1985) *Affective Education Assessment*. Manchester Education Committee (SERIS), Manchester.

Libby, J.D., Polloway, E.A. and Smith, J.D. (1983) Lesch-Nyan syndrome: A review. *Education and Training of the Mentally Retarded*, **18**(3), 226–31.

Page, T.J., Finney, J.W., Parrish, J.M. and Iwata, B.A. (1983) Assessment and reduction of food stealing in Prader Willi children. *Applied Research in Mental Retardation*, **4**(3), 219–28.

Palmer, S. and Horn, S. (1978) Feeding problems in children, in *Pediatric Nutrition in Developmental Disorders*, (eds S. Palmer and S. Ekval), Charles C. Thomas, Springfield, Illinois, pp. 107–29.

Utley, B.L., Halvoet, J.F. and Barnes, K. (1977) Handling, positioning and feeding the physically handicapped, in *Educational Programming for the Severely and Profoundly Handicapped*, (ed F. Sontag), Council for Exceptional Children, Reston, Virginia, pp. 279–99.

Richmond, G., Rugh, J.D., Dolfi, R. and Wasilewsky, J.W.

(1984) Survey of bruxism in an institutionalised mentally retarded population. *American Journal of Mental Deficiency*, **88**(4), 418–21.

Singh, N.N. and Bakker, L.W. (1984) Suppression of pica by overcorrection and physical restraint: A comparative study. *Journal of Autism and Developmental Disorders*, **14**(3), 331–41.

Wurtele, S.K., King, A.C. and Drabman, R.S. (1984) Treatment package to reduce SIB in a Lesch-Nyan patient. *Journal of Mental Deficiency*, **28**(3), 227–34.

Vomiting and scavenging behaviour

Foxx, R.M. and Martin, E.D. (1975) Treatment of scavenging behaviour (coprophagy and pica) by overcorrection. *Behaviour Research and Therapy*, **13**, 153–62.

Hinds, R. and Oliver, C. (1985) Chronic vomiting in people who are mentally handicapped. *Mental Handicap*, **13**(4), 152–4.

Jackson, G.M., Johnson, C.R., Ackron, G.S. and Crowley, R. (1975) Food satiation as a procedure to decelerate vomiting. *American Journal of Mental Deficiency*, **80**(2), 223–7.

Smith, A.L. Jr., Piersel, W.C., Philbeck, R.W. and Gross, E.J. (1983) The elimination of mealtime food stealing and scavenging behavior in an institutionalised severely mentally retarded adult. *Mental Retardation*, **21**(6), 255–9.

Assessment

Coupe, J., Aherne, P., Crawford, N. *et al.* (1987) *Assessment of Early Feeding and Drinking Skills.* Manchester Education Committee (SERIS), Manchester.

Hogg, J. and Raynes, N.V. (1987) *Assessment in Mental Handicap: A Guide to Assessment Practices and Checklists.* Croom Helm, London.

Shackelton-Bailey, M.J. (1980) *Hampshire Assessement for Living with Others.* Hampshire County Council, Winchester.

Types of treatment

Barrett, R.P. (1986) *Severe Behavior Disorders in the Mentally Retarded: Nondrug Approaches to Treatment.* Plenum Press, New York.

Gadow, K.D. and Poling, A.G. (1988) *Pharmacotherapy and Mental Retardation*. Taylor and Francis, London.

Glaser, B.A. and Morreau, L.E. (1986) Effects of interdisciplinary team review on the use of antipsychotic agents with severely and profoundly mentally retarded persons. *American Journal of Mental Deficiency*, **90**(4), 371–9.

Gunn, M. (1985) The law and mental handicap: 6. Consent to treatment. *Mental Handicap*, **13**(2), 70–2.

Hall, R.V. and Hall, M.C. (1980) *How to Use Planned Ignoring (Extinction)*. H and H Enterprises, Lawrence, Kansas.

McGee, J., Menolascino, F.J., Hobbs, D.C. and Menosek, P.E. (1987) *Gentle Teaching: A Non-Aversive Approach for Helping Persons with Mental Retardation*. Human Sciences Press, New York.

Thompson, S.B.N. (1990b) Talking about sex . . . .*Therapy Weekly*, **17**(13), 8.

Feeding

Crump, I.M. (1987) *Nutrition and Feeding of the Handicapped Child*. College Hill Press, Boston, Massachusetts.

Hewitt, K. and Burden, P. (1984) Behavioural management of food regurgitation: Parents and therapists. *Mental Handicap*, **12**(4), 168–9.

Lobato, D., Carlson, E.I. and Barrera, R.A. (1986) Modified satiation reducing ruminative behaviour without excessive weight gain. *Applied Research in Mental Retardation*, **7**(3), 337–47.

Morris, S.E. (1977) *Program Guidelines for Feeding Problems*. Childcraft Education Corporation, Edison, New Jersey.

O'Neil, P.M., White, J.L., King, C.R. Jr. and Carek, D.J. (1979) Controlling childhood rumination through differential reinforcement of other behavior. *Behavior Modification*, **3**(3), 355–72.

Rast, J., Johnston, J.M., Allen, J.E. and Drum, C. (1985) Effects of nutritional and mechanical properties of food on ruminative behavior. *Journal of Experimental Analysis of Behavior*, **44**(2), 195–206.

Rast, J., Johnston, J.M., Drum, C. and Conrin, J. (1981) The relation of food quantity to rumination behavior. *Journal of Applied Behavior Analysis*, **14**(2), 121–30.

Thompson, S.B.N. and Gittins, D.K. (1989a) Finding the right incentive. *Therapy Weekly*, **16**(18), 8.

Tierney, D. and Jackson, H.J. (1984) Psychosocial treatments of rumination disorder: A review of the literature. *Australian and New Zealand Journal of Developmental Disabilities*, **10**(2), 81–112.

Warner, J. (1981a) *Feeding Check List*. Winslow Press, Buckingham.

Warner, J. (1981b) *Helping the Handicapped Child with Early Feeding*. Winslow Press, Buckingham.

Outcome

Davis, W.B., Wieseler, N.A. and Hanzel, T.E. (1983) Reduction of rumination and out-of-seat behavior and generalization of treatment effects using a non-intrusive method. *Journal of Music Therapy*, **20**(3), 115–31.

Jackson, H.J. and Boag, P.G. (1981) The efficacy of self-control procedures as motivational strategies with mentally retarded persons: A review of the literature and guidelines for future research. *Australian Journal of Developmental Disabilities*, **7**(2), 65–79.

Matson, J.L. and McCartney, J.R. (1981) *Handbook of Behavior Modification with the Mentally Retarded*. Plenum Press, New York.

Palmer, S., Thompson, R.J. Jr. and Linscheid, T.R. (1975) Applied behavior analysis in the treatment of childhood feeding problems. *Developmental Medicine and Child Neurology*, **17**, 333–9.

Whitehead, W.E., Drescher, V.M., Morrill-Cobin, E. and Catalo, M.S. (1985) Rumination syndrome in children treated by increased holding. *Journal of Paediatric Gastroenterology and Nutrition*, **4**, 550–6.

Research

Ball, T.S., Hendricksen, H. and Clayton, J.A. (1974) A special feeding technique for chronic regurgitation. *American Journal of Mental Deficiency*, **78**(4), 486–93.

Cole, A. (1990) Teaching people how to manage their own 'special' diets: Some lessons from practice. *Mental Handicap*, **18**(4), 156–9.

Conrin, J., Pennypacker, H.S., Johnston, J. and Rast, J. (1982) Differential reinforcement of other behaviors to treat chronic rumination of mental retardates. *Journal of Behavior Therapy and Experiemental Psychiatry*, **13**(4), 325–9.

Friedin, B.D. and Johnson, H.K. (1979) Treatment of retarded child's faeces smearing and coprophagic behavior. *Journal of Mental Deficiency Research*, **23**(1), 55–61.

Hinds, R. and Oliver, C. (1985) Chronic vomiting in people who are mentally handicapped. *Mental Handicap*, **13**(4), 152–4.

Jackson, H.J. and King, N.J. (1982) The therapeutic management of an autistic child's phobia using laughter as the anxiety inhibitor. *Behavioural Psychotherapy*, **10**(4), 364–9.

Johnston, J.M., Greene, K.S., Rawal, A., Vazin, T. and Winston, M. (1991) Effects of caloric level on ruminating. *Journal of Applied Behavior Analysis*, **24**(3), 597–603.

Thompson, S.B.N. (1992b) Tips to trigger memory. *Therapy Weekly*, **19**(7), 7.

Thompson, S.B.N. and Gittins, D.K. (1989b) Using a pethna to increase the independence in feeding of a woman with profound mental handicap. *International Journal of Rehabilitation Research*, **12**(2), 204–7.

Thompson, S.B.N. and Muir, J. (1993) Monitoring behaviour, diet and anthropometric changes to explain low weight gain in clients with a severe learning disability. *British Journal of Developmental Disabilities*, **xxxix**, 1(76), 60–71.

Thompson, S.B.N., North, N.J. and Pentland, B. (1992) Clinical management of a man with complex partial seizures and a severe head injury. *Brain Injury*, **6**(3), 293–8.

Thompson, S.B.N., Smith, L. and Muir, J. (1992) The proof of the pudding. *Therapy Weekly*, **19**(16), 7.

Thompson, S.B.N. (1992d) Doubting dementia in Down's syndrome and other forms of learning disability? *The Psychologist*, (in press).

For further information on learning disabilities/mental handicap contact:

British Institute of Learning Disabilities, Stourport House, Foley Industrial Park, Stourport Road, Kidderminster, Worcestershire DY11 7QG.

How to eat a more healthy diet

Most dairy produce is high in fat, particularly full cream milk, cheese and whole milk yoghurt. Butter and margarine are almost pure fat. Butter and polyunsaturated margarine contain the same amount of fat and the same number of calories so there is no benefit in changing from one to the other. It is better to reduce your total fat intake. One way to cut down on fat is to use a low fat spread. The following is a useful guideline:

1 oz butter = 23 g fat = 210 cals
1 oz polyunsaturated margarine = 23 g fat = 210 cals
1 oz low fat spread = 11.5 g fat = 104 cals

Here are some useful tips on how to reduce fat in your diet:

1. Choose low fat milk, e.g. skimmed or semi-skimmed.
2. Avoid frying foods, grill or bake instead.
3. Use butter or margarine sparingly.
4. Eat reduced fat yoghurt and cheese.
5. Use natural yoghurt in preference to cream for savoury dishes.
6. Buy lean cuts of meat.
7. Remove visible fat before or after cooking.
8. Try meals using beans, lentils and peas.
9. Use more fish or chicken (without the skin).
10. Avoid, or eat only on special occasions, foods that are particularly high in fat such as: pastries, cakes, biscuits, salad cream, cheese spread, meat paste, peanut butter, toffee, chocolate, mayonnaise.

HOW TO EAT LESS SUGAR

Generally, about half the sugar we eat is from adding sugar to drinks, cereals, in puddings and baking. The remainder is from chocolate, sweets, fizzy drinks, jams, tinned fruit and sweetened breakfast cereals. We also take in sugar from some savoury foods such as tomato ketchups, baked beans, soups, sauces and pickles. Sugar is a major contributor to tooth decay, especially when eaten between meals. In particular, the following 'hidden' sugars may be found on food labels and can be avoided (or cut down): dextrose, fructose, glucose, lactose, maltose, sucrose, caramel, honey, molasses, treacle and syrup.

Here are some useful tips on how to reduce sugar in your diet:

1. Try sugar-free fizzy drinks and squashes, unsweetened fruit juices or even water with meals.
2. Cut down on sweets and chocolates. Avoid eating them between meals.
3. Eat unsweetened breakfast cereals preferably with higher fibre.
4. Eat plain biscuits.
5. Reduce or cut out sugar on cereals and in drinks. Sometimes sweeteners help but do not remove the tendency for a 'sweet tooth'.
6. Cut down the amount of sugar in favourite recipes.
7. Choose low sugar varieties of jams, baked beans and instant desserts.
8. Eat more sugar-free or low sugar snacks such as fresh fruit.
9. Use fruit tinned in natural juice in preference to syrup.
10. Keep special treats (like cakes) for special occasions only.

Here are some examples of how much sugar is in our foods:

Coke (1 can)	7 teaspoonfuls
Lucozade (1 sml bottle)	9 teaspoonfuls
Ribena (1 tablespoonful)	3.5 teaspoonfuls
Liquorice (4 oz sml box)	18 teaspoonfuls
Dolly mixtures (4 oz sml box)	20 teaspoonfuls
Mars bar (Fun size)	3 teaspoonfuls
Mars bar (Std size)	10 teaspoonfuls
Milk chocolate (Sml bar)	7 teaspoonfuls
Toffees (4 oz)	16 teaspoonfuls

Boiled sweets (4 oz) .... 20 teaspoonfuls
Chocolate biscuit (fully coated) .... 3 teaspoonfuls
Ice cream (Indiv. block) .... 1.5 teaspoonfuls
Jelly (average helping) .... 3 teaspoonfuls

HOW TO EAT LESS SALT

Too much salt may lead to high blood pressure which can lead to heart disease, stroke and kidney failure. Salt can also increase the amount of fluid retained by your body. Most of the salt we eat we add ourselves, both in cooking and at the table. Adding salt to your food becomes a habit. However, some foods are already very salty, e.g. bacon, cheese, smoked fish, canned meats such as gammon, tongue, corned beef. Canned vegetables also have salt added to them and so do many butters and margarines. Other products often eaten between meals also contain salt: crisps, nuts, salted crackers. Sea salt, although containing a few minerals, is still salt and should be cut down in your diet.

Here are some useful tips on how to reduce salt in your diet:

1. Reduce the amount of salty foods you eat. Look for fish canned in tomato juice for a change and cottage cheese instead of Cheddar, for example.
2. Use unsalted or slightly salted varieties of butter and margarine.
3. Use fewer stock cubes and meat extracts.
4. Avoid salted snacks such as crisps, salted nuts or peanut butter.
5. Choose crackers without a coating of salt.
6. Look for vegetables canned without added salt or use fresh or frozen vegetables.
7. Do not add salt to food at the table.
8. Cut down on salt in cooking.
9. Try using herbs and spices in preference to salt.
10. Try making meals that use spices instead of salt for their flavour, e.g. a vegetable curry.

HOW TO EAT MORE FIBRE

Fibre is the indigestible material in foods of plant origin. It is the outer covering of cereal grains and the edible skins and pips of fruit and vegetables. Fibre is passed through the body unchanged. It is undigested and provides bulk to keep our system working and our internal muscles functioning properly. The undigested fibre works like a sponge soaking up fluid, making the contents of the bowel softer and easier to pass, so preventing constipation. Some medical conditions are thought to be caused (or aggravated) by a lack of fibre in our diets: irritable bowel syndrome, constipation and gall stones. An increase in the fibre in your diet should also be accompanied with an adequate fluid intake, e.g. eight cups of fluid a day, and this change in diet should be made gradually over time to allow your digestive system to adapt to the change.

Here are some useful tips on how to eat more fibre in your diet:

1. Eat high fibre breakfast cereal, such as porridge, bran flakes, muesli.
2. Use wholemeal flour in baking. Start by using equal amounts of white and wholemeal flour in the recipe (e.g. for cakes, pastry, scones).
3. Eat wholemeal bread or, second best, granary or high fibre white bread.
4. Try wholemeal digestive or bran biscuits; wholemeal crackers, crispbreads and oatcakes.
5. Use wholemeal pasta.
6. Use brown rice instead of white rice.
7. Eat more potatoes with their skins, especially baked or boiled potatoes (but avoid chips and roast potatoes).
8. Eat raw vegetables and salads.
9. Eat fresh fruit (and the skins as well) or tinned fruits in natural juice.
10. Try meals based on beans, lentils and peas, or soups with wholemeal bread.

Here are some examples of how much fibre is in our foods:

1 slice wholemeal bread	2.5 g fibre
1 med. size jacket potato	5 g fibre
1 portion root vegetable (carrot)	2 g fibre
1 portion green vegetables	1.5 g fibre
1 piece of fruit (apple/orange)	2.5 g fibre
1 digestive biscuit	1 g fibre
1 Shredded Wheat	5 g fibre

2 Weetabix .... 5 g fibre
All-bran (average bowl) .... 11 g fibre
Bran flakes (average bowl) .... 4 g fibre
Muesli (average bowl) .... 5 g fibre
Cornflakes (average bowl) .... 1 g fibre
Porridge (average bowl) .... 2 g fibre

SOURCES OF IMPORTANT VITAMINS AND MINERALS

Vitamin/mineral	*Source*	*In the body*
Vitamin B complex:		
a) Vitamin B (thiamin)	Wholegrain cereals; nuts; meats; fish; pulses; yeast extract	Assists in breakdown of foods to give energy
b) Vitamin B_2 (riboflavin)	Liver; milk; eggs	
c) Vitamin B_{12} (folic acid)	Green vegetables; liver; meat; eggs; yeast extract	Blood formation
d) Nicotinic acid	Wholegrain cereals; meat; fish; liver; pulses	Efficient functioning of nervous system
Vitamin C	Citrus fruit; fruit juice; potatoes	Aids iron absorption; helps to combat infections, healing of wounds
Vitamin D	Oily fish (e.g. herring sardines, pilchards); eggs; yoghurt; some breakfast cereals; fortified margarines and evaporated milk	Maintains structure of bones and teeth
Calcium	Cheese; milk; yoghurt; fish; pulses; dark green vegetables	Maintains structure of bones and teeth
Iron	Liver; kidney; red meat; wholemeal bread; dried fruit	Formation of red blood cells

References

Abbey, S.E., Toner, B.B., Garfinkel, P.E., Kennedy, S.H. and Kaplan, A.S. (1990) Self-report symptoms that predict major depression in patients with prominent physical symptoms. *International Journal of Psychiatry and Medicine*, **20**(3), 247–58.

Abdallah, A.H., Roby, D.M., Boeckler, W.H. and Riley, C.C. (1976) Role of dopamine in the anorexigenic effect of DITA: Comparison with d-amphetamine. *European Journal of Pharmacology*, **40**, 39–44.

Abraham, S., Collins, C. and Nordsiech, M. (1960) Relationship of childhood weight status to morbidity in adults. *Health Report*, HMSO, London, 273–84.

Abraham, S. and Llewellyn-Jones, D. (1984) *Eating Disorders: The Facts*. Oxford University Press, Oxford.

Abramson, E.E. (1973) A review of behavioural approaches to weight control. *Behaviour Research and Therapy*, **11**, 547–56.

Agras, W.S. (1987) *Eating Disorders: Management of Obesity, Bulimia and Anorexia Nervosa*. Pergamon, Oxford.

Agras, W.S., Barlow, D.H., Chapin, H.N., Abel, G.G. and Leitenberg, H. (1974) Behaviour modification of anorexia nervosa. *Archives of General Psychiatry*, **30**, 279–86.

Agras, W.S. and Kraemer, H.C. (1983) The treatment of anorexia nervosa: Do different treatments have different outcomes? in *Eating and Its Disorders*, (eds A.J. Stunkard and E. Stellor), Raven, New York, pp. 286–302.

Ahola, S. (1982) Unexplained parotid enlargement. A clue to occult bulimia. *Connecticut Medicine*, **46**, 185–6.

Alden, J.F. (1977) Gastric and jejuno-ileal bypass. *Archives of Surgery*, **112**, 799.

Allen, G.S. (1977) A double blind clinical trial of diethylpropion hydrochloride, mazindol and placebo in the treatment of exogenous obesity. *Current Therapy and Research*, **22**, 678.

Allenbeck, P., Hallberg, D. and Espmark, S. (1976) Body image – an apparatus for measuring disturbances in estimation of size and shape. *Journal of Psychosomatic Research*, **20**, 583–9.

Altshuler, K.Z. and Weiner, M.F. (1985) Anorexia nervosa and depression: A dissenting view. *American Journal of Psychiatry*, **142**, 328–32.

Aman, M.G. (1985) Drugs in mental retardation: Treatment or strategy? *Australian and New Zealand Journal of Developmental Disabilities*, **10**(4), 215–26.

Aman, M.G. and Singh, N.N. (1983) Pharmacological intervention, in *Handbook of Mental Retardation*, (eds J.L. Matson and J.A. Mulick), Pergamon Press, New York, pp. 317–37.

American Psychiatric Association (1980) *Task Force on Nomenclature and Statistics. Diagnostic and Statistical Manual of Mental Disorders*, 3rd edn. American Psychiatric Association, Washington DC.

American Psychiatric Association (1987) *Diagnostic and Statistical Manual of Mental Disorders 69*, revised 3rd edn. American Psychiatric Association, Washington DC.

Andersen, A.E. and Mickalide, A.D. (1983) Anorexia nervosa in the male: An underdiagnosed disorder. *Psychosomatics*, **24**, 1066–75.

Andersen, A.E., Morse, C. and Santmeyer, K. (1984) Inpatient treatment for anorexia nervosa, in *Handbook of Psychotherapy for Anorexia Nervosa*, (eds D.M. Garner and P.E. Garfinkel), Guildford Press, New York, pp. 313–43.

Andersen, M.S. (1928) Insulin som understotteles-middel ved fedekure. *Ugeskr Laeger*, **90**, 1013–17.

Anderson, E.C. and Langham, W.H. (1959) Average potassium concentration of the human body as a function of age. *Science*, **130**, 713–14.

Andres, R. (1980) Effect of obesity on total mortality. *International Journal of Obesity*, **4**, 381–6.

Apfelbaum, M. (1987) The mechanisms of weight regulation, in *Body Weight Control. The Physiology, Clinical Treatment and Prevention of Obesity*, (eds A.E. Bender and L.J. Brookes), Churchill Livingstone, Edinburgh, pp. 26–35.

Army Individual Test Battery (1944) *Manual of Directions and*

Scoring. War Department, Adjutant General's Office, Washington DC.

Ashwell, M.A. and Etchell, L. (1974) Attitude of the individual to his own body weight. *British Journal of Preventive and Social Medicine*, **28**, 127–32.

Askevold, F. (1975) Measuring body image. *Psychotherapy and Psychosomatics*, **26**, 71–7.

Ayllon, T. (1963) Intensive treatment of psychotic behaviour by stimulus satiation and food reinforcement. *Behaviour Research and Therapy*, **1**, 53–61.

Azima, H., Lemieux, M. and Azima, F.J. (1962) Isolement sensoriel: Étude psychopathologique et psychoanalytique de la régression et du schema corporel. *Evolutions dans la Psychiatrie (Paris)*, **27**, 259–80.

Azrin, N.H. and Armstrong, P.M. (1973) The 'mini-meal' – a method for teaching eating skills to the profoundly retarded. *Mental Retardation*, **11**(1), 9–13.

Azrin, N.H., Jammer, J.P. and Besalel, V.A. (1986) Vomiting reduction by slower food intake. *Applied Research in Mental Retardation*, **7**(4), 409–13.

Bachrach, A.J., Erwin, W.J. and Mohr, J.P. (1965) The control of eating behavior in an anorexic by operant conditioning techniques, in *Case Studies in Behavior Modification*, (eds L.P. Ullman and L. Krasner), Holt, Rhinehart and Winston, New York, pp. 153–63.

Bacon, S.J. (1974) Arousal and the range of cue utilization. *Journal of Experimental Psychology*, **102**, 81.

Ball, T.S., Henricksen, H. and Clayton, J.A. (1974) A special feeding technique for chronic regurgitation. *American Journal of Mental Deficiency*, **78**(4), 486–93.

Barcai, A. (1977) Lithium in adult anorexia nervosa: A pilot report on two patients. *Acta Psychiatrica Scandinavica*, **55**, 97–101.

Bardwick, J. (1971) *Psychology of Women: A Study of Bio-Cultural Conflicts*. Harper and Row, New York.

Barry, V.C. and Klawans, H.L. (1976) On the role of dopamine in the pathophysiology of anorexia nervosa. *Journal of Neurotransmission*, **38**, 107–22.

Baxter, L.R., Phelps, M.E. and Mazziotta, J.C. (1987) Local cerebral glucose metabolic rates in obsessive–compulsive disorder. *Archives of General Psychiatry*, **44**, 211–18.

Beck, A.T. (1967) Depression: Clinical, Experimental and Theoretical Aspects. Harper and Row, New York.

Beck, A.T. (1976) Cognitive Therapy and the Emotional Disorders. International Universities Press, New York.

Beck, A.T., Rush, A.J., Shaw, B.F. and Emery, G. (1979) Cognitive Therapy for Depression: A Treatment Manual. Guildford Press, New York.

Beck, A.T., Ward, C., Mendelsohn, M., Mock, M. and Erbaugh, J. (1961) An inventory for measuring depression. Archives of General Psychiatry, 120, 561–71.

Becker, J.V., Turner, S.M. and Sajwaj, T.E. (1978) Multiple behavioral effects of the use of lemon juice with a ruminating toddler-aged child. Behavior Modification, 2, 267–78.

Beech, H.R. and Vaughan, M. (1978) Behavioural Treatment of Obsessional States. Wiley, London.

Behar, D., Rapoport, J.L. and Berg, L.J. (1984) Computerized tomography and neuropsychological test measures in adolescents with obsessive–compulsive disorder. American Journal of Psychiatry, 141, 363–8.

Bemis, K.M. (1978) Current approaches to the etiology and treatment of anorexia nervosa. Psychological Bulletin, 85, 593–617.

Benady, D.R. (1970) Cyproheptadine hydrochloride (periactin) and anorexia nervosa: A case report. British Journal of Psychiatry, 117, 681–2.

Bender, A.E. and Brookes, L.J. (1987) Body Weight Control. The Physiology, Clinical Treatment and Prevention of Obesity. Churchill Livingstone, Edinburgh.

Benn, R.J. (1971) Some mathematical properties of weight for height indices as measures of adiposity. British Journal of Preventive and Social Medicine, 25, 42–50.

Bennett, D. (1960) The body concept. Journal of Mental Science, 106, 56–75.

Benton, A.L. (1968) Differential behavioral effects in frontal lobe disease. Neuropsychologia, 6, 53–60.

Benton, A.L. and Hamsher, K. de S. (1976) Multilingual Aphasia Examination. University of Iowa, Iowa.

Benton, A.L., Hamsher, K. de S., Varney, N.R. and Spreen, O. (1983) Contributions to Neuropsychological Assessment. Oxford University Press, New York.

Ben Tovim, D.I., Walker, M.K., Fok, D. and Yapp, E. (1989)

An adaptation of the Stroop Test for measuring shape and food concerns in eating disorders: A quantitative measure of psychopathology? *International Journal of Eating Disorders*, **8**, 681.

Berg, E.A. (1948) A simple objective test for measuring flexibility in thinking. *Journal of General Psychology*, **39**, 15–22.

Berger, S. and Cohen, M. (1982) *The Southampton Diet*. Simon and Schuster, New York.

Bernard, J.L. (1968) Rapid treatment of gross obesity by operant techniques. *Psychological Reports*, **23**, 663–6.

Bernstein, I.C. (1972) Anorexia nervosa: 94-year-old woman treated with electroshock. *Minneapolis Medicine*, **55**, 552–3.

Berscheid, E., Walster, E. and Bohrnstedt, G. (1973) The happy American body: A survey report. *Psychology Today*, **November**, 119–23; 128–31.

Beumont, P.J.V. (1977) Further categorization of patients with anorexia nervosa. *Australian and New Zealand Journal of Psychiatry*, **11**, 223–6.

Beumont, P.J.V. (1985) Nutritional conselling in anorexia nervosa, in *Handbook of Eating Disorders*, (eds P.J.V. Beumont, G.D. Burrows and R. Casper), Elsevier, Amsterdam.

Beumont, P.J.V., Beardwood, C.J. and Russell, G.F.M. (1972) The occurrence of the syndrome of anorexia nervosa in male subjects. *Psychological Medicine*, **2**, 216–31.

Beumont, P.J.V., Burrows, G.D. and Casper, R.C. (1987) *Handbook of Eating Disorders. Part 1: Anorexia and Bulimia Nervosa*. Elsevier, Amsterdam.

Beumont, P.J.V., Chambers, T.L., Rouse, L. and Abraham, S.F. (1981) The diet composition and nutritional knowledge of patients with anorexia nervosa. *Journal of Human Nutrition*, **35**, 265–73.

Beumont, P.J.V., George, G.C.W. and Smart, D.E. (1976) Dieters, vomiters, and purgers in anorexia nervosa. *Psychological Medicine*, **6**, 617–22.

Bhanji, S. (1979) Anorexia nervosa: Physicians' and psychiatrists' opinions and practice. *Journal of Psychosomatic Research*, **23**, 7–11.

Bhanji, S. and Mattingly, D. (1988) *Medical Aspects of Anorexia Nervosa*. Wright, London.

Biederman, J., Herzog, D.B., Rivinus, T.M. *et al.* (1985) Amitriptyline in the treatment of anorexia nervosa: A double-blind placebo-controlled study. *Journal of Clinical Psychopharmacology*, **5**, 10–16.

Binder, L.M. (1982) Constructional strategies on complex figure drawings after unilateral brain damage. *Journal of Clinical Neuropsychology*, **4**, 51–8.

Björntorp, P. (1981) Adipocyte precursor cells, in *Recent Advances in Obesity Research*, (eds P. Björntorp, M. Cairella and A.N. Howard), John Libbey, London, p. 58.

Björntorp, P. (1983) The role of adipose tissue in human obesity, in *Obesity*, (ed M.R.C. Greenwood), Churchill Livingstone, New York, pp. 17–24.

Björntorp, P., Cairella, M. and Howard, A.N. (1981) *Recent Advances in Obesity Research*. John Libbey, London.

Bjurulf, P. (1959) Atherosclerosis and body build with special reference to size and number of subcutaneous fat cells. *Acta Medica Scandinavica (Supplement)*, 166.

Black, F.W. and Strub, R.L. (1976) Constructional apraxia in patients with discrete missile wounds of the brain. *Cortex*, **12**, 212–20.

Blackburn, I.M. and Davidson, K.M. (1990) *Cognitive Therapy for Depression and Anxiety: A Practitioner's Guide*. Blackwell, Oxford.

Bliss, E.L. and Hardin Branch, C.H. (1960) *Anorexia Nervosa: Its History, Psychology, and Biology*. Hoeber, New York.

Bloch, A. (1989) Questions by adolescents about dieting. *Harefuah*, **117**(12), 257–9.

Blonz, E.R. and Stern, J.S. (1981) Obesity and fat diets, in *Controversies in Nutrition*, (ed L. Ellenbogen), Churchill Livingstone, New York, pp. 105–24.

Bogen, J.E., DeZure, R., Tenhouten, W.D. and March, J.F. (1972) The other side of the brain IV: The A/P ratio. *Bulletin of the Los Angeles Neurological Societies*, **37**, 49–61.

Bond, D.D. (1949) Anorexia nervosa. *Rocky Mountain Medical Journal*, **46**, 1012–19.

Borgström, B. and Wollesen, C. (1981) Effect of fenfluramine and related compounds on the pancreatic colipase/lipase system. *FEBS Letters*, **126**, 25–8.

Borjeson, M. (1976) The aetiology of obesity in children. *Acta Paediatrica Scandinavica*, **65**, 279–87.

Borsini, F., Bendotti, C. and Carli, M. (1979) The roles of brain noradrenaline and dopamine in the anorectic activity of diethylpropion in rats: A comparison with d-amphetamine. *Research in Community Chemistry, Pathology and Pharmacology,* **26**, 3–11.

Boskind-Lodahl, M. (1976) Cinderella's stepsisters: A feminist perspective on anorexia nervosa and bulimia. *Signs,* **2**, 342–56.

Boskind-Lodahl, M. (1978) The definition and treatment of bulimarexia: The gorging/purging syndrome of young women. *Dissertation Abstracts International,* **38**, 717A.

Boskind-White, M. (1984) *Bulimarexia: The Binge/Purge Cycle.* W.W. Norton, London.

Bossert, S., Schnabel, E. and Krieg, J.C. (1989) Effects and limitations of cognitive behaviour therapy in bulimia in-patients. *Psychotherapy and Psychosomatics,* **51**(2), 77–82.

Boszormenyi-Nagy, I. and Spark, G. (1973) *Invisible Loyalties.* Harper and Row, New York.

Bowden, P.K., Touyz, S.W., Rodriguez, P.J., Hensley, R. and Beumont, P.J.V. (1989) Distorting patient or distorting instrument? Body shape disturbance in patients with anorexia nervosa and bulimia. *British Journal of Psychiatry,* **155**, 196–201.

Branch, C.H. and Eurman, L.J. (1980) Social attitudes toward patients with anorexia nervosa. *American Journal of Psychiatry,* **137**, 631–2.

Bray, G.A. (1976a) Definitions, measurements and classification of the syndromes of obesity. *International Journal of Obesity,* **2**, 99–112.

Bray, G.A. (1976b) *The Obese Patient. Major Problems in Internal Medicine, Volume 9.* W.B. Saunders, Philadelphia.

Bray, G.A. (1976c) The risks and disadvantages of obesity, in *The Obese Patient,* (ed G.A. Bray), W.B. Saunders, Philadelphia, pp. 215–50.

Bray, G.A. (1978) *Recent Advances in Obesity Research.* Newman, London.

Bray, G.A. (1983) The Prader Willi syndrome. A study of 40 patients and a review of the literature. *Medicine,* **62**, 59–80.

Bray, G.A. (1987) Factors leading to obesity: Physical (including metabolic) factors and disease states, in *Body Weight Control. The Physiology, Clinical Treatment and Prevention of Obesity,* (eds A.E. Bender and L.J. Brookes), Churchill Livingstone, Edinburgh, pp. 53–61.

Bray, G.A., Davidson, M.B. and Drenick, E.J. (1972) Obesity: A serious symptom. *Annals of Internal Medicine*, **77**, 779–95.

Bray, G.A. and York, D.A. (1971) Genetically transmitted obesity in rodents. *Physiological Reviews*, **51**, 598–646.

Bray, G.A. and York, D.A. (1979) Hypothalamic and genetic obesity in experimental animals. An automatic and endocrine hypothesis. *Physiological Reviews*, **59**, 719–809.

Brook, C.G.D., Huntley, R.M.C. and Slack, J. (1975) Influence of heredity and environment in determination of skinfold thickness in children. *British Medical Journal*, **2**, 1719–21.

Brook, C.G.D., Lloyd, J.K. and Wolf, O.H. (1972) Relation between age of onset of obesity and size and number of adipose cells. *British Medical Journal*, **2**, 25.

Brotman, A.W., Herzog, D.B. and Woods, S.W. (1984) Antidepressant treatment of bulimia: The relationship between bingeing and depressive symptomatology. *Journal of Clinical Psychiatry*, **45**, 7–9.

Bruch, H. (1957) *The Importance of Overweight*. W.W. Norton, New York.

Bruch, H. (1962) Perceptual and conceptual disturbances in anorexia nervosa. *Psychosomatic Medicine*, **24**, 187–94.

Bruch, H. (1965) Anorexia nervosa and its differential diagnosis. *Journal of Nervous and Mental Disorders*, **141**, 555.

Bruch, H. (1971) Anorexia nervosa in the male. *Psychosomatic Medicine*, **33**, 31–47.

Bruch, H. (1973) *Eating Disorders*. Basic Books, New York.

Bruch, H. (1975) Anorexia nervosa, in *American Handbook of Psychiatry Volume 4*, (ed M.F. Reiser), Basic Books, New York.

Bruch, H. (1977) Depressive factors in adolescent eating disorders, in *Phenomenology and Treatment of Depression*, (eds W.E. Fann, I. Karacan, A.D. Pokorny and R.L. Williams), Spectrum, New York, pp. 143–52.

Bruch, H. (1978) *The Golden Cage*. Open Books, London.

Bruch, H. (1979) Anorexia nervosa. *Key*, **7**, 60.

Bruch, H. (1980) Anorexia nervosa: Therapy and theory. *American Journal of Psychiatry*, **139**, 1531–8.

Brumberg, J.J. (1988) *Fasting Girls: The Emergence of Anorexia Nervosa as a Modern Disease*. Harvard University Press, Cambridge, Massachusetts.

Brunzell, J.D. and Miller, N.E. (1981) Atherosclerosis in

inherited and acquired disorders of plasma lipoprotein metabolism, in *Lipoproteins, Atherosclerosis and Coronary Heart Disease*, (eds N.E. Miller and B. Lewis), Elsevier, Amsterdam, pp. 73–88.

Bryce-Smith, D. (1986) Environmental chemical influences on behaviour and mentation. *Chemistry Society Review*, **15**, 99–123.

Bryce-Smith, D. and Simpson, R.I.D. (1984) Anorexia, depression, and zinc deficiency. *Lancet*, **ii**, 1162.

Butler, N. (1988) An overview of anorexia nervosa, in *Anorexia and Bulimia Nervosa*, (ed D. Scott), Croom Helm, London, pp. 3–23.

Button, E.J. (1985) Construing the anorexic, in *Personal Construct Theory and Mental Health: Theory, Research and Practice*, (ed E.J. Button), Croom Helm, London.

Button, E.J. and Whitehouse, A. (1981) Subclinical anorexia nervosa. *Psychological Medicine*, **11**, 509–16.

Buvat, J. and Buvat-Herbaut, M. (1977) La sexualité de l'anorectique mental(e). *Nouvelle Presse Medicale*, **6**, 859–61.

Buvat-Herbaut, M., Hebbinckuys, P., Lemaire, A. and Buvat, J. (1983) Attitudes towards weight, body image, eating, menstruation, pregnancy, and sexuality in 81 cases of anorexia compared with 288 normal control school girls. *International Journal of Eating Disorders*, **2**, 45–59.

Cabanac, M. (1971) Physiological role of pleasure. *Science*, **173**, 1103–7.

Cabanac, M. and Duclaux, R. (1970) Obesity: Absence of satiety aversion to sucrose. *Science*, **168**, 496–7.

Cairns, A., Shalet, S., Marshall, A.J. and Hartog, M. (1977) A comparison of phenformin and metformin in the treatment of maturity onset obese diabetes. *Diabete et Metabolisme*, **3**, 183.

Caldwell, P. (1991) Stimulating people with profound handicaps. How can we work together? *British Journal of Mental Subnormality*, **37**(73), 92–100.

Campbell, C.J., Bhalla, I.P., Steele, H.M. and Duncan, L.J.P. (1977) A controlled trial of phentermine in obese diabetic patients. *Practitioner*, **218**, 851.

Canning, H. and Mayer, J. (1966) Obesity – its possible effect on college acceptance. *New England Journal of Medicine*, **275**, 1171–4.

Carey, R.J. (1976) Effects of selective forebrain depletions of norepinephrine and serotonin on the activity and food intake effects of amphetamine and fenfluramine. *Pharmacology and Biochemistry of Behavior*, **5**, 519–23.

Carrier, J. (1939) *L'Annorexie Mentale*. Libraire E. François, Paris.

Caspary, W.F. (1978) Sucrose malabsorption in man after ingestion of alpha-glucosidehydrolase inhibitor. *Lancet*, **1**, 1231–3.

Casper, R.C. (1982) Treatment approaches in anorexia nervosa. *Adolescent Psychiatry*, **10**, 86–100.

Casper, R.C. (1983) On the emergence of bulimia nervosa as a syndrome: A historical view. *International Journal of Eating Disorders*, **2**, 3–16.

Casper, R.C., Eckert, E.D., Halmi, K.A. *et al.* (1980) Bulimia: Its incidence and clinical importance in patients with anorexia nervosa. *Archives of General Psychiatry*, **37**, 1030–5.

Casper, R.C., Offer, D. and Ostrov, E. (1981) The self-image of adolescents with acute anorexia nervosa. *Journal of Pediatrics*, **98**, 656–61.

Castelli, W.Y., Doyle, J.P., Gordon, T. *et al.* (1977) HDL cholesterol and other lipids in coronary heart disease – The Cooperative Lipoprotein Phenotyping Study. *Circulation*, **55**, 767–72.

Cautela, J.R. (1966) Treatment of compulsive behavior by covert sensitisation. *Psychological Records*, **16**, 33–41.

Cautela, J.R. (1967) Covert sensitisation. *Psychological Reports*, **20**, 459–68.

Cautela, J.R. (1972) The treatment of over-eating by covert conditioning. *Psychotherapy: Theory, Research and Practice*, **9**, 211–16.

Cesar, F.P., Leme, C.E., Ohnuma, L.Y., Palomino, C.R.P. and Wajchenberg, B.L. (1980) Mechanism of action of phenethylbiguanide (phenformin) in man. IV. Effect of phenethylbiguanide (PBG) on glucose tolerance and lactate dynamics in obese non-diabetic and chemical diabetic subjects. *Metabolism and Clinical Experimentation*, **29**, 270–8.

Chaitow, L. (1983) *Relaxation and Meditation Techniques*. Thorsons, London.

Channon, S., Helmsley, D. and de Silva, P. (1988) Selective processing of food words in anorexia nervosa. *British Journal of Clinical Psychology*, **27**, 259.

Chapman, J.M., Coulson, A.H., Clark, V.A. and Raymond, E. (1971) The differential effect of serum cholesterol, blood pressure and weight on the incidence of myocardial infarction and angina pectoris. *Journal of Chronic Diseases*, **23**, 631–45.

Charalambous, B.M., Webster, D.J.T. and Mir, M.A. (1984) Elevated skeletal muscle sodium-potassium-ATPase in human obesity. *Clinician Chemica Acta*, **141**, 189–95.

Chen, Y. and Silverstone, T. (1990) Lithium and weight gain. *International Clinical Psychopharmacology*, **5**(3), 217–25.

Clarke, B.F. and Campbell, I.W. (1977) Comparison of metformin and chlorpropamide in non obese, maturity onset diabetics uncontrolled by diet. *British Medical Journal*, **2**, 1576.

Clarke, M.G. and Palmer, R.L. (1983) Eating attitudes and neurotic symptoms in university students. *British Journal of Psychiatry*, **142**, 299–304.

Clineschmidt, B.V. (1979) MK-212: A serotonin-like agonist in the CNS. *General Pharmacology*, **10**, 287–90.

Clow, F.E. (1932) Anorexia nervosa. *New England Journal of Medicine*, **207**, 613–17.

Cobb, J. (1983) Behaviour therapy in phobic and obsessional disorders. *Psychiatric Developments*, **1**, 351–65.

Cohen, A.R. (1959) Some implications of self-esteem for social influence, in *Personality and Persuasibility*, (eds C.I. Hovland and I.L. Janis), Yale University Press, New Haven, pp. 102–20.

Cohen, E.A., Gelfand, D.M. and Dodd, D.K. (1980) Self-control practices associated with weight loss maintenance in children and adolescents. *Behavior Therapy*, **11**, 26–37.

Cole, A. (1990) Teaching people how to manage their own 'special' diets: Some lessons from practice. *Mental Handicap*, **18**(4), 156–9.

Collingwood, T.R. and Willett, L. (1971) The effects of physical training upon self-concept and body attitudes. *Journal of Clinical Psychology*, **27**, 411–12.

Comai, K. and Sullivan, A.C. (1980) Antiobesity activity of pluronic L-101. *International Journal of Obesity*, **4**, 33–42.

Comai, K., Triscari, J. and Sullivan, A.C. (1978) Comparative effects of amphetamine and fenfluramine on lipid biosynthesis and absorption in the rat. *Biochemistry and Pharmacology*, **27**, 1987–94.

Comstock, G.W. and Stone, R.W. (1972) Changes in body

weight and subcutaneous fatness related to smoking habits. *Archives of Environmental Health*, **24**, 271–6.

Connor-Greene, P. (1987) An educational group treatment program for bulimia. *Journal of the American College of Health*, **35**, 229–31.

Connors, M.E., Johnson, C.L. and Stuckey, M.K. (1984) Treatment of bulimia with brief psychoeducational group therapy. *American Journal of Psychiatry*, **141**, 1512–16.

Cooper, P. and Cooper, Z. (1989) Behavioural treatment of bulimia nervosa. *International Journal of Eating Disorders*, **8**, 87–92.

Cooper, S.J. and Sweeney, K.F. (1980) Effects of spiperone alone in combination with anorectic agents on feeding parameters in the rat. *Neuropharmacology*, **19**, 997–1003.

Cooper, Z., Cooper, P.J. and Fairburn, C.G. (1989) The validity of the eating disorder examination and its subscales. *British Journal of Psychiatry*, **154**, 807–12.

Copley, J. (1991) Child dieters risk anorexia, study shows. *The Scotsman*, **12 April**, 3.

Cottrell, D.J. and Crisp, A.H. (1984) Anorexia nervosa in Down's syndrome – a case report. *British Journal of Psychiatry*, **138**, 244–7.

Craik, F.I.M. (1977) Age differences in human memory, in *Handbook of the Psychology of Aging*, (eds J.E. Birren and K.W. Schaie), Van Nostrand, New York.

Crisp, A.H. (1967) Anorexia nervosa. *Hospital Medicine*, **1**, 713–18.

Crisp, A.H. (1977) The differential diagnosis of anorexia nervosa. *Proceedings of the Royal Society of Medicine*, **70**, 686.

Crisp, A.H. (1980a) *Anorexia Nervosa: Let Me Be*. Academic Press, London.

Crisp, A.H. (1980b) Sleep, activity and mood. *British Journal of Psychiatry*, **137**, 1–7.

Crisp, A.H. (1981) Anorexia nervosa at a normal weight! The abnormal weight control syndrome. *International Journal of Psychiatry and Medicine*, **11**, 203–4.

Crisp, A.H. (1983) Anorexia nervosa. *Britsh Medical Journal*, **287**, 855–8.

Crisp, A.H. (1984) Treatment of anorexia nervosa: What can be the role of psychopharmacological agents? in *The Psychobiology of Anorexia Nervosa*, (eds K.M. Pirke and D. Ploog), Springer-Verlag, Berlin, pp. 148–60.

Crisp, A.H., Harding, B. and McGuinness, B. (1974) Anorexia nervosa: Psychoneurotic characteristics of patients: Relationship to prognosis. A quantitative study. *Journal of Psychosomatic Research*, **18**, 167–73.

Crisp, A.H. and Toms, D.A. (1972) Primary anorexia nervosa or weight phobia in the male: Report on 13 cases. *British Medical Journal*, **i**, 334–8.

Curtis-Prior, P.B., Oblin, A.R. and Tan, S. (1980) Antihypertriglyceridaemic activity of some phenylethylamine anorectic compounds. *International Journal of Obesity*, **4**, 111–19.

Czyzyk, A., Tawecki, J., Sadowski, J., Ponilowska, I. and Szczepanik, Z. (1968) Effect of biguanides on intestinal absorption of glucose. *Diabetes*, **17**, 492–8.

Dally, P.J. (1981) Treatment of anorexia nervosa. *British Journal of Hospital Medicine*, **25**, 434–40.

Dally, P.J. and Gomez, J. (1980) *Obesity and Anorexia Nervosa: A Question of Shape*. Faber and Faber, London.

Dally, P.J., Gomez, J. and Isaacs, A.J. (1979) *Anorexia Nervosa*. Heinemann, London.

Dally, P.J., Oppenheim, G.B. and Sargant, W. (1958) Anorexia nervosa. *British Medical Journal*, **ii**, 633–4.

Danforth, E. Jr. and Landsberg, L. (1983) Energy expenditure and its regulation, in *Obesity*, (ed M.R.C. Greenwood), Churchill Livingstone, New York, pp. 103–21.

Danowski, T.S. (1967) Diabetes mellitus and obesity: Phenformin hydrochloride as a research tool. *Metabolism and Clinical Experimentation*, **16**, 865–9.

Davis, P.K. and Curo, A.J. (1980) Chronic vomiting and rumination in intellectually normal and retarded individuals: Review and evaluation of behavioral research. *Behavior Research in Severe Developmental Disability*, **1**, 31–59.

Day, S. and Hollins, S. (1985) The role of the dietician, in *Mental Handicap*, (eds M. Craft, J. Bicknell and S. Hollins), Baillière-Tindall, London.

Decourt, J. (1951) Nosologie de l'annorexie mentale. *Presse Médecine*, **59**, 797.

DeLuise, M., Blackburn, G.L. and Flier, J.S. (1980) Reduced activity in the red-cell sodium–potassium pump in human obesity. *New England Journal of Medicine*, **303**, 1017–22.

Deneux, A., Sans, P., LeClech, H.G. and Messak, E. (1977) Three cases of mental anorexia in men. *Revue de Neuropsychiatrie de l'Ouest (Rennes)*, **14**, 83–95.

Department of Health and Social Security (1981) *Care in the Community: A Consultative Document on Moving Resources for Care.* DHSS, London.

Deutsche Gesellschaft für Ernährung (DGE) (1984) *Ernährungsbericht 1984.* DGE, Frankfurt.

DeVeaugh-Geiss, J., Katz, R., Landau, P., Goodman, W. and Rasmussen, S. (1990) Clinical predictors of treatment response in obsessive–compulsive disorder: Exploratory analyses from multicenter trials of chlomipramine. *Psychopharmacology Bulletin,* **26,** 54–9.

DeWys, W.D. (1977) Changes in taste sensation in cancer patients: Correlation with caloric intake, in *The Chemical Senses and Nutrition,* (eds M.R. Kare and O. Maller), Academic Press, New York.

DiNicola, V.F., Roberts, N. and Oke, L. (1989) Eating and mood disorders in young children. *Psychiatric Clinics of North America,* **12**(4), 873–93.

Dinoff, M., Rickard, H.C. and Colwick, J. (1972) Weight reduction through successive contracts. *American Journal of Orthopsychiatry,* **42,** 110–13.

Dobbins III, W.O., Herrero, B.A. and Mansbach, C.M. (1968) Morphologic alterations associated with neomycin induced malabsorption. *American Journal of Medical Science,* **255,** 63–77.

Dobrzanski, S. and Doggett, N.S. (1979) The effect of propranolol phentolamine and pimozide on drug-induced anorexia in the mouse. *Psychopharmacology,* **66,** 297–300.

Dodrill, C.B. (1978) A neuropsychological battery for epilepsy. *Epilepsia,* **19,** 611–23.

Dolecek, R. and Janstova, V. (1985) Long-term effect of pizotifen treatment on growth hormone levels of underweight children, including those with anorexia nervosa. *Pharmatherapeutica,* **4,** 81–7.

Down, J.L. (1866) Observations on an ethnic classification of idiots. *London Hospital Reports,* London Hospitals, London.

Drewe, E.A. (1974) The effect of type and area of brain lesion on Wisconsin Card Sorting Test performance. *Cortex,* **10,** 159–70.

Drewnowski, A. (1981) *Cognitive Aspects of Taste Perception in Obesity.* Paper presented at Eastern Psychological Association Meeting, New York.

Drewnowski, A. (1983) Cognitive structure in obesity in dieting, in *Obesity*, (ed M.R.C. Greenwood), Churchill Livingstone, New York, pp. 87–101.

Drumm, D.A. and Schade, D.S. (1986) How communication disorders destabilise diabetes. *Clinical Diabetes*, **Jan/Feb**, 16–22.

Dubois, A., Gross, H.A. and Ebert, W.H. (1980) Bethanecol stimulated gastric emptying and acid output in anorexia nervosa patients. *Digestive Disorders Science*, **25**, 716.

Dubois, R. (1913) De l'annorexie mentale comme predom de la demence precoce. *Annales de Médecine Psychologie*, **4**, 431.

Duhault, J., Beregi, L. and du Boistesselin, R. (1979) General and comparative pharmacology of fenfluramine. *Current Medical Research Opinion (Supplement)*, **6**, 3–14.

Eckert, E.D., Goldberg, S.C., Casper, R.C. and Halmi, K.A. (1979) Cyproheptadine in anorexia nervosa. *British Journal of Psychiatry*, **134**, 67–70.

Edwards, S. and Stevens, R. (1991a) Peripherally administered 5-hydroxytryptamine elicits the full behavioral sequence of satiety. *Physiology and Behavior*, **50**, 1075–7.

Edwards, S. and Stevens, R. (1991b) Effects of the peripheral 5-HT$_2$ antagonist xylamidine on consumatory behaviors. *Psychobiology*, **19**(3), 243–6.

Eisler, I. (1988) Family-therapy approaches to anorexia, in *Anorexia and Bulimia Nervosa*, (ed D. Scott), Croom Helm, London, pp. 95–107.

Elder, G.H. (1969) Appearance and education in marriage mobility. *American Sociological Revue*, **34**, 519–33.

Elkin, T.E., Hersen, M., Eisler, R.M. and Williams, J.G. (1973) Modification of caloric intake in anorexia nervosa: An experimental analysis. *Psychological Reports*, **32**, 75–8.

Ellis, A. (1962) *Reason and Emotion in Psychotherapy*. Lyle Stuart, New York.

Epstein, L.H. and Wing, R.R. (1987) Behavioral treatment of childhood obesity. *Psychological Bulletin*, **101**(3), 331–42.

Erber, J.T., Botwinick, J. and Storandt, M. (1981) The impact of memory on age differences in Digit Symbol performance. *Journal of Gerontology*, **36**, 586–90.

Erichsen, A. (1987) *Anorexia Nervosa: The Broken Circle*. Faber and Faber, London.

Estes, W.K. (1974) Learning theory and intelligence. *American*

Psychologist, **41**, 1036–42.

Eysenck, H.J., Arnold, W.J. and Meili, R. (1975) *Encyclopedia of Psychology, Volume One: A–K*. Fontana, Suffolk.

Eysenck, M.W. (1979) Anxiety, learning and memory: A reconceptualization. *Journal of Research and Personality*, **13**, 363.

Fairburn, C.G. (1981) A cognitive–behavioral approach to the treatment of bulimia. *Psychological Medicine*, **11**, 707–11.

Fairburn, C.G. (1982) Binge eating and its management. *British Journal of Psychiatry*, **141**, 631–3.

Fairburn, C.G. (1985) Cognitive–behavioural treatment for bulimia, in *Handbook of Psychotherapy for Anorexia Nervosa and Bulimia*, (eds D.M. Garner and P.E. Garfinkel), Guildford Press, New York.

Fairburn, C.G. and Cooper, P.J. (1982) Self-induced vomiting and bulimia nervosa: An undetected problem. *British Medical Journal*, **284**, 1153–5.

Fairburn, C.G. and Cooper, P.J. (1988) Eating disorders, in *Cognitive–Behavioural Approaches to Adult Psychiatric Disorders: A Practical Guide*, (eds K. Hawton, P. Salkovskis, J. Kirk and D.M. Clarke), Oxford University Press, Oxford.

Fairburn, C.G. and Steel, J.M. (1980) Anorexia nervosa in diabetes mellitus. *British Medical Journal*, **280**, 1167–8.

Faloon, W.W., Paes, I.C. and Woolfolk, D. (1966) Effect of neomycin and kanamycin upon intestinal absorption. *Annals of the New York Academy of Science*, **132**, 879–87.

Falstein, E.I., Feinstein, S.C. and Judas, I. (1956) Anorexia nervosa in the male child. *American Journal of Orthopsychiatry*, **26**, 751–72.

Faust, F.M., Johnson, P.R., Stern, J.S. and Hirsch, J. (1978) Diet-induced adipocyte number increase in adult rats: A new model of obesity. *American Journal of Physiology*, **235**, E279.

Favell, J.E. and Cannon, P.R. (1976) Evaluation of entertainment materials for severely retarded persons. *American Journal of Mental Deficiency*, **81**, 357–61.

Federni, P. (1926) Some variations in ego feeling. *International Journal of Psychoanalysis*, **7**, 434–44.

Feighner, J.P., Robins, E., Guze, S.B. *et al.* (1972) Diagnostic criteria for use in psychiatric research. *Archives of General Psychiatry*, **26**, 57–63.

Ferster, C.B., Nurnberger, J.I. and Levitt, E.E. (1962) The control of eating. *Journal of Mathetics*, **1**, 87–109.

Fichter, M.M. (1990) *Bulimia Nervosa: Basic Research, Diagnosis and Therapy*. Wiley and Sons, Chichester.

Fichter, M.M. and Keeser, W. (1980) Behavioural treatment of an anorexic male: Experimental analysis generalisation. *Behaviour Analysis and Modification*, **4**, 152–68.

Finkelstein, B.A. (1972) Parenteral hyperalimentation in anorexia nervosa. *Journal of the American Medical Association*, **219**, 217.

Fisher, S. (1951) *Body Experience in Fantasy and Behaviour*. Appleton-Century-Crofts, New York.

Fisher, S. and Cleveland, S.E. (1958) *Body Image and Personality*. Dover Publications Inc., New York.

Fitzgibbon, M.L. and Kirschenbaum, D.S. (1990) Heterogeneity of clinical presentation among obese individuals seeking treatment. *Addictive Behaviour*, **15**(3), 291–5.

Flor-Henry, P., Yeudall, L.T. and Koles, Z.J. (1979) Neuropsychological and power spectral EEG investigations of the obsessive–compulsive syndrome. *Biological Psychiatry*, **14**, 119–30.

Foa, E.B. (1979) Failures in treating obsessive–compulsives. *Behaviour Research and Therapy*, **17**, 169–76.

Folkins, C.H. and Sime, W.E. (1981) Physical fitness training and mental health. *American Psychology*, **36**, 373–89.

Forbes, G.B., Gallup, J. and Hursh, J.B. (1961) Estimation of total body fat from potassium-40 content. *Science*, **133**, 101–2.

Foreyt, J.P. (1977) *Behavioral Treatments of Obesity*. Pergamon Press, New York.

Foreyt, J.P. and Kennedy, W.A. (1971) Treatment of overweight by aversion therapy. *Behaviour Research and Therapy*, **9**, 29–34.

Fox, C.F. (1981) Neuropsychological correlates of anorexia nervosa. *International Journal of Psychiatry in Medicine*, **11**(3), 285–90.

Fox, R.A., Hartney, C.W., Rotatori, A.F. and Kurpiers, E.M. (1985) Incidence of obesity among retarded children. *Education and Training of the Mentally Retarded*, **20**(3), 175–81.

Francis, A. and Clarkin, J.F. (1981) No treatment as the prescription of choice. *Archives of General Psychiatry*, **38**, 542–5.

Frazier, S.H. (1965) Anorexia nervosa. *Diseases of the Nervous System*, **26**, 155–9.

Freeman, C.P.L., Barry, F., Dunkeld-Turnbull, J. and

Henderson, A. (1988) Controlled trial of psychotherapy for bulimia nervosa. *British Medical Journal*, **296**, 521–4.

Freeman, R.J., Thomas, C.D., Solyom, L. and Koopman, R.F. (1985) Clinical and personality correlates of body size overestimation in anorexia nervosa and bulimia nervosa. *International Journal of Eating Disorders*, **4**, 439–56.

Frerichs, H., Daweke, H. and Gries, F. (1973) A novel pancreatic amylase inhibitor (Bay d 7791). Experimental studies on rats and clinical observations in normal and obese diabetic and non-diabetic subjects. *Diabetologia*, **9**, 68.

Freud, S. (1918) *Aus der Geschichte einer Infantilen Neurose*, translated in *The Standard Edition of the Complete Psychological Works of Sigmund Freud Volume XVII*, (ed J. Stracey), Hogarth Press, London, 1955.

Friar Williams, E. (1977) *Notes of a Feminist Therapist*. Brunner/Mazel, New York.

Fryer, J.H. (1962) Studies of body composition in men aged 60 and over, in *Biological Aspects of Aging*, (ed N.W. Shock), Columbia University Press, New York, pp. 57–78.

Galbraith, L. and Wilson, A. (1992) Adolescent obesity – A new treatment programme in Ninewells Hospital, Dundee. *BPS Scottish Branch Newsletter*, **14**, 10–12.

Gallo, L. and Randel, A. (1981) Chronic vomiting and its effect on the primary dentition: Report of a case. *Journal of Dentistry in Children*, **48**, 383–4.

Gambert, S.R., Garthwaite, T.L., Pontzer, C.H. (1981) Running elevates plasma beta-endorphin immunoreactivity and ACTH in untrained human subjects. *Proceedings of the Society of Experimental Biology and Medicine*, **168**, 1–4.

Gambrill, E.D. and Richey, C.A. (1975) An assertion inventory for use in assessment and research. *Behaviour Research and Therapy*, **6**, 550–61.

Garattini, S., Caccia, S. and Mennini, T. (1979) Biochemical pharmacology of the anorectic drug fenfluramine: A review. *Current Medical Research Opinion*, **6**, 15–27.

Garattini, S. and Samanin, R. (1978) *Central Mechanisms of Anorectic Drugs*. Raven Press, New York.

Gardner, J. and Williams, E. (1974) *The Drinking Man's Diet*. Cameron and Co., San Francisco.

Garfinkel, P.E. (1985) *Handbook of Psychotherapy for Anorexia Nervosa and Bulimia Nervosa*. Guildford Press, London.

Garfinkel, P.E. and Garner, D.M. (1982) *Anorexia Nervosa: A Multi-dimensional Perspective.* Brunner/Mazel, New York.

Garfinkel, P.E. and Garner, D.M. (1984) Perceptions of the body in anorexia nervosa, in *The Psychobiology of Anorexia Nervosa*, (eds K.M. Pirke and D. Ploog), Springer-Verlag, Berlin.

Garfinkel, P.E., Moldofsky, H. and Garner, D.M. (1977) Prognosis in anorexia nervosa as influenced by clinical features, treatment and self perception. *Canadian Medical Association Journal*, **117**, 1041–5.

Garfinkel, P.E., Moldofsky, H. and Garner, D.M. (1980) The heterogeneity of anorexia nervosa: Bulimia as a distinct subgroup. *Archives of General Psychiatry*, **37**, 1036–40.

Garn, S.M., Bailey, S.M., Cole, P.E. and Higgins, I.T.T. (1977) Level of education, level of income, and level of fatness in adults. *American Journal of Clinical Nutrition*, **30**, 721–5.

Garner, D.M. (1986) Cognitive–behavioural therapy for eating disorders. *Clinical Psychologist*, **39**, 36–9.

Garner, D.M. and Bemis, K.M. (1982) A cognitive–behavioural approach to anorexia nervosa. *Cognitive Therapy and Research*, **6**, 123–50.

Garner, D.M. and Bemis, K.M. (1985) Cognitive therapy for anorexia nervosa, in *Handbook of Psychotherapy for Anorexia Nervosa and Bulimia*, (eds D.M. Garner and P.E. Garfinkel), Guildford Press, New York.

Garner, D.M. and Garfinkel, P.E. (1979) The eating attitudes test: An index of the symptoms of anorexia nervosa. *Psychological Medicine*, **9**, 273–9.

Garner, D.M. and Garfinkel, P.E. (1981) Body image in anorexia nervosa,: Measurement theory and clinical implications. *International Journal of Psychiatry in Medicine*, **11**, 263–84.

Garner, D.M., Garfinkel, P.E. and Olmsted, M.P. (1983) An overview of the socio-cultural factors in the development of anorexia nervosa, in *Anorexia Nervosa: Recent Developments*, (eds P.L. Darby, P.E. Garfinkel and D.V. Coscina), Alan R. Liss, New York, pp. 65–82.

Garner, D.M., Garfinkel, P.E., Schwartz, D. and Thompson, M. (1980) Cultural expectations of thinness in women. *Psychological Reprints*, **47**, 483–91.

Garner, D.M., Garfinkel, P.E., Stancer, H.C. and Moldofsky,

H. (1976) Body image disturbances in anorexia nervosa and obesity. *Psychosomatic Medicine*, **38**, 327–37.

Garner, D.M., Olmsted, M.P., Bohr, V. and Garfinkel, E. (1982) The eating attitudes test: Psychometric features and clinical correlates. *Psychological Medicine*, **12**, 871–8.

Garner, D.M., Olmsted, M.P. and Polivy, J. (1983) Development and validation of a multidimensional eating disorder inventory for anorexia nervosa and bulimia. *International Journal of Eating Disorders*, **2**, 15–34.

Garrison, R.J., Kannel, W.B., Feinleib, M. *et al.* (1978) Cigarette smoking and HDL cholesterol: The Framingham offspring study. *Atherosclerosis*, **30**, 17–25.

Garrod, A.E. (1902) The incidence of alkaptonuria: A study of chemical individuality. *Lancet*, **2**, 1616–20.

Garrow, J.S. (1988) *Obesity and Related Diseases*. Churchill Livingstone, London.

Garrow, J.S. and Gardiner, G.T. (1981) Maintenance of weight loss in obese patients after jaw wiring. *British Medical Journal*, **860**, 858–60.

Gartner, A.F., Marcus, R.N., Halmi, K. and Loranger, A.W. (1989) DSM-III-R personality disorders in patients with eating disorders. *American Journal of Psychiatry*, **146**(12), 1585–91.

Gaudoin, T. (1991) Life after the wonder drug. *Harpers and Queen*, **December**, 108–12.

Gellert, E., Girgus, J. and Cohen, J. (1971) Children's awareness of their bodily appearance: A developmental study of factors associated with the body percept. *General Psychological Monographs*, **84**, 109–74.

Gillie, O., Price, A. and Robinson, S. (1982) *The Sunday Times Self-Help Directory*. **September 9**, 7–8.

Giuora, A.Z. (1967) Dysorexia: A psychopathological study of anorexia nervosa. *American Journal of Psychiatry*, **124**, 391–3.

Glamour magazine (1984) Feeling fat in a thin society: 33 000 women tell how they feel about their bodies. *Glamour*, **February**, 198–201; 251–2.

Glick, Z. and Bray, G.A. (1981) Effect of acarbose on food intake of rats maintained on high carbohydrate and high fat diets. *Federal Proceedings*, **40**, 916.

Glick, Z., Teague, R. and Bray, G.A. (1981) Brown adipose tissue: Thermic response increased by a single low protein meal. *Science*, **213**, 1125–7.

Glosser, G., Butters, N. and Kaplan, E. (1977) Visuo-perceptual processes in brain damaged patients on the digit symbol substitution test. *International Journal of Neuroscience*, **7**, 59–66.

Glucksman, M.L. and Hirsch, J. (1969) The response of obese patients to weight reduction III: The perception of body size. *Psychosomatic Medicine*, **31**, 1–7.

Golay, A., Schutz, Y. and Meyer, H.U. (1982) Glucose-induced thermogenesis in non-diabetic and diabetic obese subjects. *Diabetes*, **31**, 1023–8.

Goldberg, S.C., Halmi, K.A., Eckert, E.D., Casper, R.C. and Davis, J.M. (1979) Cyproheptadine in anorexia nervosa. *British Journal of Psychiatry*, **134**, 67–70.

Goldblatt, P.B., Moore, M.F. and Stunkard, A.J. (1965) Social factors in obesity. *Journal of the American Medical Association*, **192**, 1039–44.

Goldiamond, I. (1965) Self-control procedures in personal behavior problems. *Psychological Reports*, **17**, 851–68.

Golding, W. (1960) *Lord of the Flies*. Penguin, London.

Goldrick, R.B. and McLoughlin, G.M. (1970) Lipolysis and lipogenesis from glucose in human fat cells of different sizes. *Journal of Clinical Investigation*, **49**, 1213.

Goodman, W.K. (1989) The Yale–Brown Obsessive–Compulsive Scale II. Validity. *Archives of General Psychiatry*, **46**(11), 1012–16.

Goodsitt, A. (1983) Self-regulatory disturbances in eating disorders. *International Journal of Eating Disorders*, **2**, 51–60.

Gordon, R.A. (1990) *Anorexia and Bulimia: Anatomy of a Social Epidemic*. Blackwell, Oxford.

Grant, D.A. and Berg, E.A. (1948) A behavioral analysis of degree of reinforcement and ease of shifting in a Weigl-type card-sorting problem. *Journal of Experimental Psychology*, **38**, 404–11.

Green, C.W., Reid, D.H., White, L.K. *et al.* (1988) Identifying reinforcers for persons with profound handicaps: Staff opinion versus systematic assessment of preferences. *Journal of Applied Behavior Analysis*, **21**(1), 31–43.

Green, H. (1979) Adipose conversion: A program of differentiation. *INSERM*, **87**, 15.

Green, R.S. and Rau, J.H. (1974) Treatment of compulsive eating disturbances with anticonvulsant medication. *American Journal of Psychiatry*, **131**, 428–32.

Green, R.T. (1977) Negative reinforcement as an unrewarding concept – a plea for consistency. *Bulletin of the British Psychological Society*, **30**, 219–22.

Greene, K.S., Johnston, J.M., Rossi, M. *et al.* (1991) The effects of peanut butter on ruminating. *American Journal of Mental Retardation*, **95**(6), 631–45.

Greenwood, M.R.C. (1983) *Obesity*. Churchill Livingstone, New York.

Griffen, W.O., Young, V.L. and Stevenson, C.C. (1977) A prospective comparison of gastric and jejuno-ileal bypass procedures for morbid obesity. *Annals of Surgery*, **186**, 500–9.

Grinker, J. (1973) Behavioral and metabolic consequences of weight reduction. *Journal of the American Dietetic Association*, **62**, 30–4.

Grinker, J. (1978) Obesity and sweet taste. *American Journal of Clinical Nutrition*, **31**, 1078–87.

Grinker, J., Most, J. and Hirsch, J. (1980) *Long-term Follow-up of the Effects of a Residential Weight Loss Program*. Third International Congress on Obesity, Rome.

Gronwall, D.M.A. (1977) Paced auditory serial-addition task: A measure of recovery from concussion. *Perceptual and Motor Skills*, **44**, 367–73.

Gronwall, D.M.A. and Sampson, H. (1974) *The Psychological Effects of Concussion*. Auckland University Press, Auckland, New Zealand.

Gronwall, D.M.A. and Wrightson, P. (1974) Delayed recovery of intellectual function after minor head injury. *Lancet*, **ii**, 1452.

Gronwall, D.M.A. and Wrightson, P. (1981) Memory and information processing capacity after closed head injury. *Journal of Neurology, Neurosurgery and Psychiatry*, **44**, 889–95.

Gross, H.A., Ebert, M.H., Faden, V.B. *et al.* (1981) A double-blind controlled trial of lithium carbonate in primary anorexia nervosa. *Journal of Clinical Psychopharmacology*, **1**, 376–81.

Grosse, M.E. and Wright, B.D. (1985) Validity and reliability of true-false tests. *Educational and Psychological Measurement*, **45**, 1–11.

Guidano, V.F. and Liotti, G. (1983) *Cognitive Processes and Emotional Disorders: A Structural Approach to Psychotherapy*. Guildford Press, New York.

Gull, W.W. (1874) Anorexia nervosa. *Translations in Clinical*

Sociology, **7**, 22–8; reprinted in *Evolution of Psychosomatic Concepts. Anorexia Nervosa: A Paradigm*, (eds R.M. Kaufman and M. Heiman), International Universities Press, New York, 1964.

Gwirtsman, H., Roy-Byrne, P., Yager, J. and Gerner, R. (1983) Neuroendocrine abnormalities in bulimia. *American Journal of Psychiatry*, **140**, 559–63.

Hall, A. (1982) Deciding to stay an anorectic. *Postgraduate Medical Journal*, **58**, 641–7.

Halle, M. (1992) Appetite for life. *Sunday Times Magazine*, **1 March**, 49.

Halmi, K.A., Eckert, E., Lodu, T.J. and Cohen, J. (1986) Anorexia nervosa: Treatment efficacy of cyproheptadine and amitriptyline. *Archives of General Psychiatry*, **43**, 117–81.

Halmi, K.A. and Falk, J.R. (1983) Behavioural and dietary discriminators of menstrual function in anorexia nervosa, in *Anorexia Nervosa: Recent Developments in Research*, (ed P.L. Darby), Academic Press, New York, pp. 323–29.

Halmi, K.A., Falk, J.R. and Schwartz, E. (1981) Binge eating and vomiting: A survey of a college population. *Psychological Medicine*, **9**, 429–48.

Hamsher, K. de S., Halmi, K.A. and Benton, A.L. (1981) Prediction of outcome in anorexia nervosa from neuropsychological status. *Psychiatry Research*, **4**(1), 79–88.

Haraczkiewicz, E. and Vasselli, J.R. (1981) Effect of intestinal glucosidase inhibition upon the development of sucrose induced obesity in rats. *Federal Proceedings*, **40**, 916.

Hards, B., Thompson, S.B.N. and Bate, R. (1986) A program of therapeutic interest. *Therapy Weekly*, **12**(31), 7.

Harmatz, M.G. and Lapuc, P. (1968) Behavior modification of overeating in a psychiatric population. *Journal of Consulting and Clinical Psychology*, **32**, 583–7.

Harper, G. (1983) Varieties of parenting failure in anorexia nervosa: Protection and parentectomy, revisited. *Journal of the American Academy of Child Psychiatry*, **22**, 134–9.

Harper, G. (1984) Anorexia nervosa: What kind of disorder? The 'Consensus' Model, myths and clinical implications. *Paediatric Annals*, **13**, 812–28.

Harris, B., Young, J. and Hughes, B. (1986) Comparative effects of seven antidepressant regimes on appetite, weight and carbohydrate preference. *British Journal of Psychiatry*, **148**,

590–2.

Harris, M.B. (1969) Self-directed program for weight control: A pilot study. *Journal of Abnormal Psychology*, **74**, 263–70.

Harris, M.B. and Smith, S.D. (1982) Beliefs about obesity: Effects of age, ethnicity, sex and weight. *Psychological Reports*, **51**, 1047–55.

Harris, M.B. and Smith, S.D. (1983) The relationship of age, sex, ethnicity and weight to stereotypes of obesity and self-perception. *International Journal of Obesity*, **7**, 361–71.

Harrower, A.D.B., Yapp, P.L., Nairn, I.M. *et al.* (1977) Growth hormone, insulin, and prolactin secretion in anorexia nervosa and obesity during bromocriptine treatment. *British Medical Journal*, **ii**, 156–9.

Hasan, M. and Tibbetts, R. (1977) Primary anorexia nervosa (weight phobia) in males. *Postgraduate Medical Journal*, **53**, 146–51.

Hasler, J. (1982) Parotid enlargement. A presenting sign in anorexia nervosa. *Oral Surgery, Oral Medicine and Oral Pathology*, **53**, 567–73.

Hathcock, J.N. and Coon, J. (1978) *Nutrition and Drug Interrelations*. Academic Press, New York.

Hay, G. and Leonard, J. (1979) Anorexia nervosa in males. *Lancet*, **2**, 574–5.

Hayslip, B. Jr. and Kennelly, K.J. (1980) *Short-term Memory and Crystalized–Fluid Intelligence in Adulthood*. Paper presented at American Psychological Association Convention, Montreal, Canada, September 1980.

Heald, F.P., Hunt, E.D. Jr., Schwartz, R. *et al.* (1963) Measures of body fat and hydration in adolescent boys. *Pediatrics*, **31**, 226–39.

Heffner, S.M., Stern, M.P., Mitchell, B.D., Hazuda, H.P. and Patterson, J.K. (1990) Incidence of type II diabetes in Mexican Americans predicted by fasting insulin and glucose levels, obesity, and body-fat distribution. *Diabetes*, **39**(3), 283–8.

Hemmes, R.B., Pack, H.M. and Hirsch, J. (1979) Chronic ingestion of L-DOPA dramatically reduces body weight of the genetically obese Zucker rat. *Federal Proceedings*, **38**, 277.

Hemmes, R.B., Pack, H.M. and Hirsch, J. (1980) Peripheral administration of 6-hydroxydopamine (60HDA) blocks the weight reducing effect of chronic L-DOPA ingestion. *Federal*

Proceedings, **39**, 782.

Henderson, M. and Freeman, C.P.L. (1987) A self-rating scale for bulimia. *British Journal of Psychiatry*, **150**, 18–24.

Hermreck, A.S., Jewell, W.R. and Hardin, C.R. (1976) Gastric bypass for morbid obesity. *Surgery, Gynaecology and Obstetrics*, **80**, 498.

Herzog, D.B. (1984) Are anorexic and bulimic patients depressed? *American Journal of Psychiatry*, **4**, 1594–7.

Herzog, D.B. and Copeland, P.M. (1985) Eating disorders. *New England Journal of Medicine*, **313**(5), 295–303.

Herzog, D.B., Norman, D.K., Gordon, C. and Pepose, M. (1984) Sexual conflict and eating disorders in 27 males. *American Journal of Psychiatry*, **141**, 989–90.

Hewitt, K. and Burden, P. (1984) Behavioural management of food regurgitation: Parents and therapists. *Mental Handicap*, **12**(4), 168–9.

Hillard, J.R. and Hillard, P.J.A. (1984) Bulimia, anorexia nervosa and diabetes – deadly combinations. *Psychiatric Clinics of North America*, **7**, 367–79.

Hindler, C.G. and Norris, D.L. (1986) A case of anorexia nervosa with Klinefelter's syndrome. *British Journal of Psychiatry*, **149**, 659–60.

Hinds, R. and Oliver, C. (1985) Chronic vomiting in people who are mentally handicapped. *Mental Handicap*, **13**(4), 152–4.

Hirsch, J. and Gallian, E. (1978) Method for the determination of adipose cell size in man and animals. *Journal of Lipid Research*, **9**, 110.

Hirsch, J. and Goldrick, R.B. (1964) Serial studies on the metabolism of human adipose tissue. I. Lipogenesis and free fatty acid uptake and release in small aspirated samples of subcutaneous fat. *Journal of Clinical Investigation*, **43**, 1776.

Hirsch, J. and Han, P.W. (1969) Cellularity of rat adipose tissue: effects of growth, starvation and obesity. *Journal of Lipid Research*, **10**, 77.

Hirsch, J and Knittle, J.L. (1970) Cellularity of obese and non-obese human adipose tissue. *Federal Proceedings*, **29**, 1516.

Hirschenfang, S. (1960) A comparison of WAIS scores of hemiplegic patients with and without aphasia. *Journal of Clinical Psychology*, **16**, 351.

Hoage, C.M. (1989) The use of an in-session structured eating in the outpatient treatment of bulimia, in *The Experiential Therapies for Eating Disorders*, (eds L. Hornyak and E. Baker), Guildford Press, New York.

Hodas, G., Liebman, R. and Collins, M.J. (1982) Pediatric hospitalization in the treatment of anorexia nervosa, in *The Psychiatric Hospital and The Family*, (ed H.T. Harbin), Spectrum Publications, Jamaica, New York, pp. 131–41.

Hogg, J. (1982) Reduction of self-induced vomiting in a multiply handicapped girl by 'lemon juice' and concomitant changes in social behaviour. *British Journal of Clinical Psychology*, **21**, 227–8.

Holden, N.L. (1990) Is anorexia nervosa an obsessive–compulsive disorder? *British Journal of Psychiatry*, **157**, 1.

Hollin, C. and Lewis, V. (1988) Cognitive–behavioural approaches to anorexia and bulimia, in *Anorexia and Bulimia Nervosa*, (ed D. Scott), Croom Helm, London, pp. 108–22.

Hollobaugh, S.L., Rao, M.B. and Kruger, F.A. (1970) Studies on the site and mechanism of action of phenformin. I. Evidence for significant 'non-peripheral' effects of phenformin on glucose metabolism in normal subjects. *Diabetes*, **19**, 45–9.

Homme, L.E. (1965) Perspectives in Psychology: XXIV. Control of coverants, the operants of the mind. *Psychological Reports*, **15**, 501–11.

Horan, J.J. and Johnson, R.G. (1971) Coverant conditioning through a self-management application of the Premack Principle: Its effect on weight reduction. *Journal of Behavioral Therapy and Experimental Psychiatry*, **2**, 243–9.

Hornak, N. (1983) Group treatment for bulimia: Bulimics Anonymous. *Journal of the College of Studies in Personnel*, **24**, 461–3.

Horney, K. (1950) *Neurosis and Human Growth: The Struggle Towards Self-Realization*. W.W. Norton, New York.

Howard, A.N., Grant, A.M. and Mills, I.H. (1978) Treatment of obesity with very low calorie liquid-formula diet: An inpatient/outpatient comparison using skimmed milk protein as the chief protein source. *International Journal of Obesity*, **2**, 321.

Hsu, L.K.G. (1980) Outcome of anorexia nervosa. A review of literature (1954 to 1978). *Archives of General Psychiatry*, **37**, 1041–6.

Hsu, L.K.G. (1984) Treatment of bulimia with lithium. *American Journal of Psychiatry*, **141**, 1260–2.

Hsu, L.K.G., Crisp, A.H. and Harding, B. (1979) Outcome of anorexia nervosa. *Lancet*, **i**, 61–5.

Hsu, L.K.G. and Holder, D. (1986) Bulimia nervosa: Treatment and short-term outcome. *Psychological Medicine*, **16**, 65–70.

Hsu, L.K.G. and Sobkiewicz, T.A. (1989) Bulimia nervosa: A four- to six-year follow-up study. *Psychological Medicine*, **19**(4), 1035–8.

Hudson, J.I., Laffer, P.S., and Pope, H.G. (1982) Bulimia related to affective disorder by family history to the dexamethasone suppression test. *American Journal of Psychiatry*, **137**, 695–8.

Hudson, J.I., Pope, H.G., Jonas, J.M. and Yurgelun-Todd, D. (1985) Treatment of anorexia nervosa with antidepressants. *Journal of Clinical Psychopharmacology*, **5**, 17–23.

Hudson, J.I., Wentworth, S.M., Hudson, M.S. and Pope, H.G. (1985) Prevalence of anorexia nervosa and bulimia among young diabetic women. *Journal of Clinical Psychiatry*, **46**, 88–9.

Hudson, K.D. (1977) The anorectic and hypotensive effect of fenfluramine in obesity. *Journal of the Royal College of General Practitioners*, **27**, 497.

Hulley, S.B., Rosenman, R.H., Bawol, R.D. and Brand, R.J. (1980) Epidemiology as a guide to clinical decisions. The association between triglyceride and coronary heart disease. *New England Journal of Medicine*, **302**, 1383–9.

Hulse, S.H., Egeth, H. and Deese, J. (1981) *The Psychology of Learning*, 5th edn. McGraw-Hill, Tokyo.

Huon, G.F. (1984) *Validation of a Self-help Treatment Program for Bulimia*. Paper presented at the International Conference on Eating Disorders, Swansea, Wales.

Huon, G.F. and Brown, L.B. (1984) Bulimia: The emergence of a syndrome. *Australian and New Zealand Journal of Psychiatry*, **8**, 113–26.

Hutson, W.R. and Wald, A. (1990) Gastric emptying in patients with bulimia nervosa and anorexia nervosa. *American Journal of Gastroenterology*, **85**(1), 41–6.

Innes, J.A., Watson, M.L., Ford, M.J. *et al.* (1977) Plasma fenfluramine levels, weight loss and side effects. *British Medical Journal*, **2**, 1322.

Insel, T.R., Donnelly, E.G.F. and Lalakea, M.L. (1983)

Neurological and neuropsychological studies of patients with obsessive–compulsive disorder. *Biological Psychiatry*, **18**, 741–51.

Iselin, H.U., Ravussin, E. and Maeder, E. (1978) Effect of a new glycoside–hydrolase inhibitor (Bay g 5421) on plasma glucose, fructose, IRI and FFA levels and on carbohydrate utilization during an oral glucose tolerance test. *Diabetologia*, **15**, 242.

Janda, L.H. and Rimm, D.C. (1972) Covert sensitisation in the treatment of obesity. *Journal of Abnormal Psychology*, **80**, 37–42.

Jeffrey, D.B., Christensen, E.R. and Pappas, J.P. (1973) Developing a behavioral program and therapist manual for the treatment of obesity. *Journal of the American College Health Association*, **21**, 455–9.

Jessner, L. and Abse, D.W. (1960) Regressive forces in anorexia nervosa. *British Journal of Medical Psychology*, **33**, 301–12.

Joffe, S.N. (1981) Surgical management of morbid obesity. *Gut*, **22**, 248.

Johanson, A.J. and Knorr, N.J. (1977) L-dopa as treatment for anorexia nervosa, in *Anorexia Nervosa*, (ed R.A. Vigersky), Raven, New York, pp. 363–72.

Johnson, C.L. and Connors, M.E. (1987) Treatment of bulimia: A review, in *Handbook of Eating Disorders. Part 1: Anorexia Nervosa and Bulimia Nervosa*, (eds P.J.V. Beumont, G.D. Burrows and R.C. Casper), Elsevier, Amsterdam, pp. 299–317.

Johnson, C.L. and Larson, R. (1982) Bulimia: An analysis of moods and behavior. *Psychosomatic Medicine*, **44**, 333–45.

Johnson, C.L., Lewis, C. and Hagman, J. (1984) The syndrome of bulimia; review and synthesis, in *The Psychiatric Clinics of North America*, (ed F.E.F. Larocca), W.B. Saunders, Philadelphia, pp. 247–73.

Johnson, C.L., Stuckey, M.K. and Lewis, L.D. (1982) Bulimia. A descriptive survey of 316 cases. *International Journal of Eating Disorders*, **2**, 3–18.

Johnson, C.L., Stuckey, M.K. and Mitchell, J. (1983) Psychopharmacological treatment of anorexia nervosa and bulimia. *Journal of Nervous and Mental Disease*, **171**, 524–34.

Johnson, D., Firth, D. and Davey, G.C.L. (1978) Vibration and praise as reinforcers for mentally handicapped people. *Mental Retardation*, **16**, 339–42.

Johnson, W.G., Schlundt, D.G., Kelly, M.L. and Ruggiero, L. (1984) Exposure with response prevention and energy regulation in the treatment of bulimia. *International Journal of Eating Disorders*, **3**, 37–46.

Johnston, J.M., Greene, K.S., Rawal, A., Vazin, T. and Winston, M. (1991) Effects of caloric level on ruminating. *Journal of Applied Behavior Analysis*, **24**(3), 597–603.

Johnston, J.M., Greene, K.S., Vazin, T. *et al.* (1990) Effects of food consistency on ruminating. *Psychological Reports*, **40**, 609–18.

Jolliffe, N. (1963) *Reduce and Stay Reduced*, 3rd edn. Simon and Schuster, New York.

Jonas, J. and Gold, M. (1987) Treatment of antidepressant-resistant bulimia with naltrexone. *International Journal of Psychiatry and Medicine*, **16**, 305–9.

Jourard, S.M. and Secord, P.F. (1955) Body cathexis and the ideal female figure. *Journal of Abnormal and Social Psychology*, **50**, 243–6.

Jung, R.T., Gurr, M.J., Robinson, M.P. and James, W.P.T. (1978) Does adipose hypercellularity in obesity exist? *British Medical Journal*, **2**, 319.

Kanner, L. (1972) *Child Psychiatry*. Charles C. Thomas, Springfield, Illinois.

Karris, L. (1977) Prejudice against obese renters. *Journal of Social Psychology*, **101**, 159–60.

Kasvikis, Y.G., Tsakiris, F., Marks, I.M., Basaglu, M. and Nashirvani, H.F. (1986) Past history of anorexia nervosa in women with obsessive–compulsive disorder. *International Journal of Eating Disorders*, **11**, 1069–75.

Katzman, M., Weiss, L. and Wolchik, S. (1986) Speak, don't eat! Teaching women to express their feelings. *Women and Therapy*, **5**, 143–57.

Kay, D.W. and Shapira, K. (1972) Psychiatric observations on anorexia. *Advancements in Psychosomatic Medicine*, **7**, 277–99.

Kelly, J., Alheid, G.F., Newberg, A. and Grossman, S.P. (1977) GABA stimulation and blockade in the hypothalamus and midbrain: Effect on feeding and their locomotor activity. *Pharmacology and Biochemistry of Behavior*, **7**, 537–41.

Kempner, W. (1949) The treatment of heart and kidney disease and of hypertensive and arteriosclerotic vascular disease with the rice diet. *Annals of Internal Medicine*, **31**, 821–56.

Kempner, W., Newborg, B.C., Peschel, R.L. and Styler, J.S.

(1975) Treatment of massive obesity with rice/reduction diet program. *Archives of Internal Medicine*, **135**, 1575–84.

Kendell, R.E., Hall, D.J., Hailey, A. and Babigan, H.M. (1973) The epidemiology of anorexia nervosa. *Psychological Medicine*, **3**(2), 200–3.

Kennedy, S.H., Piran, N. and Garfinkel, P.E. (1985) Monoamine oxidase inhibitor therapy for anorexia nervosa and bulimia: A preliminary trial of isocarboxazid. *Journal of Clinical Psychopharmacology*, **5**, 279–85.

Kennedy, W.A. and Foreyt, J.P. (1968) Control of eating behavior in an obese patient by avoidance conditioning. *Psychological Reports*, **22**, 571–6.

Kerry, R.J., Leibling, L.I. and Owen, G. (1970) Weight changes in lithium responders. *Acta Psychiatrica Scandinavica*, **46**, 238–43.

Keup, U. and Puls, W. (1975) Metabolic studies with an amylase inhibitor (Bay e 4609). *Archives of Pharmacology (Supplement)*, **287**, R85.

Keys, A. (1980a) *Seven Countries: A Multivariate Analysis of Death and Coronary Heart Disease*. Harvard University Press, Cambridge, Massachusetts.

Keys, A. (1980b) Overweight, obesity, coronary heart disease and mortality. *Nutrition Review*, **38**, 297–307.

Keys, A., Brozek, J. and Henschel, A. (1950) *The Biology of Human Starvation, Volume 1*. University of Minnesota Press, Minneapolis.

Kingsley, R.G. and Wilson, G.T. (1977) Behavior therapy for obesity: A comparative investigation of long-term efficacy. *Journal of Consulting and Clinical Psychology*, **45**, 288–98.

Kirkley, B.G., Agras, W.S. and Weiss, I.I. (1986) Necessity of dietary management in eating disorders, in *Annual Series of European Research in Behaviour Therapy*, (ed W. Vandereycken), Swets and Zeitlinger, Lisse.

Kirkley, B.G., Schneider, J.A., Agras, W.S. and Bachman, J.A. (1985) Comparison of two group treatments for bulimia. *Journal of Consultancy in Clinical Psychology*, **53**, 43–8.

Kissebah, A.H.N., Vydelingum, R., Murray, D.J. *et al.* (1982) Relation of body fat distribution to metabolic complications of obesity. *Journal of Clinical Endocrinology and Metabolism*, **54**, 254–60.

Klemperer, E. (1954) Changes in body image in hypnoanalysis.

Journal of Clinical and Experimental Hypnosis, **2**, 157–62.

Klyde, B.J. and Hirsch, J. (1979) Increased cellular proliferation in adipose tissue of adult rats fed a high-fat diet. *Journal of Lipid Research*, **20**, 705.

Knox, W.E. (1958) Sir Archibald Garrod's 'inborn errors of metabolism'. II. Alkaptonuria. *American Journal of Human Genetics*, **10**, 95–124.

Knox, W.E. (1960) An evaluation of the treatment of phenyl-ketonuria with diets low in phenylalanine. *Journal of Paediatrics*, **26**, 1–11.

Kolb, C. (1975) Disturbances of body image, in *American Handbook of Psychiatry, Volume 4*, (ed S. Arieti), Basic Books, New York, pp. 810–31.

Korman, M. and Blumberg, S. (1963) Comparative efficiency of some tests of cerebral damage. *Journal of Consulting Psychology*, **27**, 303–9.

Kraepelin, E. (1920) Symptoms of mental disease. *Zentblischen Neurologische und Psychiatrische*, **2**.

Krivacek, D. and Powell, J. (1978) Negative preference management: Behavioural suppression using Premack's punishment hypothesis. *Education and Treatment of Children*, **1**(4), 5–13.

Kron, L., Katz, J.L., Gorzynski, G. and Weiner, H. (1978) Hyperactivity in anorexia nervosa: A fundamental feature. *Comparative Psychiatry*, **19**, 433–40.

Kronfol, Z., Hamsher, K. de S., Digre, K. and Waziri, R. (1978) Depression and hemispheric functions: Changes associated with unilateral ECT. *British Journal of Psychiatry*, **132**, 560–7.

Kronig, M. (1986) Case report of successful treatment of bulimia with isocarboxazid. *American Journal of Psychiatry*, **45**, 217–22.

Lacey, J.H. (1983) The patient's attitude to food, in *Clinical Reactions to Food*, (ed M.H. Lessof), Wiley, New York, pp. 35–58.

Laccy, J.H. and Crisp, A.H. (1980) Hunger, food intake and weight: The impact of clomipramine on a refeeding anorexia nervosa population. *Postgraduate Medical Journal*, **56**, 79–85.

Laessle, R.G., Bossert, S., Hank, G., Hahlweg, K. and Pirke, K.M. (1990) Cognitive performance in patients with bulimia nervosa: Relationship to intermittent starvation. *Biological Psychiatry*, **27**(5), 549–51.

Laessle, R.G., Schweiger, U., Daute-Herold, U. et al. (1988) Nutritional knowledge in patients with eating disorders. *International Journal of Eating Disorders*, **7**(1), 1–10.

Lambley, P. (1983) *How to Survive Anorexia*. Frederick Muller, London.

Lambley, P. and Scott, D. (1988) An overview of bulimia nervosa, in *Anorexia and Bulimia Nervosa*, (ed D. Scott), Croom Helm, London, pp. 24–36.

Larocca, F.E.F. (1984) *The Psychiatric Clinics of North America*. W.B. Saunders, Philadelphia.

Larsson, B., Björntorp, P. and Tibblin, G. (1981) The health consequences of moderate obesity. *International Journal of Obesity*, **5**, 97–116.

Lasègue, C. (1873) De l'annorexie hystérique. *Archives Générals de Medecine*, reprinted in *Evolution of Psychosomatic Concepts. Anorexia Nervosa: A Paradigm*, (eds R.M. Kaufman and M. Heiman), International Universities Press, New York, 1964.

Laube, H., Fouladfar, M., Aubell, R. and Schmitz, H. (1980) Effect of glucosidase inhibitor, Bay g 5421 (acarbose), on the blood glucose in obese diabetic patients type 2 (NIDDM). *Arzneimittelforsch*, **30**, 1154–7.

Lawrence, M. (1984) *The Anorexic Experience*. The Women's Press, London.

Lawson, J.S., Marshall, W.L. and McGrath, P. (1979) The social self-esteem inventory. *Education and Psychological Measurement*, **39**, 803–11.

Leclair, N. and Berkowitz, B. (1983) Counselling concerns for the individual with bulimia. *Personnel Guidance Journal*, **2**, 353–5.

Lefcourt, H.M. (1966) Internal versus external control of reinforcement. *Psychological Bulletin*, **65**, 206–20.

Leibowitz, S.F. and Rossakis, C. (1979) L-DOPA feeding suppression: Effect on catecholamine neurons of the perifornical lateral hypothalamus. *Psychopharmacology*, **61**, 273–80.

Leitenberg, H., Gross, J., Peterson, and Rosen, J.C. (1984) Analysis of an anxiety model and the process of change during exposure plus response prevention treatment of bulimia nervosa. *Behavior Therapy*, **15**, 3–20.

Lemonnier, D. (1972) Effect of age, sex and site in cellularity of the adipose tissue in mice and rats rendered obese by a high fat diet. *Journal of Clinical Investigation*, **51**, 2907.

Leon, G.R. (1982) Personality and behavioral correlates of obesity, in *Psychological Aspects of Obesity: A Handbook*, (ed B.R. Wolman), Reinhold, New York, pp. 15–29.

Lerner, R.M. (1973) The development of personal space schemata toward body build. *Journal of Psychology*, **84**, 229–35.

Lerner, R.M. and Gelbert, E. (1969) Body identification, preference, and aversion in children. *Developmental Psychology*, **5**, 256–462.

Lerner, R.M. and Korn, S.J. (1972) The development of body build stereotypes in males. *Child Development*, **43**, 908–20.

Levitt, J. (1986) Treating adults with eating disorders by using an inpatient approach. *Health and Social Work*, **11**, 133–40.

Levitz, L.S. and Stunkard, A.J. (1974) A therapeutic coalition for obesity: Behavior modification and patient self-help. *American Journal of Psychiatry*, **131**, 423–7.

Lew, E.A. and Garfinkel, P.E. (1979) Variations in mortality by weight among 750000 men and women. *Journal of Chronic Disorders*, **32**, 226–32.

Lewis, H.L. and MacGuire, M.P. (1985) Review of a group for parents of anorexics. *Journal of Psychiatric Research*, **19**(2), 453–8.

Lezak, M.D. (1979a) *Behavioral Concomitants of Configurational Disorganisation*. Paper presented at Seventh Annual Meeting of the International Neuropsychological Society, New York.

Lezak, M.D. (1979b) Recovery of memory and learning functions following traumatic brain injury. *Cortex*, **15**, 63–70.

Lezak, M.D. (1983) *Neuropsychological Assessment*, 2nd edn. Oxford University Press, New York.

Libby, D.G. and Phillips, E. (1979) Eliminating rumination behavior in a profoundly retarded adolescent: An exploratory study. *Mental Retardation*, **17**, 94–5.

Lick, J. and Bootzin, R. (1971) *Covert Sensitization for the Treatment of Obesity*. Paper presented at Midwestern Psychological Association, Detroit, Michigan.

Liebman, R., Minuchin, S. and Baker, L. (1974) An integrated treatment program for anorexia nervosa. *American Journal of Psychiatry*, **131**, 432–6.

Linn, R. and Stuart, S.L. (1977) *The Last Chance Diet*. Bantam Books, New York.

Loevinger, J. and Wessler, R. (1970) *Measuring Ego Development*. Jossey-Bass, San Francisco.

Loganbill, C. and Koch, M. (1983) Eating disorder group. *Journal of the College of Studies in Personnel*, **24**, 174–275.

Logue, A.W. (1986) *The Psychology of Eating and Drinking*. Freeman, New York.

Long, C.G. and Cordle, C.G. (1982) Psychological treatments of binge-eating and self-induced vomiting. *British Journal of Medical Psychology*, **55**, 139–45.

Long, C.J. and Brown, D.A. (1979) *Analysis of Temporal Cortex Dysfunction by Neuropsychological Techniques*. Paper presented at American Psychological Association Convention, New York.

Lopez-Virella, M.F.L., Stone, P.G. and Colwell, J.A. (1977) Serum high density lipoprotein in diabetic patients. *Diabetologia*, **13**, 285–91.

Lucas, A.R., Duncan, J.W. and Piens, V. (1976) The treatment of anorexia nervosa. *American Journal of Psychiatry*, **133**, 1034–8.

Luria, A.R. (1973) *The Working Brain: An Introduction to Neuropsychology*. Basic Books, New York.

Lutjens, A. and Smit, J.L. (1977) Effect of biguanide treatment in obese children. *Helvetia Paediatrica Acta*, **31**, 473–80.

Luxemberg, J.S., Swedo, S.E. and Flament, M.E. (1987) Neuroanatomical abnormalities in obsessive–compulsive disorder detected with quantitative X-ray computed tomography. *American Journal of Psychiatry*, **145**, 1089–93.

Maddox, G.L., Beck, K.W. and Liederman, V.R. (1968) Overweight as social deviance and disability. *Journal of Health and Social Behavior*, **9**, 287–798.

Maddox, G.L. and Leiderman, V.R. (1969) Overweight as a social disability. *Journal of Medical Education*, **44**, 214–20.

Maiman, L.A., Wang, V.L., Becker, M.H., Finlay, T. and Simonson, M. (1979) Attitudes towards obesity and the obese among professionals. *Journal of the American Dietetic Association*, **74**, 331–6.

Malcolm, R., O'Neil, P.M. and Hirsch, A.A. (1980) Taste hedonics and thresholds in obesity. *International Journal of Obesity*, **4**, 203–12.

Malone, G.L. and Armstrong, B.K. (1985) Treatment of anorexia nervosa in a young adult patient with diabetes mellitus. *Journal of Nervous and Mental Disease*, **173**, 509–11.

Maloney, M.J. and Farrell, M.K. (1980) Treatment of severe weight loss in anorexia nervosa with hyperalimentation and psychotherapy. *American Journal of Psychiatry*, **137**, 310–14.

Mann, R.A. (1972) The behavior-therapeutic use of contingency contracting to control an adult behavior problem: Weight control. *Journal of Applied Behavior Analysis*, **5**, 99–109.

Manno, B. (1972) Weight reduction as a function of the timing of reinforcement in a covert aversive conditioning paradigm. *Diss Abstracts International*, **32(7-B)**, 4221.

Manno, B. and Marston, A.R. (1972) Weight reduction as a function of negative covert reinforcement (sensitisation) versus positive covert reinforcement. *Behaviour Research and Therapy*, **10**, 201–7.

Marks, H.H. (1960) Influence of obesity in morbidity and mortality. *Bulletin of the New York Academy of Science*, **36**, 296–312.

Marks, I.M., Hodgson, R.J. and Rachman, S. (1975) Treatment of chronic obsessive–compulsive neurosis by *in vivo* exposure: A two-year follow-up and issues in treatment. *British Journal of Psychiatry*, **127**, 349–64.

Martin, J.E. (1989a) Bulimia: A literature review. *British Journal of Occupational Therapy*, **52**, 138–42.

Martin, J.E. (1989b) The role of body image in the development of bulimia. *British Journal of Occupational Therapy*, **52**, 262–5.

Martin, J.E. (1990) Bulimia: A review of the medical, behavioural and psychodynamic models of treatment. *British Journal of Occupational Therapy*, **53**(12), 495–500.

Mason, E.E. (1981) Surgical treatment of obesity. *Major Problems in Clinical Surgery*, **26**, 1–493.

Mattingly, D. and Bhanji, S. (1982) The diagnosis of anorexia nervosa. *Journal of the Royal College of Physicians of London*, **16**, 191–4.

Mavissakalian, M. (1982) Anorexia nervosa treated with response prevention and prolonged exposure. *Behaviour Research and Therapy*, **20**, 27–31.

Mawson, A.R. (1974) Anorexia nervosa and the regulation of intake: A review. *Psychological Medicine*, **4**, 289–308.

Mazel, J. (1981) *The Beverly Hills Diet*. Macmillan, New York.

McConaghy, M. and Blaszcynski, A. (1988) Imaginal desensitisation: A cost-effective treatment in two shoplifters and a binge-eater resistant to previous therapy. *Australian and New Zealand Journal of Psychiatry*, **2**, 78–82.

McCrea, C.W., Summerfield, A. and Rosen, B. (1982) Body image: A selective review of existing measurement techniques. *British Journal of Medical Psychology*, **55**, 225–33.

McCullagh, E.P. and Tupper, W.R. (1940) Anorexia nervosa. *Annals of Internal Medicine*, **14**, 817–38.

McFie, J. (1975) *Assessment of Organic Intellectual Impairment*. Academic Press, London.

McGee, J., Menolascino, F.J., Hobbs, D.C. and Menosek, P.E. (1987) *Gentle Teaching: A Non-Aversive Approach for Helping Persons with Mental Retardation*. Human Sciences Press, New York.

McKenzie, K., Thompson, S.B.N. and Weeks, D.J. (1991) *Your Memory Manual: A Self-Help Guide to Help People Overcome Everyday Memory Difficulties*. Lothian Health Board, Edinburgh.

McReynolds, W.T. (1982) Toward a psychology of obesity: Review of research on the role of personality and level of adjustment. *International Journal of Eating Disorders*, **2**, 37–57.

Mehrabian, A. (1987) *Eating Characteristics and Temperament: General Measures and Interrelationships*. Springer-Verlag, New York.

Mehrabian, A., Nahum, I.V. and Duke, V. (1986) Individual difference correlates and measures of predisposition to obesity and to anorexia. *Imagination, Cognition and Personality*, **5**, 339–55.

Mehrabian, A. and Riccioni, M. (1986) Measures of eating-related characteristics for the general population: Relationships and temperament. *Journal of Personality Assessment*, **50**, 610–29.

Mental Handicap in Wales Applied Research Unit (1985) *Introductory Leaflet*. Mental Handicap in Wales Applied Research Unit, Cardiff.

Merl, H. (1989) Systemic family therapy in a case of anorexia nervosa in a boy: A case report within the scope of final interventions. *Psychotherapy, Psychosomatics and Medical Psychology*, **39**(12), 444–51.

Messerli, P., Seron, X. and Tissot, R. (1979) Quelques aspects des troubles de la programmation dans le syndrome frontal. *Archives Suisse de Neurologie, Neurochirurgie, et de Psychiatrie*,

125, 23–35.

Metropolitan Life Insurance Company (1959) New weight standards for men and women. *Statistical Bulletin,* **40**, 1–4.

Meyer, V. and Crisp, A.H. (1964) Aversion therapy in two cases of obesity. *Behaviour Research and Therapy,* **2**, 143–7.

Meynen, G.E. (1970) A comparative study of three treatment approaches with the obese: relaxation, covert sensitization and modified systematic desensitization. *Diss Abstracts International,* **31(5-B),** 3998.

Miceli, G., Caltagirone, C., Gainotti, G., Masullo, C. and Silveri, M.C. (1981) Neuropsychological correlates of localized cerebral lesions in non-aphasic brain-damaged patients. *Journal of Clinical Neuropsychology,* **3**, 53–63.

Michael, J. (1975) Positive and negative reinforcement, a distinction that is no longer necessary; or a better way to talk about bad things, in *Behavior Analysis: Areas of Research and Application,* (eds E. Ramp and G. Semb), Prentice Hall, Englewood Cliffs, New Jersey, pp. 31–44.

Miller, E. and Hague, F. (1975) Some characteristics of verbal behaviour in presenile dementia. *Psychological Medicine,* **5**, 255–9.

Miller, N.E., Forde, O.H., Thelle, D.S. and Mjös, O.D. (1977) High-density lipoprotein and coronary heart disease: A prospective case-control study. *Lancet,* **1**, 965–7.

Mills, I.H. (1978) The disease of coping. *Practitioner,* **217**, 529–38.

Mills, I.H. and Medlicott, L. (1984) The basis of naloxone treatment in anorexia nervosa and the metabolic reponses to it, in *The Psychobiology of Anorexia Nervosa,* (eds K.M. Pirke and D. Ploog), Springer-Verlag, Berlin, pp. 161–71.

Mintz, I.L. (1983) Anorexia nervosa and bulimia in males, in *Fear of Being Fat: The Treatment of Anorexia Nervosa and Bulimia,* (eds C.P. Wilson, C.C. Hogan and I.L. Mintz), Jason Aronson, New York.

Minuchin, S., Rosman, B.L. and Baker, L. (1978) *Psychosomatic Families: Anorexia Nervosa in Context.* Harvard University Press, Cambridge, Massachusetts.

Mitchell, J.E. and Groat, R. (1984) A placebo-controlled, double-blind trial of amitriptyline in bulimia. *Journal of Clinical Psychopharmacology,* **4**, 186–93.

Mitchell, J.E., Pyle, R.L., Eckert, E.D. *et al.* (1990) A comparison study of structured intensive group psychotherapy in the treatment of bulimia nervosa. *Archives of General Psychiatry*, **47**(2), 149–57.

Mitchell, J.E., Pyle, R.L., Hatsukami, D. and Boutacoff, L. (1984) The dexamethasone suppression test in patients with bulimia. *Journal of Clinical Psychiatry*, **45**, 508–11.

Mizes, J.S. and Fleece, E.L. (1984) *On the Use of Progressive Relaxation in the Treatment of Bulimia: A Replication and Extension*. Paper presented at the Annual Meeting of the Society of Behavioural Medicine, Philadelphia.

Mizes, J.S. and Klesger, R.C. (1989) Validity, reliability, and factor structure of the anorectic cognitions questionnaire. *Addictions and Behaviour*, **14**(5), 589–94.

Mizes, J.S. and Lohr, J.M. (1983) The treatment of bulimia (binge eating): A quasi-experimental investigation of the effects of stimulus narrowing, self-reinforcement, and self-control relaxation. *International Journal of Eating Disorders*, **2**, 59–65.

Montgomery, S.A. (1979) Depressive symptoms in acute schizophrenia. *Progress in Neuropsychopharmacology*, **3**(4), 429–33.

Montgomery, S.A. and Asberg, M. (1979) A new depression scale designed to be sensitive to change. *British Journal of Psychiatry*, **134**, 382–9.

Monti, P.M., McCrady, B.S. and Barlow, D.H. (1977) Effect of positive reinforcement, informational feedback, and contingency contracting on a bulimic anorexic female. *Behavior Therapy*, **8**, 258–64.

Moore, C.H. and Crum, B.C. (1969) Weight reduction in a chronic schizophrenic by means of operant conditioning procedures: A case study. *Behaviour Research and Therapy*, **7**, 129–31.

Moore, R., Mills, I.H. and Forster, A. (1981) Naloxone in the treatment of anorexia nerovsa: Effect on weight gain and lipolysis. *Journal of the Royal Society of Medicine*, **74**, 129–31.

Morgan, H.G. and Haywood, A.E. (1988) Clinical assessment of anorexia nervosa. The Morgan-Russell Outcome Assessment Schedule. *British Journal of Psychiatry*, **152**, 367–71.

Morgan, H.G. and Russell, G.F.M. (1975) Value of family background and clinical features as predictors of long-term outcome in anorexia nervosa: Four-year follow-up study of

41 patients. *Psychological Medicine*, **5**, 355–71.

Morgan, M. and Thompson, S.B.N. (1989) Bridging the gap. *Therapy Weekly*, **15**(40), 10.

Morton, R. (1689) *Pathisiologica – or a Treatise of Consumption*. Smith and Walford, London.

Moss, F.A. (1924) Note on building likes and dislikes in children. *Journal of Experimental Psychology*, **7**, 475–8.

Mrosovsky, N. and Powley, T.L. (1977) Set points for body weight and fat. *Behavioral Biology*, **20**, 205–23.

Munn, N.L. (1956) *Psychology: The Fundamentals of Human Adjustment*. Houghton Mifflin, Boston.

Munro, J.F. (1979) *The Treatment of Obesity*. MTP Press, Lancaster.

Murstein, B.I. and Leipold, W.D. (1961) The role of learning motor abilities in the Wechsler-Bellevue Digit Symbol test. *Educational Psychological Measurement*, **21**, 103–12.

Myerson, B. and Adler, W. (1982) *I Love New York Diet*. William Morrow, New York.

Nagler, W. and Androff, A. (1990) Investigating the impact of deconditioning anxiety on weight loss. *Psychological Reports*, **66**(2), 595–600.

Nathan, D.M., Singer, D.E., Hurxthal, K. and Goodson, J.D. (1984) The clinical information value of the glycosylated haemoglobin assay. *New England Journal of Medicine*, **310**, 341–6.

National Center for Health Statistics (1981) Plan and operation of the National Health and Nutrition Examination Survey, 1976–1980. *Vital and Health Statistics*, **1**(15), 81–1317, Public Health Service, Washington DC.

Nedergaard, J. and Lindberg, O. (1981) The brown fat cell. *International Review of Cytology*, **74**, 187–254.

Nelson, H.E. and O'Connell, A. (1978) Dementia: The estimation of premorbid intelligence levels using the New Adult Reading Test. *Cortex*, **14**, 234–44.

Nemiah, J.C. (1959) Anorexia nervosa: Fact and theory. *American Journal of Digestive Diseases*, **3**, 249–74.

Nestler, J.E., Powers, L.P., Matt, D.W. *et al* (1991) A direct effect of hyperinsulinemia on serum sex hormone-binding globulin levels in obese women with the polycystic ovary syndrome. *Journal of Clinical Endocrinology and Metabolism*, **71**(1), 83–9.

Neuman, P. and Halvorsen, P. (1983) *Anorexia Nervosa and Bulimia: A Handbook for Counsellors and Therapists*. Van Nostrand Reinhold, New York.

Newcombe, F. (1969) *Missile Wounds of the Brain*. Oxford University Press, London.

Newman, H.H., Freeman, F.N. and Holzinger, K.H. (1937) *Twins: A Study of Heredity and Environment*. University of Chicago Press, Chicago.

Nicolle, G. (1938) Prepsychotic anorexia. *Proceedings of the Royal Society of Medicine*, **32**, 153.

Nidetch, J. and Heilman, J.R. (1972) *The Story of Weight Watchers*. New American Library, New York.

Nisbett, R.E. (1972) Hunger, obesity, and the ventromedial hypothalamus. *Psychological Review*, **79**, 433–53.

Nogami, Y. and Yabana, F. (1977) On kibarashi-gui (binge-eating). *Folia Psychiatrica et Neurologica Japonica*, **31**, 159–66.

Novak, L.P. (1963) Age and sex differences in body density and creatinine excretion of high school children. *Annals of the American Academy of Science*, **110**, 545–77.

Novin, D., Wyrwicka, W. and Bray, G.A. (1976) *Hunger: Basic Mechanisms and Clinical Implications*. Raven Press, New York.

Nunes-Correa, J., Pereira, E., Carreiras, F. and Gardete Correia, L. (1980) Stopping biguanide therapy. *Lancet*, **1**, 427.

Nylander, I. (1971) The feelings of being fat and dieting in a school population: Epidemiologic interview investigation. *Acta Sociomedica Scandinavicà*, **3**, 17–26.

Ohwaki, S. and Zingarelli, G. (1988) Feeding clients with severe multiple handicaps in a skilled nursing care facility. *Mental Retardation*, **26**, 21–4.

Oliver, B.E. (1986) Exclusion diets in mental handicap practice. *Mental Handicap*, **14**(3), 94–8.

Ollendick, T.H. (1979) Behavioral treatment of anorexia nervosa: A five year study. *Behavior Modification*, **3**, 124–35.

Orbach, S. (1978) *Fat is a Feminist Issue: How to Lose Weight Permanently – Without Dieting*. Paddington Press, London.

Orbach, S. (1984) *Fat is a Feminist Issue 2: How to Free Yourself from Feeling Obsessive about Food*. Hamlyn, London.

Orbach, S. (1985) Visibility/invisibility: Social considerations in anorexia nervosa – a feminist perspective, in *Theory and Treatment of Anorexia Nervosa and Bulimia*, (ed S.W. Emmett), Brunner/Mazel, New York, pp. 127–38.

Ordman, A. and Kirschenbaum, D. (1985) Cognitive–behavioural therapy for bulimia: An initial outcome study. *Journal of Consulting and Clinical Psychology*, **53**, 305–11.

Orshansky, M. (1965) Who's who among the poor: A demographic view of poverty. *Social Security Bulletin*, **28**, 3–32.

Osterreith, P.A. (1944) Le test de copie d'une figure complexe. *Archives de Psychologie*, **30**, 206–356.

Pace, C.M., Ivanic, M.T., Edwards, G.L., Iwata, B.A. and Page, T.J. (1985) Assessment of stimulus preference and reinforcer value with profoundly retarded individuals. *Journal of Applied Behavior Analysis*, **18**(3), 249–55.

Paffenbarger, R.S. and Wing, A.L. (1969) Chronic disease in former college students. *American Journal of Epidemiology*, **90**, 527–36.

Page, T.J., Finney, J.W., Parrish, J.M. and Iwata, B.A. (1983a) Assessment and reduction of food stealing in Prader Willi children. *Applied Research in Mental Retardation*, **4**(3), 219–28.

Page, T.J., Stanley, A.E., Richman, G.S., Deal, R.M. and Iwata, B.A. (1983b) Reduction of food theft and maintenance of weight loss in a Prader Willi adult. *Journal of Behavior Therapy and Experimental Psychiatry*, **14**(3), 261–8.

Palmer, R.L. (1979) Dietary chaos syndrome: A useful new term? *British Journal of Medical Psychology*, **52**, 187–90.

Palmer, R.L. (1982) *Anorexia Nervosa: A Guide to Sufferers and Families*. Penguin Books, Middlesex.

Parizkova, J. (1961) Total body fat and skinfold thickness in children. *Metabolism*, **10**, 794–807.

Parker, R. and Mauger, S. (1976) Self-starvation. *Spare Rib*, **28**, 7.

Parsons, O.A. (1975) Brain damage in alcoholics: Altered states of unconsciousness, in *Alcohol Intoxication and Withdrawal, Experimental Studies No. 2*, (ed M.M. Gross), Plenum, New York.

Patel, D.P. and Stowers, J.M. (1964) Phenformin in weight reduction of obese diabetics. *Lancet*, **2**, 282–4.

Patton, G.C., Wood, K. and Johnson-Sabine, E. (1986) Physical illness: A risk factor in anorexia nervosa. *British Journal of Psychiatry*, **149**, 756–9.

Paykel, E.S., Mueller, P.S. and de la Vergne, P.M. (1973) Amitriptyline, weight gain and carbohydrate craving: A side-effect. *British Journal of Psychiatry*, **123**, 501–7.

Pell, S. and Alonzo, A.O. (1963) Acute myocardial infarction in a large industrial population. *Journal of the American Medical Association*, **185**, 117–24.

Penick, S.B. (1970) The use of amphetamine in obesity. *Psychiatric Opinion*, **1**, 27–30.

Penick, S.B., Filion, R., Fox, S. and Stunkard, A.J. (1971) Behavior modification in the treatment of obesity. *Psychosomatic Medicine*, **33**, 49–55.

Perret, E. (1974) The left frontal lobe of man and the suppression of habitual responses in verbal categorical behaviour. *Neuropsychologia*, **12**, 323–30.

Pertschuk, M.J., Forster, J., Buzby, G. and Mullen, J.L. (1981) The treatment of anorexia nervosa with total perenteral nutrition. *Biology and Psychiatry*, **16**, 53–60.

Peters, G., Besseghir, K., Kasermann, H.P. and Peters-Haefeli, L. (1979) Effects of drug on ingestive behavior. *Pharmacological Therapy*, **5**, 485–503.

Peveler, R.C. and Fairburn, C.G. (1989) Anorexia nervosa in association with diabetes mellitus – a cognitive–behavioural approach to treatment. *Behaviour Research and Therapy*, **27**(1), 95–9.

Peyre, F., Martinez, R., Calache, M., Verdoux, H. and Bourgeois, M. (1989) New validation of the Montgomery and Asberg Depression Scale (MADRS) on a sample of 147 hospitalized depressed patients. *Annals of Medical Psychology (Paris)*, **147**(7), 762–7.

Pierloot, R.A. and Houben, M.E. (1978) Estimation of body dimensions in anorexia nervosa. *Psychological Medicine*, **8**, 317–24.

Pierloot, R.A., Vandereycken, W. and Verhaest, S. (1982) An inpatient treatment program for anorexia nervosa patients. *Acta Psychiatrica Scandinavica*, **66**, 1–8.

Pitts, F.N. and Guze, S.B. (1963) Anorexia nervosa and gonadal dysgenesis (Turner's syndrome). *American Journal of Psychiatry*, **119**, 1100–2.

Plantey, F. (1977) Pimozide in treatment of anorexia nervosa. *Lancet*, **i**, 1105.

Pooling Project Research Group (1978) Relationship of blood pressure, serum cholesterol, smoking habit, relative weight, and ECG abnormalities to incidence of major coronary events: Final report of the Pooling Project. *Journal of Chronic*

Diseases, **31**, 201–306.

Pope, H.G., Hudson, J., Jonas, J. and Yurgelun-Todd, D. (1983) Bulimia treated with imipramine: A placebo-controlled double-blind study. *American Journal of Psychiatry*, **140**, 554–8.

Premack, D. (1959) Towards empirical behaviour laws: 1. Positive reinforcement. *Psychological Review*, **66**(4), 219–33.

Premack, D. (1971) Catching up with commonsense or two sides of a generalisation: Reinforcement and punishment, in *The Nature of Reinforcement*, (ed R. Glaser), Academic Press, New York.

Presland, J.L. (1989) *Overcoming Difficult Behaviour: A Guide and Source-book for Helping People with Severe Mental Handicaps*. BIMH Publications, Kidderminster.

Printen, K.J. and Mason, E.E. (1977) Gastric bypass for morbid obesity in patients more than 50 years of age. *Surgery, Gynaecology and Obstetrics*, **144**, 192.

Pritikin, N. and McGrady, P. Jr. (1979) *The Pritikin Program for Diet and Exercise*. Grosset and Dunlap, New York.

Puls, W. and Keup, U. (1973) Influence of an alpha-amylase inhibitor (Bay d 7791) on blood glucose, serum insulin and NEFA in starch loading tests in rats, dogs and man. *Diabetologia*, **9**, 97–101.

Puls, W., Keup, U. and Krause, H.P. (1977) Glucosidase inhibition. A new approach to the treatment of diabetes, obesity and hyperlipoproteinaemia. *Naturwissenschaften*, **64**, 536–7.

Pyke, S. and Agnew, N. McK. (1963) Digit Span performance as a function of noxious stimulation. *Journal of Consulting Psychology*, **27**, 281.

Pyle, R.L., Halvorsen, P., Neuman, P. and Goff, G. (1983) The incidence of bulimia in freshman college students. *International Journal of Eating Disorders*, **2**, 75–86.

Pyle, R.L., Mitchell, J.E. and Eckert, E.D. (1981) Bulimia: A report of 34 cases. *Journal of Clinical Psychiatry*, **2**, 60–4.

Pyle, R.L., Mitchell, J.E., Eckert, E.D., Hatsukami, D.K. and Goff, G.M. (1984) The interruption of bulimic behaviors: A review of three treatment programs. *Psychiatric Clinics of North America*, **7**, 275–86.

Rabavilas, A.D., Boulougouris, J.C. and Stefanis, C. (1976) Duration of flooding sessions in the treatment of obsessive–

compulsive patients. *Behaviour Research and Therapy*, **14**, 349–55.

Rachman, S., Cobb, J., Grey, S. *et al.* (1979) Behavioural treatment of obsessive–compulsive disorders with and without clomipramine. *Behaviour Research and Therapy*, **17**, 467–78.

Rachman, S., Hodgson, R. and Marzillier, J. (1970) Treatment of an obsessional compulsive disorder by modelling. *Behaviour Research and Therapy*, **8**, 385–92.

Ramier, A-M. and Hecaen, H. (1970) Rôle respectif des atteintes frontales et de la latéralisation lésionnelle dans les déficits de la 'fluence verbale'. *Revue Psychologique*, **123**, 17–22.

Rapoff, M.A., Altman, K. and Christophersen, E.R. (1980) Suppression of self-injurious behavior: Determining the least restrictive alternative. *Journal of Mental Deficiency*, **24**, 37–47.

Rast, J., Johnston, J.M., Allen, J.E. and Drum, C. (1985) Effects of nutritional and mechanical properties of food on ruminative behavior. *Journal of Experimental Analysis of Behavior*, **44**(2), 195–206.

Rau, J.H., Struve, F.A. and Green, R.S. (1979) Electroencephalographic correlates of compulsive eating. *Clinical Electroencephalography*, **10**, 180–8.

Redmond, D.E., Swann, A. and Heninger, G.R. (1976) Phenoxybenzamine in anorexia nervosa. *Lancet*, **ii**, 307.

Reh, M. (1953) Fettzellgrösse beim Menschen und Abhängigkeit vom Ernährungszustand. *Virchows Archives (Pathologische Anatomie)*, **324**, 234.

Reitan, R.M. (1955) Investigation of the validity of Halstead's measure of biological intelligence. *Archives of Neurology and Psychiatry*, **73**, 28–35.

Reitan, R.M. (1958) Validity of the Trail Making Test as an indication of organic brain damage. *Perceptual and Motor Skills*, **8**, 271–6.

Reitan, R.M. and Tarshes, E.L. (1959) Differential effects of lateralized brain lesions on the Trail Making Test. *Journal of Nervous and Mental Disease*, **129**, 257–62.

Reitman, E.E. and Cleveland, S.E. (1964) Changes in body image following sensory deprivation in schizophrenia and control groups. *Journal of Abnormal Social Psychology*, **68**, 168–76.

Rey, A.L. (1941) L'examen psychologique dans les cas d'encéphalopathie traumatique. *Archives de Psychologie*, **28**(112), 286–340.

Rey, A.L. (1964) *L'examen Clinique de Psychologie*. Presses Universitaires de France, Paris.

Richfield, E.K., Twyman, R. and Berent, S. (1987) Neurological syndrome following bilateral change to the head of the caudate nuclei. *Annals of Neurology*, **22**, 768–71.

Richter, J. (1992) Reflux disease. *International Journal of Hospital Medicine*, **X**(5), 49.

Rimm, A.A., Werner, L.H., Bernstein, R. and van Yserloo, B. (1972) Diabetes and obesity in 73 532 women. *Obesity Bariatric Medicine*, **1**, 77–84.

Roberts, E., Chase, T. and Towers, D. (1976) *GABA in Nervous System Function*. Raven Press, New York.

Roberts, S.W. (1977) *Nutrition Assessment Manual*. University of Iowa, Iowa.

Robinson, A.L., Heaton, R.K., Lehman, R.A.W. and Stilson, D.W. (1980) The utility of the Wisconsin Card Sorting Test in detecting and localizing frontal lobe lesions. *Journal of Consulting and Clinical Psychology*, **48**, 605–14.

Robinson, P., Checkley, S. and Russell, G. (1985) Suppression of eating by fenfluramine in patients with bulimia nervosa. *British Journal of Psychiatry*, **146**, 168–76.

Rodin, G.M., Daneman, D., Johnson, L.E., Kenshole, A. and Garfinkel, P.E. (1985) Anorexia nervosa and bulimia in female adolescents with insulin-dependent diabetes mellitus: A systematic study. *Journal of Psychiatric Research*, **19**, 381–4.

Rodin, J., Moskowitz, H.R. and Bray, G.A. (1976) Relationship between obesity, weight loss and taste responsiveness. *Psychological Bulletin*, **17**, 591–7.

Rollins, N. and Piazza, E. (1978) Diagnosis of anorexia nervosa: A critical reappraisal. *Journal of the American Academy of Child Psychiatry*, **17**, 126–37.

Ronsard, N. (1975) *Cellulite*. Bantam Books, New York.

Roper, G., Rachman, S. and Hodgson, R. (1973) An experiment on obsessional checking. *Behaviour Research and Therapy*, **11**, 271–8.

Rosen, J.C. and Leitenberg, H. (1982) Bulimia nervosa: Treatment with exposure and response prevention. *Behavior Therapy*, **13**, 117–24.

Rosenberg, M. (1979) Conceiving the Self. Basic Books, New York.

Rosenvinge, J.H. and Mouland, S.O. (1990) Outcome and prognosis of anorexia nervosa. A retrospective study of 41 subjects. British Journal of Psychiatry, 156, 92–7.

Rosmark, B., Berne, C., Holmgren, S. et al. (1986) Eating disorders in patients with insulin-dependent diabetes. Journal of Clinical Psychiatry, 47, 547–50.

Rothenberg, A. (1990) Adolescence and eating disorder: The obsessive–compulsive syndrome. Psychiatric Clinics of North America, 13(3), 469–88.

Rozin, P. and Kalat, J. (1971) Specific hungers and poison avoidance and adaptive specializations of learning. Psychological Review, 78, 459–86.

Russell, D.M.C., Freedman, M.L., Feighlin, D.H.I. et al. (1983) Delayed gastric emptying and improvement with domperidone in a patient with anorexia nervosa. American Journal of Psychiatry, 140, 1235–6.

Russell, G.F.M. (1978) The present status of anorexia nervosa. Psychological Medicine, 7, 363.

Russell, G.F.M. (1979) Bulimia nervosa: An ominous variant of anorexia nervosa. Psychological Medicine, 9, 429–48.

Russell, G.F.M. (1985) Do drugs have a place in the management of anorexia nervosa? in Psychopharmacology and Food, (eds M. Sandler and T. Silverstone), Oxford University Press, Oxford, pp. 146–61.

Ryle, J.A. (1936) Anorexia nervosa. Lancet, ii, 893–9.

Rzechorzek, A. (1979) Cognitive dysfunctions resulting from unilateral frontal lobe lesions in man, in Brain Impairment: Proceedings of the 1978 Brain Impairment Workshop, (eds M. Molloy, G.V. Stanley and K.W. Walsh), University of Melbourne, Melbourne.

Sabine, E., Yonace, A., Farrington, K., Barratt, K. and Wakeling, A. (1983) Bulimia nervosa: A placebo-controlled double-blind therapeutic trial of mianserin. British Journal of Pharmacology, 15, 1955–2025.

Sachs, L.B. and Ingram, G.L. (1972) Covert sensitization as a treatment for weight control. Psychological Reports, 30, 971–4.

Safai-Kutti, S. and Kutti, J. (1984) Zinc supplementation and anorexia nervosa. American Journal of Clinical Nutrition, 44, 581–2.

Safai-Kutti, S. and Kutti, J. (1986) Zinc and anorexia nervosa. *Annals of Internal Medicine*, **100**, 317–18.

Sakurazawa, N. (1965) *Macrobiotics*. Award Books, New York.

Salans, L.B., Cushman, S.W. and Weismann, R.E. (1973) Studies on human adipose tissue. Adipose cell size and number in non-obese and obese patients. *Journal of Clinical Investigation*, **52**, 929.

Saleh, J.W. and Lebwohl, P. (1980) Metoclopramide-induced gastric emptying in patients with anorexia nervosa. *American Journal of Gastroenterology*, **74**, 127–32.

Salkovskis, P.M. and Warwick, H.M.C. (1985) Cognitive therapy of obsessive–compulsive disorder: Treating treatment failures. *Behavioural Psychotherapy*, **13**, 243–55.

Samanin, R., Caccia, S. and Bendotti, C. (1980) Further studies on the mechanism of serotonin-dependent anorexia in rats. *Psychopharmacology*, **68**, 99–104.

Samanin, R., Mennini, T., Ferraris, A., Bendotti, C. and Borsini, F. (1980) Repeated treatment with d-fenfluramine or methergoline alters cortex binding of 3-H-serotonin and serotonergic sensitivity in rats. *European Journal of Pharmacology*, **61**, 203–6.

Sanghvi, I.S., Singer, G., Friedman, E. and Gershon, S. (1975) Anorexigenic effects of d-amphetamine and L-DOPA in the rat. *Pharmacology and Biochemistry of Behavior*, **3**, 81–6.

Sarason, S.B. and Doris, J. (1969) *Psychological Problems in Mental Deficiency*. Harper and Row, New York.

Sarason, S.B. and Gladwin, T. (1958) Psychological and cultural problems in mental subnormality: A review of research. *Genetic Psychology Monographs*, **57**, 3–290.

Saul, S., Dekker, A. and Watson, C. (1981) Acute gastric dilation with infarction and perforation. Case report. *Gut*, **22**, 978–83.

Saunders, D.R. (1960) A factor analysis of the Information and the Arithmetic items in the WAIS. *Psychological Reports*, **6**, 367–83.

Savage, C. (1955) Variations in ego feeling induced by d-lysergic acid diethylamide (LSD-25). *Psychoanalysis Review*, **42**, 1–16.

Schaeffer, E.J., Anderson, D.W., Danner, R.N., Brewer, H.B. Jr. and Blackwelder, W.C. (1978) Plasma triglycerides in regulation of HDL cholesterol levels. *Lancet*, **2**, 391–2.

Schilder, P. (1935) *The Image and Appearance of the Human Body*. Kegan Paul, Trench and Trubner, London.

Schliessener-Stropp, B. (1985) Bulimia: A review of the literature. *Psychological Bulletin*, **95**, 247–57.

Schmidt, D.D., Frommer, W. and Junge, B. (1977) Alpha-glucosidase inhibitors. New complex oligosaccharides of microbial origin. *Naturwissenschaften*, **64**, 535–6.

Schneider, J. and Agras, S. (1985) A cognitive–behavioural group treatment of bulimia. *British Journal of Psychiatry*, **146**, 66–9.

Schneiderman, L. (1956) The estimation of one's own body traits. *Journal of Social Psychology*, **44**, 89–99.

Schwartz, R.C. (1982) Bulimia and family therapy. A case study. *International Journal of Eating Disorders*, **2**, 75–82.

Schwartz, R.C., Barrett, M.J. and Saba, G. (1984) Family therapy for bulimia, in *Handbook of Psychotherapy for Anorexia Nervosa and Bulimia*, (eds D.M. Garner and P.E. Garfinkel), Guildford Press, New York, pp. 280–307.

Schwartz, R.S. and Brunzell, J.D. (1981) Increase in adipose tissue lipoprotein lipase activity with weight loss. *Journal of Clinical Investigation*, **67**, 1425–30.

Schweiger, U., Laessle, R.G. and Pirke, K.M. (1986) Necessity of dietary management in eating disorders, in *Annual Series of European Research in Behaviour Therapy*, (ed W. Vandereycken), Swets and Zeitlinger, Lisse.

Scott, C. (1991) Are our kids growing up too fast? *Me Magazine*, **29 July**, 12–13.

Scott, D. (1988) *Anorexia and Bulimia Nervosa: Practical Approaches*. Croom Helm, London.

Screenivasan, U. (1978) Anorexia nervosa in boys. *Canadian Psychiatric Association Journal*, **23**, 159–62.

Seaver, R.L. and Binder, H.J. (1972) Anorexia nervosa and other anorectic states in man. General clinical considerations. *Advancements in Psychosomatic Medicine*, **7**, 257–76.

Secord, P.F. (1953) Objectification of word association procedures by the use of homonyms: Measure of body cathexis. *Journal of Personality*, **3**, 479–95.

Seguin, E. (1866) *Idiocy: Its Treatment by the Physiological Method*. William Wood, New York.

Seltzer, C.C. and Mayer, J. (1965) A simple criterion of obesity. *Postgraduate Medicine*, **38**(2), A101–A107.

Selvini Palazzoli, M.S. (1974) *Self-starvation: From the Intra-psychic to the Transpersonal Approach to Anorexia Nervosa.* Chaucer, London.

Sergent, J. and Liebman, R. (1984) Outpatient treatment of anorexia nervosa. *Psychiatric Clinics of North America*, **7**(2), 235–45.

Shargill, N.S., Ohshima, K., Bray, G.A. and Chan, T.M. (1984) Muscle protein turnover in the perfused hindquarters of lean genetically obese-diabetic (db/db) mice. *Diabetes*, **33**, 1160–4.

Sheer, D.E. (1956) Psychometric studies, in *Studies in Topectomy*, (eds N.D.C. Lewis, C. Landis and H.E. King), Grune and Stratton, New York.

Sherman, A.A. (1981) Obesity and sexism: Parental child preferences and attitudes toward obesity. MA thesis, Psychology Department, University of Cincinnati.

Shisslak, C., Crago, M., Schnaps, L. and Swain, B. (1986) Interactional group therapy for anorexic and bulimic women. *Psychotherapy*, **23**, 598–607.

Silk, D.B.A. (1983) Parenteral feeding, in *Nutritional Support in Hospital Practice*, (ed D.B.A. Silk), Blackwell, Oxford.

Silverstone, J.T. (1970) Obesity and social class. *Psychotherapy and Psychosomatics*, **18**, 266–330.

Silverstone, J.T., Stark, J.E. and Buckle, R.M. (1966) Hunger during total starvation. *Lancet*, **1**, 1343–4.

Silverstone, T., Fincham, J., Wells, B. and Kyriakides, M. (1980) The effect of the dopamine receptor blocking drug pimozide on the stimulant and anorectic actions of dextro-amphetamine in man. *Neuropharmacology*, **19**, 1235–7.

Simat, B.M., Maynard, R.R. and From, A.H.L. (1983) Is the erythrocyte sodium pump altered in human obesity? *Journal of Clinical Endocrinology and Metabolism*, **56**, 925–9.

Sjöström, L., Björntorp, P. and Vrana, J. (1971) Microscopic fat cell size measurements on frozen-cut adipose tissue in comparison with automatic determination of osmium-fixed fat cells. *Journal of Lipid Research*, **12**, 521.

Skidmore, C. (1985) Eating disorders: A comparison between schools in the private and public sector. The search for a familial transmission pattern. MA (Honours) psychology thesis, University of Edinburgh.

Slade, P.D. (1985) *A Review of Body Image Studies in Anorexia Nervosa and Bulimia Nervosa.* Proceedings of the International

Conference on Anorexia Nervosa and Related Disorders, Swansea, Wales.

Slade, P.D. and Russell, G.F. (1973) Awareness of body dimensions in anorexia nervosa: Cross-sectional and longitudinal studies. *Psychological Medicine*, **3**(2), 188–99.

Slagerman, M. and Yager, J. (1989) Multiple family group treatment for eating disorders: A short term program. *Psychiatric Medicine*, **7**(4), 269–83.

Small, A. (1984) The contribution of psychodiagnostic test results toward understanding anorexia nervosa. *International Journal of Eating Disorders*, **3**, 47–60.

Smeets, P.M. (1970) Withdrawal of social reinforcers as a means of controlling rumination and regurgitation in a profoundly retarded person. *Training in Schools Bulletin*, **67**, 158–67.

Smith, A. (1966) Intellectual functions in patients with lateralized frontal tumors. *Journal of Neurology, Neurosurgery, and Psychiatry*, **29**, 52–9.

Smith, A. (1967) Consistent sex differences in a specific (decoding) test performance. *Educational and Psychological Measurement*, **27**, 1077–83.

Smith, A.L. Jr., Piersel, W.C., Philbeck, R.W. and Gross, E.J. (1983) The elimination of mealtime food stealing and scavenging behavior in an institutionalised severely mentally retarded adult. *Mental Retardation*, **21**(6), 255–9.

Smith, L.H. Jr. (1976) *The Obese Patient*. W.B. Saunders, Philadelphia.

Snaith, R.P. (1981) *Clinical Neurosis*. Oxford University Press, Oxford.

Society of Actuaries (1960) Build and blood pressure study. *Society of Actuaries (Chicago)*, **1**, 1–268.

Solyom, L., Freeman, R.J. and Miles, J.E. (1982) A comparative psychometric study of anorexia nervosa and obsessive neurosis. *Canadian Journal of Psychiatry*, **27**, 282.

Sorlie, P., Gordon, D. and Kannel, W.B. (1980) Body build and mortality. The Framingham study. *Journal of the American Medical Association*, **243**, 1828–31.

Sorrell, V.F. and Burcher, S.K. (1976) Gastric bypass for morbid obesity. *New Zealand Medical Journal*, **84**, 96.

Spitz, H.H. (1972) Note on immediate memory for digits: Invariance over the years. *Psychological Bulletin*, **78**, 183–5.

Spreen, O. and Benton, A.L. (1965) Comparative studies of some psychological tests for cerebral damage. *Journal of Nervous and Mental Disease*, **140**, 323–33.

Staffieri, J.R. (1967) A study of social stereotype of body image in children. *Journal of Personality and Social Psychology*, **7**, 101–4.

Stern, J.S. (1983) Diet and exercise, in *Obesity*, (ed M.R.C. Greenwood), Churchill Livingstone, New York, pp. 65–84.

Stern, R.S., Lipsedge, M. and Marks, I. (1973) Obsessive ruminations: A controlled trial of a thought-stopping technique. *Behaviour Research and Therapy*, **11**, 659–62.

Stern, S. (1986) The dynamics of clinical management in the treatment of anorexia nervosa and bulimia: An organising theory. *International Journal of Eating Disorders*, **5**, 233–54.

Stevens, E.V. and Salisbury, J.D. (1984) Group therapy for bulimic adults. *American Journal of Orthopsychiatry*, **54**, 156–61.

Stevenson, R.W. and Solyom, L. (1990) The aphrodisiac effect of fenfluramine: Two case reports of a possible side effect to the use of fenfluramine in the treatment of bulimia. *Journal of Clinical Psychopharmacology*, **10**(1), 69–71.

Stewart, D.E., Robinson, E., Goldbloom, D.S. and Wright, C. (1990) Infertility and eating disorders. *American Journal of Obstetrics and Gynaecology*, **163**(4), 1196–9.

Stewart, J., Walsh, B.T., Wright, L., Roose, S. and Glassman, A. (1984) An open trial of monoamine oxidase inhibitors in bulimia. *Journal of Clinical Psychiatry*, **45**, 508–11.

Stollak, G.E. (1967) Weight loss obtained under different experimental procedures. *Psychotherapy: Theory, Research and Practice*, **4**, 61–4.

Strangler, R.S. and Printz, A.M. (1980) DSM-III: Psychiatric diagnosis in a university population. *American Journal of Psychiatry*, **137**, 937–40.

Strasser, M. and Giles, G. (1988) Ethical considerations, in *Anorexia and Bulimia Nervosa*, (ed D. Scott), Croom Helm, London, pp. 204–12.

Strauss, J. and Ryan, R.M. (1988) Cognitive dysfunction in eating disorders. *International Journal of Eating Disorders*, **7**(1), 19–27.

Strober, M. (1980) Personality and symptomatological features in young non-chronic anorexia nervosa patients. *Journal of*

Psychosomatic Research, **4**, 353–9.

Strober, M. (1981) The significance of bulimia in juvenile anorexia nervosa: An exploration of possible etiological factors. *International Journal of Eating Disorders*, **1**, 28–43.

Strober, M. (1983) An empirically-derived typology of anorexia nervosa, in *Anorexia Nervosa: Recent Developments*, (eds P.L. Darby, P.E. Garfinkel, D.M. Garner and D.V. Coscina), Alan R. Liss, New York, pp. 185–98.

Strober, M., Salkin, B., Burroughs, J. and Morrell, W. (1982) Validity of the bulimia-restrictor distinction in anorexia nervosa. Parental personality characteristics and family psychiatric morbidity. *Journal of Nervous and Mental Diseases*, **170**, 545–51.

Stroop, J.R. (1935) Studies of interference in serial verbal reactions. *Journal of Experimental Psychology*, **18**, 643–62.

Strupp, B.J., Weingartner, H., Kaye, W. and Gwirtsman, H. (1986) Cognitive processing in anorexia nervosa: A disturbance in automatic information processing. *Neuropsychobiology*, **15**, 89–94.

Stuart, R.B. (1967) Behavioural control of overeating. *Behaviour Research and Therapy*, **5**, 357–65.

Stuart, R.B. and Davis, B. (1972) *Slim Chance in a Fat World: Behavioral Control of Obesity*. Research Press, Champaign, Illinois.

Stunkard, A.J. (1958) The management of obesity. *New York State Journal of Medicine*, **58**, 79–87.

Stunkard, A.J. (1991) Meaning of the term bulimia. *American Journal of Psychiatry*, **148**(9), 1274.

Stunkard, A.J. and McLaren-Hume, M. (1959) The results of treatment for obesity. *Diseases of the Nervous System*, **30**, 669–74.

Stunkard, A.J., Rickels, K. and Hesbacher, P. (1973) Fenfluramine in the treatment of obesity. *Lancet*, **1**, 503.

Sturmey, P., Woods, D. and Crisp, A.G. (1984) Validation of the Pethna toy through changes in collateral behaviours. Unpublished (available from authors: Department of Clinical Psychology, Olive Mount Hospital, Wavertree, Liverpool).

Sullivan, A.C., Baruth, H.W. and Cheng, L. (1980) Recent advances in the design and development of antiobesity agents. *Annual Reports in Medicine and Chemistry*, **15**, 172–81.

Sullivan, A.C. and Comai, K. (1978) Pharmacological treatment of obesity. *International Journal of Obesity*, **2**, 167–89.

Swanson, D.W. and Dinello, F. (1969) Therapeutic starvation in obesity. *Diseases of the Nervous System*, **30**, 669–74.

Swift, W., Camp, B., Bushnell, N. and Bargman, G. (1984) Ego development in anorexia inpatients. *International Journal of Eating Disorders*, **3**, 73–80.

Swift, W. and Letven, R. (1984) Bulimia and the basic fault: A psychoanalytic interpretation of the binge–vomiting syndrome. *Journal of the American Academy of Child Psychiatry*, **23**, 489–97.

Sykes, D., Currie, K. and Gross, M. (1987) The use of group therapy in the treatment of bulimia. *International Journal of Psychosomatics*, **34**, 7–10.

Sykes, J.B. (1977) *The Concise Oxford Dictionary of Current English*. Oxford University Press, Oxford.

Szmukler, G.I. and Russell, G.F.M. (1983) Diabetes mellitus, anorexia nervosa and bulimia. *British Journal of Psychiatry*, **142**, 305–8.

Taipale, V., Larkio-Miettinen, K., Valanne, E., Morren, R. and Aukee, M. (1972) Anorexia nervosa in boys. *Psychosomatics*, **13**, 236–40.

Talland, G.A. (1965) *Deranged Memory*. Academic Press, New York.

Tanner, J.M. and Whitehouse, R.H. (1962) Standards for subcutaneous fat in British children. Percentiles for thickness of skinfolds over triceps and below scapula. *British Medical Journal*, **5276**, 446–50.

Tarnower, H. and Baker, S.S. (1978) *The Complete Scarsdale Medical Diet*. Rawson, New York.

Tarter, R.E. and Parsons, O.A. (1971) Conceptual shifting in chronic alcoholics. *Journal of Abnormal Psychology*, **77**, 71–5.

Taylor, E.M. (1959) *The Appraisal of Children with Cerebral Deficits*. Harvard University Press, Cambridge, Massachusetts.

Theander, S. (1970) Anorexia nervosa: A psychiatric investigation of 44 female cases. *Acta Psychiatrica Scandinavica (Supplement)*, **214**, 1–194.

Thomas, A. (1981) The girl who'll eat anything. . . . *Woman*, **29 July**, 52–3.

Thompson, G.R., Barrowman, J., Gutierrez, L. and Dowling, R.H. (1971) Action of neomycin on the intraluminal phase of lipid absorption. *Journal of Clinical Investigation*, **50**, 319–23.

Thompson, S.B.N. (1982) Does informational influence affect the interpretation of photographic stimuli with human content? BA (Honours) psychology dissertation, Plymouth Polytechnic.

Thompson, S.B.N. (1983a) Organised diversion can work against patients. *Therapy Weekly*, **10**(1), 7.

Thompson, S.B.N. (1983b) Training surface personnel: Implications from a recent study. *Nautical Magazine*, **229**(4), 16–17.

Thompson, S.B.N. (1983c) Training influences on maritime personnel. *Nautical Magazine*, **230**(3), 18–19.

Thompson, S.B.N. (1984a) Computer-assisted visual feedback as a potential prognostic tool for adult hemiplegia in occupational therapy. Postgraduate Diploma in Information Systems dissertation PD/20/1984, School of Information Science, Portsmouth Polytechnic.

Thompson, S.B.N. (1984b) Investigacion psicologica con personal de superficie de la marina. *La Revista Psicologia General Y Aplicada*, **39**(1), 193–4.

Thompson, S.B.N. (1985) Computerised therapy for leg injuries. *Therapy Weekly*, **12**(11), 4.

Thompson, S.B.N. (1986) Monitoring nerve impluses in leg muscles. *Therapy Weekly*, **13**(15), 4.

Thompson, S.B.N. (1987a) Testing manual dexterity. *Therapy Weekly*, **13**(38), 4.

Thompson, S.B.N. (1987b) A system for rapidly converting quadriceps contraction to a digital signal for use in micro-computer-oriented muscle therapy and stroke patient assessment schedules. *Computers in Biology and Medicine International Journal*, **17**(2), 117–25.

Thompson, S.B.N. (1987c) A microcomputer-feedback system for improving control of incompletely innervated leg muscle in adult cerebrovascular accident patients. *British Journal of Occupational Therapy*, **50**(5), 161–6.

Thompson, S.B.N. (1987d) A microcomputer-based assessment battery, data file handling and data retrieval system for the forward planning of treatment for adult stroke patients. *Journal of Microcomputer Applications*, **10**(2), 127–35.

Thompson, S.B.N. (1987e) Stroke recovery model. *Therapy Weekly*, **14**(9), 7.

Thompson, S.B.N. (1987f) A stochastic model of cerebrovascular accident prognosis. PhD thesis, School of Information Science, Portsmouth Polytechnic.

Thompson, S.B.N. (1989) Techniques for tackling anxiety. *Therapy Weekly*, **15**(49), 6.

Thompson, S.B.N. (1990a) Update on dexterity testing. *Therapy Weekly*, **16**(26), 10.

Thompson, S.B.N. (1990b) Talking about sex. . . . *Therapy Weekly*, **17**(13), 8.

Thompson, S.B.N. (1991a) Sexuality training in occupational therapy for people with a learning difficulty. *British Journal of Occupational Therapy*, **54**(8), 303–4.

Thompson, S.B.N. (1991b) Correlates of cognitive dysfunction in anorexia nervosa. MPhil thesis, Department of Clinical Psychology, University of Edinburgh.

Thompson, S.B.N. (1991c) Distorted image. *Therapy Weekly*, **18**(18), 8.

Thompson, S.B.N. (1992a) Implications from neuropsychological test results of women in a new phase of anorexia nervosa. *Eating Disorders Review*, (in press).

Thompson, S.B.N. (1992b) Tips to trigger memory. *Therapy Weekly*, **19**(7), 7.

Thompson, S.B.N. (1992c) Traitement de la dépression en rééducation cardiaque ambulatoire. *Visages de la Dépression*, **March**, 9–10.

Thompson, S.B.N. (1992d) Doubting dementia in Down's syndrome and other forms of learning disability. *The Psychologist*, (in press).

Thompson, S.B.N. (1993a) *Anorexia Nervosa: An Organic Origin?* Paper presented at XXV International Congress of Psychology at Brussels International Conference Centre, Brussels, Belgium, 19–24 July, 1992, in *Le Journal des Psychologues*, (in press).

Thompson, S.B.N. (1993b) Alzheimer's disease and Down's syndrome. *Therapy Weekly*, (in press).

Thompson, S.B.N., Blincoe, C., Eggison, P. *et al.* (1989) *Policy and Guidelines for Staff on Sexual Relationships for People with a Mental Handicap in St Margaret's Hospital; Report.* Department of Clinical Psychology, St Margaret's Hospital, Birmingham.

Thompson, S.B.N. and Coleman, M.J. (1987a) An investigation into stroke. *Therapy Weekly*, **13**(29), 7.

Thompson, S.B.N. and Coleman, M.J. (1987b) Leg-injured

patients switch on to rehabilitation. *Therapy Weekly*, **13**(48), 7.

Thompson, S.B.N. and Coleman, M.J. (1987c) A quantitative assessment of neuromuscular function for use with unilateral cerebrovascular accident patients. *International Journal of Rehabilitation Research*, **10**(3), 312–16.

Thompson, S.B.N. and Coleman, M.J. (1988a) *Making the Therapist's Prognosis of Stroke a More Scientific Process*. Paper presented at First International Convention of Human Service Information Technology Applications (HUSITA 87) on A Technology to Support Humanity, at City of Birmingham Polytechnic, Birmingham, 7–11 September, 1987, in *Information Technology and Human Services*, (eds B. Glastonbury, W. LaMendola and S. Toole), John Wiley, Chichester, pp. 68–75.

Thompson, S.B.N. and Coleman, M.J. (1988b) Occupational therapists' prognoses of their patients: Findings of a British survey of stroke. *International Journal of Rehabilitation Research*, **11**(3), 275–9.

Thompson, S.B.N. and Coleman, M.J. (1989) *An Interactive Microcomputer-based System for the Assessment and Prognosis of Stroke Patients*. Paper presented at Special European Conference of the American Society for Cybernetics on Design for Development of Social Systems at University of St Gallen, St Gallen, Switzerland, 15–19 March, 1987, in *Journal of Microcomputer Applications*, **12**(1), 33–40.

Thompson, S.B.N., Coleman, M.J. and Yates, J. (1986) Visual feedback as a prognostic tool. *Journal of Microcomputer Applications*, **9**(3), 215–21.

Thompson, S.B.N. and Gittins, D.K. (1989a) Finding the right incentive. *Therapy Weekly*, **16**(18), 8.

Thompson, S.B.N. and Gittins, D.K. (1989b) Using a pethna to increase the independence in feeding of a woman with profound mental handicap. *International Journal of Rehabilitation Research*, **12**(2), 204–7.

Thompson, S.B.N., Hards, B. and Bate, R. (1986) Computer-assisted visual feedback for new hand and arm therapy apparatus. *British Journal of Occupational Therapy*, **49**(1), 19–21.

Thompson, S.B.N., McKenzie, K. and Weeks, D.J. (1991) Aide-mémoire. *Therapy Weekly*, **18**(20), 7.

Thompson, S.B.N. and Morgan, M. (1990) *Occupational Therapy for Stroke Rehabilitation*. Chapman & Hall, London.

Thompson, S.B.N. and Muir, J. (1993) Monitoring behaviour, diet and anthropometric changes to explain low weight gain in clients with a severe learning disability. *British Journal of Developmental Disabilities*, **xxxix**, 1(76), 60–71.

Thompson, S.B.N., North, N.J. and Pentland, B. (1992) Clinical management of a man with complex partial seizures and a severe head injury. *Brain Injury*, **6**(3), 293–8.

Thompson, S.B.N., Smith, L. and Muir, J. (1992) The proof of the pudding. *Therapy Weekly*, **19**(16), 7.

Thornton, L.P. and DeBlassie, R.R. (1989) Treating bulimia. *Adolescence*, **24**(95), 631–7.

Thorpe, J.G., Schmidt, E., Brown, P.T. and Castell, D. (1964) Aversive relief therapy: A new method for general application. *Behaviour Research and Therapy*, **2**, 71–82.

Thurlby, P.L. and Trayhurn, P. (1980) Regional blood flow in genetically obese (ob/ob) mice: The importance of brown adipose tissue to the reduced energy expenditure on non-shivering thermogenesis. *Pflugers Archives*, **386**, 193–201.

Tighe, T.J. and Elliott, R. (1968) A technique for controlling behavior in natural life settings. *Journal of Applied Behavior Analysis*, **1**, 263–6.

Tolstoi, L.G. (1989) The role of pharmacotherapy in anorexia nervosa and bulimia. *Journal of the American Dietetic Association*, **89**(11), 1640–6.

Touyz, S.W. and Beumont, P.J.V. (1985) *Eating Disorders: Prevalence and Treatment*. Williams and Wilkins, Sydney.

Traub, A.C. and Orbach, J. (1964) Psychophysical studies of body image: the adjustable body-distorting mirror. *Archives of General Psychiatry*, **11**, 53–66.

Treasure, J. (1988) Psychopharmacological approaches to anorexia and bulimia, in *Anorexia and Bulimia Nervosa*, (ed D. Scott), Croom Helm, London, pp. 123–34.

Tunbridge, W.M. and Fraser, T.R. (1972) Anorexia nervosa with multiple organic disorders in a young man. *Proceedings of the Royal Society of Medicine*, **65**(11), 984–5.

Turnbull, J., Freeman, C.P.L., Barry, F. and Annandale, A. (1987) Physical and psychological characteristics of five male bulimics. *British Journal of Psychiatry*, **150**, 25–9.

Turner, P. (1979) Peripheral mechanism of action of fenfluramine. *Current Medical Research Opinion*, **6**, 101–6.

Tyler, V.O. and Straughan, J.H. (1970) Coverant control and breath holding as techniques for the treatment of obesity. *Psychological Records*, **20**, 473–8.

Upper, D. and Newton, J.G. (1971) A weight-reduction program for schizophrenic patients on a token economy unit: Two case studies. *Journal of Behavior Therapy and Experimental Psychiatry*, **2**, 113–15.

Van, R.L.R., Bayliss, C.E. and Roncari, D.A.K. (1976) Cytological and enzymological characterization of adult human adipocyte precursors in culture. *Journal of Clinical Investigation*, **58**, 699.

Vandereycken, W. (1984) Neuroleptics in the short-term treatment of anorexia nervosa: A double-blind placebo-controlled study with sulpiride. *British Journal of Psychiatry*, **144**, 288–92.

Vandereycken, W. and Meerman, R. (1984a) Anorexia nervosa: Is prevention possible? *International Journal of Psychiatric Medicine*, **14**, 191–205.

Vandereycken, W. and Meerman, R. (1984b) *Anorexia Nervosa. A Clinician's Guide to Treatment*. Walter de Gruyter, Berlin.

Vandereycken, W. and Pierloot, R. (1982) Pimozide combined with behavior therapy in the short-term treatment of anorexia nervosa. *Acta Psychiatrica Scandinavica*, **66**, 445–50.

VanItallie, T.B. (1979) Obesity: Adverse effects on health and longevity. *American Journal of Clinical Nutrition*, **32**, 2723–33.

VanItallie, T.B. (1985) Health implications of overweight and obesity in the United States. *Annals of Internal Medicine*, **103**, 983–8.

VanItallie, T.B. and Woteki, C.E. (1987) Who gets fat? in *Body Weight Control. The Physiology, Clinical Treatment and Prevention of Obesity*, (eds A.E. Bender and L.J. Brookes), Churchill Livingstone, Edinburgh, pp. 39–52.

Vardi, J., Oberman, Z. and Rabey, I. (1976) Weight loss in patients treated long-term with levo-DOPA, metabolic aspects. *Journal of Neurological Science*, **30**, 33–40.

Vernon, P.E. (1979) *Intelligence, Heredity and Environment*. Freeman, San Francisco.

Vertes, R. (1971) The should: A critical analysis. *Rational Living*, **6**, 22–5.

Vigersky, R.A. (1977) *Anorexia Nervosa*. Raven Press, New York.

Vigersky, R.A. and Loriaux, D.L. (1977) The effect of cyproheptadine in anorexia nervosa: A double-blind trial, in *Anorexia Nervosa*, (ed R.A. Vigersky), Raven Press, New York, pp. 349–56.

Visser, R.S.H. (1973) *Manual of the Complex Figure Test.* Swets and Zeitlinger, Amsterdam.

Wacker, D.P., Berg, W.K., Wiggins, B., Muldoon, M. and Cavanagh, J. (1985) Evaluation of reinforcer preferences for profoundly handicapped students. *Journal of Applied Behavior Analysis*, **18**(2), 173–8.

Wade, C. (1976) *The New Enzyme Catalyst Diet.* Parker Publishing, West Nyack, New York.

Wales, J.K. (1979) The effect of fenfluramine on obese, maturity onset diabetic patients. *Current Medical Research Opinion*, **6**, 226–35.

Walker, A.R.P. and Segal, I. (1980) The puzzle of obesity in the African black female. *Lancet*, **1**, 263.

Wall, J.H. (1959) Diagnosis, treatment and results in anorexia nervosa. *American Journal of Psychiatry*, **115**, 997–1001.

Waller, G., Calam, R. and Slade, P. (1989) Eating disorders and family interaction. *British Journal of Clinical Psychology*, **28**(3), 285–6.

Walsh, B.T., Roose, S.P. and Glassman, A.H. (1983) *Depression and Eating Disorders.* Paper presented at the Annual Meeting of the American Psychiatric Association, Washington DC.

Warah, A. (1989) Body image disturbance in anorexia nervosa. *American Journal of Psychiatry*, **34**(9), 898–905.

Wardle, J. and Beinart, H. (1981) Binge eating: A theoretical review. *British Journal of Clinical Psychology*, **20**, 97–109.

Weber, K. and Gilingham, W. (1984) Group counselling for anorexic and bulimic students. *Journal of the College of Studies in Personnel*, **25**, 276.

Wechsler, D. (1944) *The Measurement of Adult Intelligence*, 3rd edn. Williams and Wilkins, Baltimore.

Wechsler, D. (1955) *Wechsler Adult Intelligence Scale, Manual.* Psychological Corporation, New York.

Wechsler, D. (1958) *The Measurement and Appraisal of Adult Intelligence*, 4th edn. Williams and Wilkins, Baltimore.

Wechsler, D. (1981) *WAIS-R Manual.* Psychological Corporation, New York.

Weilburg, J.B., Mesula, M.M. and Weintraub, S. (1989) Focal

striatal abnormalities in a patient with obsessive–compulsive disorder. *Archives of Neurology*, **46**, 233–5.

Weinberg, J., Diller, L., Gerstman, L. and Schulman, P. (1972) Digit span in right and left hemiplegics. *Journal of Clinical Psychology*, **28**, 361.

Weingartner, H., Grafman, J., Bontelle, W., Kaye, W. and Martin, P. (1983) Forms of memory failure. *Science*, **221**, 380.

Welbourne, J. and Purgold, J. (1984) *The Eating Sickness: Anorexia, Bulimia and the Myth of Suicide by Slimming*. Harvester Press, Brighton.

Wermuth, B.M., Davis, K.L., Hollister, L.E. and Stunkard, A.J. (1977) Phenytoin treatment of the binge-eating syndrome. *American Journal of Psychiatry*, **134**, 1249–53.

Wheeler, L. and Reitan, R.M. (1963) Discriminant functions applied to the problem of predicting cerebral damage from behavioural tests: A cross-validation study. *Perceptual and Motor Skills*, **16**, 681–701.

White, W.C. and Boskind-White, M. (1981) An experimental–behavioural approach to the treatment of bulimarexia. *Psychotherapy Theory, Research and Practice*, **18**, 501–7.

Whitehouse, A.M., Freeman, C.P.L. and Annandale, A. (1988) Body size estimation in anorexia nervosa. *British Journal of Psychiatry*, **153**(Supplement 2), 23–6.

Wiener, J.M. (1976) Identical male twins discordant for anorexia nervosa. *Journal of the American Academy of Chirurgiae and Psychiatry*, **15**, 523.

Wilbom, E. (1960) The after-effects of brain injuries. *Acta Psychiatrica Neurologia Scandinavica (Supplement)*, **142**, 105–45.

Willard, S.G., Swain, B.S. and Winstead, D.K. (1989) A treatment strategy for psychogenic vomiting. *Psychiatric Medicine*, **7**(3), 59–73.

Wilson, C.P., Hogan, C.C. and Mintz, I.L. (1983) *Fear of Being Fat: The Treatment of Anorexia Nervosa and Bulimia*. Jason Aronson, New York.

Wingate, B.A. and Christie, M.J. (1978) *Ego Strength in Anorexia Nervosa and Bulimia Nervosa*. Proceedings of the International Conference on Anorexia Nervosa and Related Disorders, Swansea, Wales.

Wirtshafter, D. and Davis, J.D. (1977) Set points, settling points and the control of body weight. *Physiology and Behavior*, **19**, 75–8.

Witherly, S.A., Pangborn, R.M. and Stern, J.S. (1980) Gustatory responses and eating duration of obese and lean adults. *Appetite*, **1**, 53–63.

Witkin, H.A., Lewis, H.B., Hertzman, M. *et al.* (1954) *Personality through Perception*. Harper, New York.

Wolf, N. (1990a) The beauty myth. Part one: The cult of thinness. *The Sunday Times*, **September 9**, 7–8.

Wolf, N. (1990b) The beauty myth. Part two: Under the knife. *The Sunday Times*, **September 16**, 6–7.

Wolf, N. (1990c) *The Beauty Myth*. Chatto and Windus, London.

Wolf, W.M., Birnbrauer, J.S., Williams, J. and Lawler, J. (1966) A note on apparent extinction of the vomiting behavior of a retarded child, in *Case Studies in Behavior Modification*, (eds L.P. Ullman and L. Krasner), Holt, Rinehart and Winston, New York, pp. 364–6.

Wolfensberger, W. (1972) *The Principle of Normalization in Human Services*. National Institute on Mental Retardation, Toronto.

Wollersheim, J.P. (1970) Effectiveness of group therapy based upon learning principles in the treatment of overweight women. *Journal of Abnormal Psychology*, **76**, 462–74.

Wolpe, J. (1954) Reciprocal inhibition as the main basis of psychotherapeutic effects. *Archives in Neurological Psychiatry*, **72**, 205–26.

Woods, P. and Parry, R. (1981) PETHNA: Tailor-made toys for the severely retarded and multiply handicapped. *Apex, Journal of the British Institute of Mental Handicap*, **9**, 53–6.

Wooley, O.W., Wooley, S.C. and Dunham, R.B. (1972) Calories and sweet taste: Effects on sucrose taste in the obese and nonobese. *Physiology of Behavior*, **9**, 765–8.

Wurtman, J.J. and Wurtman, R.J. (1979) Fenfluramine and other serotonergic drugs depress food intake and carbohydrate consumption while sparing protein consumption. *Current Medical Research Opinion*, **6** (Supplement 1), 28–33.

Wurtman, J.J., Wurtman, R.J. and Growdon, L. (1981) Carbohydrate craving in obese people: Suppression by treatments affecting serotonergic transmission. *International Journal of Eating Disorders*, **1**, 2–14.

Yager, J., Landsverk, J. and Edelstein, C.K. (1989a) The uses of a self-report instrument for eating disorders diagnoses: How different are DSM-III-R vs DSM-III? *Psychiatric Medicine*, **7**(3),

83–99.

Yager, J., Landsverk, J. and Edelstein, C.K. (1989b) Help seeking and satisfaction with care in 641 women with eating disorders. I: Patterns of utilization, attributed change, and perceived efficacy of treatment. *Journal of Nervous and Mental Diseases*, **177**(10), 632–7.

Yarnall, G.D. and Dodgion-Ensor, B. (1980) Identifying effective reinforcers for a multiply handicapped student. *Education of the Visually Handicapped*, **12**(1), 11–20.

Yates, A. (1970) Current perspectives on the eating disorders. II: Treatment, outcome, and research directions. *Journal of the American Academy of Child and Adolescent Psychiatry*, **29**(1), 1–9.

Young, C.M. (1963) Body composition studies of 'older' women, thirty to seventy years of age. *Annals of the New York Academy of Science*, **110**, 589–607.

Young, C.M. (1964) Predicting specific gravity and body fatness in 'older' women. *Journal of the American Dietetic Association*, **45**, 333–9.

Young, C.M., Martin, M.E.K., Chilhan, M. *et al.* (1961) Body composition of young women. *Journal of the American Dietetic Association*, **38**, 332–40.

Young, C.M., Tensuan, R.S., Sault, F. and Holmes, F. (1963) Estimating body fat of a normal young woman. Visualizing fat pads by soft-tissue X-rays. *Journal of the American Dietetic Association*, **42**, 409–13.

Zinkland, H., Cadoret, R.J. and Widmes, R.B. (1984) Incidence and detection of bulimia in a family practice population. *Journal of Family Practice*, **18**, 555–60.

Index

Page numbers appearing in **bold** refer to figures and page numbers appearing in *italic* refer to tables.